Alternative Medicine Guide to

Chronic Fatigue, Fibromyalgia & Environmental Illness

BURTON GOLDBERG *and the Editors of*
ALTERNATIVE MEDICINE DIGEST

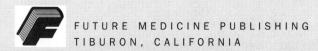

FUTURE MEDICINE PUBLISHING
TIBURON, CALIFORNIA

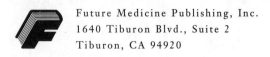

Future Medicine Publishing, Inc.
1640 Tiburon Blvd., Suite 2
Tiburon, CA 94920

Editor: Richard Leviton
Senior Editor: Stephanie Marohn
Writers: Richard Leviton & Stephanie Marohn
Associate Editor: John Anderson
Assistant Editor: Emily Rabin
Art Director: Janine White
Production Manager: Gail Gongoll
Cover and book design: Amparo Del Rio Design

Indicated images: LifeART Images Copyright©1989-1997
by TechPool Studios, Inc. USA

Manufactured in Canada

10

Library of Congress Cataloging-in-Publication Data
Goldberg, Burton, 1926-
      Alternative Medicine Guide to Chronic Fatigue, Fibromyalgia, and
Environmental Illness / Burton Goldberg and the Editors of
Alternative Medicine Digest.
            p.   cm.
      Includes bibliographical references and index.
      ISBN 1-887299-11-4 (pbk.)
      1. Chronic fatigue syndrome—Alternative treatment.
2. Fibromyalgia—Alternative treatment. 3. Environmentally induced
diseases—Alternative treatment.   I. Alternative Medicine Digest.
II. Title.   III. Title: Chronic fatigue, fibromyalgia, & environmental
illness   IV. Title: Chronic fatigue, fibromyalgia, and environmental illness
RB150.F37G643   1998
616'.0478--dc21   97-48756
                                                          CIP
Portions of this book were previously published,
in a different form, in *Alternative Medicine:
The Definitive Guide* and *Alternative Medicine Digest*.

Important Information

BURTON GOLDBERG and the editors of *Alternative Medicine Digest* are proud of the public and professional praise accorded Future Medicine Publishing's series of books. This latest book continues the groundbreaking tradition of its predecessors.

The health of you and your loved ones is important. Treat this book as an educational tool that will enable you to better understand, assess, and choose the best course of treatment when chronic fatigue, fibromyalgia, or environmental illness strikes, and how to prevent them from striking in the first place. It could save your life.

Remember that this book on chronic fatigue is different. It is not another catalog of mainstream medicine's conventional treatments and drugs used to treat this disease. This book is about *alternative* approaches to chronic fatigue–approaches generally not understood and, at this time, not endorsed by the medical establishment. We urge you to discuss the treatments described in this book with your doctor. If your doctor is open-minded, you may actually educate him or her. We have been gratified to learn that many of our readers have found their physicians to be open to new ideas.

Use this book wisely. Because many of the treatments described in this book are, by definition, alternative, they have not been investigated, approved or endorsed by any government or regulatory agency. National, state, and local laws may vary regarding the use and application of many of the treatments that are discussed. Accordingly, this book should not be substituted for the advice and care of a physician or other licensed health care professional. Pregnant women, in particular, are especially urged to consult with a physician before commencing any therapy. Ultimately, you, the reader, must take responsibility for your health and how you use the information in this book.

Future Medicine Publishing and the authors have no financial interest in any of the products or services discussed in this book, other than the citations to Future Medicine's other publications. All of the factual information in this book has been drawn from the scientific literature.

Contents

You Don't Have to Endure Chronic Fatigue

IF YOU HAVE CHRONIC FATIGUE syndrome or one of its close relatives—fibromyalgia and environmental illness—you most likely have experienced years of frustration trying to find relief from your puzzling assortment of symptoms. You may have spent years just trying to find a doctor who could tell you what's wrong with you. In the process, you probably encountered many medical professionals who dismissed your complaints as neurotic imaginings.

If you were fortunate enough to find a physician who acknowledged your problem by giving it a name, a name was likely *all* you got. Conventional medicine is usually baffled by these disorders and can only offer drugs to *temporarily* ease *some* of the symptoms: painkillers for the muscle pain of CFS and fibromyalgia; antihistamines for the allergies of CFS and environmental illness; antidepressants for the mood disorders of all three. As you probably know, most conventional drugs produce their temporary relief only at the cost of considerable side effects and toxicity.

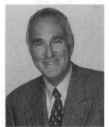

It is not only conventional physicians who have failed you. It is the whole conventional medical establishment which has spent the past decade squabbling over whether CFS even exists and, if it does, debating the number and nature of symptoms that qualify a person for the distinction of having CFS. This has been the pursuit of the U.S. government's Centers for Disease Control whose accomplishments after more than ten years of investigating CFS consist of the development of formal diagnosis criteria.

But they are no closer to discovering what causes CFS (or how to treat it) than they were when the outbreak in Incline Village, Nevada, first drew their attention in the mid-1980s to what would become an epidemic. Conventional medical research, as it does with most illnesses, seems capable only of focusing on the search for that single cause which will then yield the mythical magic bullet cure. That's not the way alternative medicine goes about dealing with a complex illness like chronic fatigue.

The good news is that you don't have to wait for the magic bullet because it will never arrive. Alternative medicine has practical solutions for you *now*. The reason is that physicians of alternative medicine know that illness is *multifactorial*. Especially in the case of such complex disorders as CFS, fibromyalgia, and environmental illness, no one cause is responsible. Multiple imbalances and deficiencies combine to produce the breakdown of the body.

Knowing this, alternative medicine physicians set about to systematically identify these factors—from viruses and yeast overgrowth to heavy metal toxicity and nutritional deficits—through precisely targeted, nontoxic tests. Once the underlying factors have been pinpointed, a treatment plan can be designed to address each one. Instead of treating symptoms, which can only produce temporary relief at best, alternative medicine goes to the root causes and so can provide a real and lasting solution to your chronic fatigue.

In addition, alternative physicians know that if you want good results, you must always consider the body as a whole. For example, if you start loading patients with supplements for their severe nutritional deficiencies without first addressing their digestive problems, it's like washing the vitamins down the drain. With faulty digestion, nutrients can't be absorbed. All the systems of the body are related and that is why holistic medical treatment is such an effective model. Holistic medicine also knows that no two people, even with the same illness, will require the same treatment. "Cookbook prescriptions" have no place in the world of alternative medicine.

In this book you will learn how over 50 alternative medicine physicians reverse CFS, environmental illness, and fibromyalgia using an individualized, holistic approach. You will read 26 case histories of people who finally found answers and solutions after years of consulting doctors and getting neither. You will discover the many factors that can contribute to the development of these disorders—factors frequently ignored or overlooked by conventional medicine.

Best of all, this book can start you on your path to *full* recovery. I'm here to tell you that you don't have to endure your illness, no matter what you've heard before. This book will show you how you can join the other success stories and leave your chronic fatigue, fibromyalgia, or environmental illness behind. God bless.

—Burton Goldberg

User's Guide

One of the features of this book is that it is interactive, thanks to the following 11 icons:

This means you can turn to the listed pages elsewhere in this book for more information on the topic.

This tells you where to contact a physician, group, or publication, or how to obtain substances mentioned in the text. This is an editorial service to our readers. Most importantly, the use of this icon empowers you right now, by giving you a source to acquire something vital to your health, quickly and easily. Whenever possible, we give you complete contact information for all substances mentioned in the text. All items are based on recommendations from the clinical practice of physicians in this book. The publisher has no financial interest in any clinic, physician, or product discussed in this book.

Many times the text mentions a medical term that requires explanation. We don't want to interrupt the text, so instead we put the explanation in the margins under this icon. This gives you the option of proceeding with the text or taking a moment to learn more about an important term. You will find some of the key definitions repeated at different places in the book so you don't have to search for the definition.

This sign tells you there may be some risks, uncertainties, side effects, or special contraindications regarding a procedure or substance. **Pay close attention to these icons.**

Here we refer you to our book, *An Alternative Medicine Definitive Guide to Cancer*, for more information on a particular topic.

Here we refer you to our best-selling book, *Alternative Medicine: The Definitive Guide*, for more information on a particular topic.

This icon will alert you to an article published in our bimonthly magazine, *Alternative Medicine Digest*, that is relevant to the topic under discussion.

This icon asks you to give a particular point special attention in your thinking. It is important to the overall discussion at hand.

This icon highlights a particularly noteworthy point and bids you to remember it.

In many cases, alternative medicine is far less expensive than conventional treatments. This icon means that the widespread acceptance of the therapy or substance under discussion could save considerable health-care money.

More research on this topic would be valuable and should be encouraged to further substantiate or clinically prove a promising possibility of benefit to many.

1

Related Epidemics

CHRONIC FATIGUE SYNDROME, FIBROMYALGIA, AND ENVIRONMENTAL ILLNESS

WHEN THE FIRST CASES of chronic fatigue syndrome (CFS) were identified in the 1980s among patients in a small Nevada town, the strange disease—marked principally by deep fatigue and muscle aches—was dubbed "Yuppie flu." It seemed to be concentrated among young, affluent white professionals. Due to this and to the seemingly subjective nature of the symptoms, CFS was the butt of jokes and its sufferers were often not taken seriously by many physicians. A decade later, CFS has become an epidemic across all ethnic and demographic barriers. It is now recognized as a severe, debilitating illness, although the dismissive attitude persists with some doctors.

> **Government health agencies have spent far too much time and attention in devising supposedly accurate descriptive terms and diagnostic categories for chronic fatigue rather than in figuring out successful ways to eliminate the problem.**

Despite the eventual recognition of the disorder, conventional medicine still does not know what *causes* chronic fatigue syndrome—blaming it variously on the Epstein-Barr virus, candidiasis (fungal overgrowth), and the herpes virus—and has no answers for treating it. Meanwhile, the number of cases continues to rise. In fact, government health agencies have spent far too much time and attention in

The Multiple Factors That Contribute to Chronic Fatigue Syndrome

■ Multiple infections (viruses, candidiasis, parasites)	See Chapter 3
■ Immune dysfunction	See Chapter 4
■ Thyroid problems	See Chapter 6
■ Toxicity (from environment, food, dental amalgams, and drugs)	See Chapters 5 & 7
■ Enzyme deficiency	See Chapter 8
■ Underlying allergies	See Chapter 9
■ Nutritional deficiency	See Chapter 10
■ Lifestyle (stress, psychological/ emotional factors)	See Chapter 11

devising supposedly accurate descriptive terms and diagnostic categories for chronic fatigue rather than in figuring out successful ways to eliminate the problem.

The U.S. Centers for Disease Control (CDC), based in Atlanta, Georgia, offers a typically conservative estimate of four to ten cases per 100,000 adults (which translates to 10,440 to 26,100 Americans),[1] but other sources place the numbers much higher. According to Murray R. Susser, M.D., a physician practicing in Santa Monica, California, chronic fatigue syndrome (also known as chronic fatigue and immune dysfunction syndrome, CFIDS) afflicts an estimated three million Americans and possibly 90 million people worldwide.

Jesse A. Stoff, M.D., coauthor of *Chronic Fatigue Syndrome: The Hidden Epidemic* and director of Integrative Medicine for Solstice Clinical Associates in Tucson, Arizona, believes it is even more widespread, estimating that the number of people with CFS in North America alone exceeds by four million the number of people with AIDS.[2] The CDC reports that 80% of diagnosed cases are women, the majority of whom are white and between the ages of 25 and 45. However, these figures reflect underreporting among nonwhite populations.[3] In addition to the United States, CFS has been reported widely in Canada, New Zealand,

Required Symptoms for a Diagnosis of Chronic Fatigue, According to the U.S. Centers for Disease Control

In March of 1988, the U.S. Centers for Disease Control (CDC) released criteria for a diagnosis of CFS, which it revised in 1994 to encompass the broader symptom spectrum of those afflicted. In order to be diagnosed with CFS, a person has to be suffering from:

1) new, unexplained, persistent or relapsing chronic fatigue which is not a consequence of exertion, not resolved by bed rest, and severe enough to significantly reduce previous daily activity; and

2) four or more of the symptoms below for at least six months

- unexplained or new headaches
- short-term memory or concentration impairment
- muscle pain
- pain in multiple joints unaccompanied by redness or swelling
- unrefreshing sleep
- postexertion malaise which lasts for longer than 24 hours
- sore throat
- tender lymph nodes in the neck or armpits.

Australia, Europe, South Africa, Russia, Japan, and Iceland.[4]

A new study probing the extent of CFS occurrence in the nonwhite population suggests that possibly 10% of that population is "highly fatigued." A survey by the San Francisco Department of Health of 16,000 residents of San Francisco revealed that 2% had suffered from unexplained fatigue for at least six months and 10% of these met the criteria for chronic fatigue syndrome as defined by the U.S. Centers for Disease Control.

When the numbers were extrapolated to all of San Francisco, it suggested that 14,600 residents were "highly fatigued, extremely tired, or exhausted," said study directors. This number was considered to be 20 times higher than previous official estimates and was consistent with similar surveys in Chicago, Illinois, and Seattle, Washington, as well as England and Australia.

The San Francisco survey also found that for every 100 whites with CFS symptoms, there were 144 African Americans and 157 Latinos, but only 64 Asians reporting the same. The symptoms were most prevalent among women, aged 30-39. No single type of job was associated with the incidence of chronic fatigue nor did it seem to cluster in households which would have suggested a contagious aspect. Contrary to earlier assumptions, the syndrome seemed to affect more people (by a factor of about 30%) with incomes under $40,000 than those with incomes exceeding this amount.[5]

In fact, fatigue in general, whether it's chronic or episodic, is increasingly a problem in the U.S. It is estimated that 24% of the general adult population of the U.S. has experienced fatigue lasting two weeks or longer; of these people, 59% to 64% reported no known medical cause. One study showed that 24% of primary care patients said they had experienced prolonged fatigue of at least one month's duration; some reported their fatigue lasted more than six months.[6]

Closely Related Severe Chronic Fatigue States

Two close relatives of chronic fatigue syndrome—fibromyalgia and environmental illness—are also becoming more prevalent. Fibromyalgia (from "fibro," connective tissue, and "myalgia," muscle pain) is a painful muscle disorder in which the thin film or tissue (myofascia) holding muscle together becomes tightened or thickened, causing pain. Fibromyalgia, also called fibrositis, shares many of the same symptoms as CFS, including debilitating fatigue, muscle and joint pain, sleeping disorders, depression, anxiety, mental confusion, and digestive problems. Jacob Teitelbaum, M.D., a specialist in the two syndromes, calls CFS the "drop-dead" flu and fibromyalgia the "aching-all-over" disease. Given the similarity that these descriptive names embody, Dr. Teitelbaum prefers to put CFS and fibromyalgia in a single category he calls severe chronic fatigue states.[7]

An estimated three to six million Americans suffer from fibromyalgia, 86% of whom are women. The level of disability caused by fibromyalgia is severe enough that 25.3% of women and 27% of men affected are unable to work, according to a recent study.[8]

The Official Definition of Fibromyalgia
In 1990, the American College of Rheumatology (ACR) established the following diagnostic criteria for fibromyalgia. According to the ACR, there must be widespread pain of at least three month's duration in 11 out of 18 tender muscle sites, as follows:

■ **Occiput** (on the head): bilateral (on both sides), at the suboccipital muscle insertion

■ **Lower Cervical**: bilateral, at the anterior aspects of the intertransverse spaces of cervical (neck) vertebrae C5-C7

■ **Trapezius** (upper back): bilateral, at the midpoint of the upper border

Symptom Chart of the Three Related Epidemics

CHRONIC FATIGUE
allergies
anxiety
brain fog and confusion
cough
decreased appetite
depression
digestive disorders
dizziness
dry eyes and mouth
general stiffness
headaches
increased thirst
irritability
joint and muscle pain
low body temperature
low-grade fever
memory loss
muscle weakness
nausea
night sweats
PMS (women)
poor concentration
prolonged fatigue
 after exertion
rashes
recurring infections

severe fatigue
sleep problems
sore throat
swollen lymph nodes
visual blurring

FIBROMYALGIA
allergies
anxiety
carpal tunnel syndrome
depression
dizziness
dry eyes alternating
 with watery eyes
dysmenorrhea (women)
exercise intolerance
fingernail ridges
general fatigue
general stiffness
headaches
heightened sensitivity
 to light, sound, smell,
 touch ("irritable
 everything syndrome")
"hurting all over"
irritability
irritable bowel symptoms

mood swings
numbness or tingling
 sensations
sensitivity to cold
sleeping disorders
tender skin
widespread muscle
 and joint pain

**ENVIRONMENTAL
ILLNESS**
anxiety
asthma
coughing or wheezing
depression
digestive problems
fatigue
headaches
infections
irritability
mood swings
multiple allergies
multiple chemical
 sensitivities
muscle pain and/or
 weakness
weight loss

■ **Supraspinatus** (shoulder blades): bilateral, at origins above the scapula near the medial border

■ **Second Rib**: bilateral, at the second costochondral junctions just lateral to the junctions on the upper surfaces

■ **Lateral Epicondyle** (top of the thigh bone, or humerus): bilateral, 2 cm distal to the epicondyle

■ **Gluteal** (buttocks): bilateral, in upper quadrants of buttocks in anterior fold of muscles

■ **Knee**: bilateral, at the medial fat pad proximal to the joint line
The symptoms of environmental illness similarly overlap with

those of both CFS and fibromyalgia. Also known as multiple chemical sensitivity, the syndrome involves numerous and extensive allergies, often to nearly everything in one's environment and to such a degree that many sufferers must isolate themselves in their homes and avoid exposure to such commonplace items as chemically treated building materials, plastics, synthetic carpets, newsprint, perfume, soap, and car exhaust, to name a few. Since the sensitivities seem to be focused on (although not limited to) manufactured products, many people view environmental illness as a response to the increasing level of toxins in our environment.

Some practitioners believe that environmental illness is an extreme extension or outcome of prolonged chronic fatigue syndrome. Shari

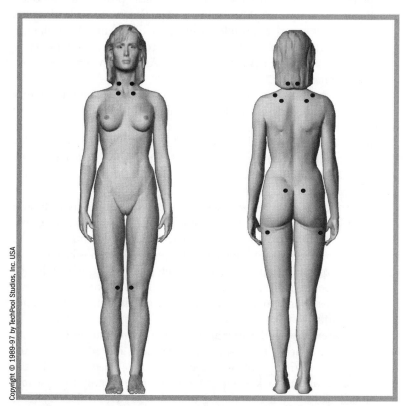

According to the American College of Rheumatology, when a patient has widespread pain of at least three months duration in 11 out of 18 tender muscle sites (as pictured above), they're diagnosed as having fibromyalgia.

The primary sufferers of CFS, fibromyalgia, and environmental illness are women and all three disorders share the dubious distinction of being poorly understood by the medical profession.

Lieberman, Ph.D., C.N.S., a nutritional specialist based in New York City, is among them. She has treated several hundred people with chronic fatigue syndrome to date and reports: "I see patients with environmental sensitivities who have come to me after three to five years of chronic fatigue. If they've only had CFS for six months, they don't tend to have environmental sensitivities."

The primary sufferers of CFS, fibromyalgia, and environmental illness are women and all three disorders share the dubious distinction of being poorly understood by the medical profession. Although fibromyalgia was first described by a physician in 1816 and classified as a distinct disorder (a painful arthritic condition) in 1904, it did not receive recognition as the debilitating condition it is until fairly recently; in 1987, the American Medical Association cited it as a disabling illness.[9]

However, a misconception in the medical community that fibromyalgia is caused by deconditioning—muscles becoming weak and limp as a result of inactivity—has added to the painful burden of those who suffer from the disorder. This blaming of the victim is singularly unhelpful to the patient's state of mind and is also medically inaccurate—most fibromyalgia sufferers were highly active people, *overachievers*, in fact, when the condition struck.

Environmental illness is less widely acknowledged as a physical disorder than fibromyalgia and CFS, but this is changing as its growing occurrence makes it a phenomenon that can no longer be ignored. All three conditions have frequently been misdiagnosed as depression and patients have often been told "it's all in your head." Some doctors still refuse to even admit the existence of the three syndromes. Fortunately, their numbers are dwindling as the number of the afflicted rises.

However, with the overlap of symptoms, it can be difficult to determine which syndrome a person has and, indeed, an individual may be suffering from all three. Alternative medicine—and the approach of this book—finds it more useful to identify the systemic imbalances which are producing the symptoms rather than try to fit the individual into one of the three conventional diagnostic categories. This approach also stems from the alternative medicine model of addressing the *sources* of illness rather than just treating symptoms; the latter practice only produces temporary relief at best. The conventional medical solution for fibromyalgia—painkillers—is a prime example of symptom-driven treatment with little understanding of causes and equally slim chances of therapeutic success.

Although this book focuses predominantly on chronic fatigue syndrome, the alternative medicine view is that the three disorders share the same cluster of underlying causes. Therefore, learning about the causes of CFS and how to address these causes in treatment (as discussed here) is equally useful for people with fibromyalgia and environmental illness. The multiple causes of the three syndromes and, therefore, the necessity for a *combination* of treatment methods, make them ideal candidates for alternative medicine's multimodal approach to healing. This means many symptoms require multiple therapies to unravel them.

Treating the Individual

As a syndrome, CFS is an array of symptoms which may appear unrelated. But according to alternative medicine, all are products of an underlying imbalance in the body produced by multiple simultaneous infections and accompanying physical, mental, and environmental factors.

Specifically, Dr. Susser states that CFS develops as a result of a combination of: nutritional deficiency; acquired toxicity (from environment, food, dental amalgams, dental infections, and/or drugs); poor stress-coping abilities; acquired systemic infections (often due to excessive use of antibiotics causing candidiasis and parasite over-

Chemical Exposure is a Factor in CFS

According to the Centers for Disease Control (CDC), exposure to toxic chemicals rules out a diagnosis of CFS. However, a recent study of 22 people who met the CDC criteria for CFS and 17 people with CFS symptoms but whose history of chemical exposure precluded a CFS diagnosis found that there was no significant difference between the two groups in terms of their blood level of chlorinated hydrocarbons, notably HCB and DDE.

Chlorinated hydrocarbons, also known as organochlorines, are chemical compounds formed by a carbon-to-chlorine bond. HCB is a widely used pesticide and DDE is a product of the metabolism of DDT, another common pesticide. Both the CFS group and the group with CFS symptoms and known chemical exposure had significantly higher organochlorine levels than the control group of 34 non-CFS subjects. The researchers concluded that toxic chemical exposure may play a causal role in CFS. They also concluded that the CDC's exclusion of a toxic exposure history from the criteria for CFS is not valid.[10]

Concise Definitions of the Three Related Epidemics

CHRONIC FATIGUE SYNDROME (CFS) is an umbrella term for a multiple symptom disorder characterized most commonly by the sudden onset of extreme, debilitating fatigue, pain in the muscles and joints, headaches, and poor concentration. The fatigue is not alleviated by rest and results in a substantial reduction in previous levels of daily activity. CFS is often cyclical, with periods of relative health followed by debilitation. Other symptoms include depression, anxiety, digestive disorders, memory loss, allergies, recurring infections, and low-grade fever. According to the U.S. Centers for Disease Control, CFS predominantly affects white women, 25-45 years old.

FIBROMYALGIA is a multiple-symptom syndrome primarily involving widespread muscle pain (myalgia) which can be debilitating in its severity. The pain seems to be caused by the tightening and thickening of the myofascia, the thin film of tissue which holds the muscle together. Typical tender sites include the neck, upper back, rib cage, hips, and knees. Other symptoms include general fatigue and stiffness, insomnia and sleeping disorders, anxiety, depression, mood swings, allergies, carpal tunnel syndrome, headaches, the sense of "hurting all over," tender skin, numbness, irritable bowel symptoms, dizziness, and exercise intolerance. Posttraumatic fibromyalgia is believed to develop after a fall, whiplash, or back strain, whereas primary fibromyalgia has an uncertain origin. The majority of fibromyalgia sufferers are women between the ages of 34 and 56.

ENVIRONMENTAL ILLNESS is a multiple-symptom, debilitating, chronic disorder involving prolonged, heightened, and often incapacitating allergies or sensitivities to numerous common substances found in one's environment. Symptoms may include headaches, fatigue, muscle pain and/or weakness, coughing or wheezing, asthma, weight loss, infections, and emotional fluctuations, depression, and irritability. The illness is sometimes referred to as "20th century disease" because patients become allergic to and functionally incompatible with many products and substances found in the modern world, such as car exhaust, synthetic carpets, plywood and other building materials, cleaning agents, office machines, and plastics, among others.

growth); and a vicious cycle of lowered immune function, allergy, more infection, and further depleted energy reserves. These factors will be explored in depth in the chapters that follow.

It is essential to understand the factors that went into creating CFS in each person because CFS is never caused by one thing alone and no two people have exactly the same causal factors. This individualizing approach is particularly important in the case of CFS because, along with fibromyalgia and environmental illness, it shares symptoms with diseases such as multiple sclerosis and lupus.[11] Misdiagnosis is common and creates additional pain and frustration, which could likely have been avoided by an *individualized* approach to the patient.

In the following section, **Jesse Stoff, M.D.**, details the multiple causes of CFS (in the context of relating a CFS case) and demonstrates that it can be successfully reversed using a treatment plan tailored to the individual's needs. Dr. Stoff's case will frame this book's approach to reversing chronic fatigue syndrome. The chapters that follow will be extensions and commentaries on Dr. Stoff's insights and protocols.

The "Whole Patient" Approach to Chronic Fatigue Syndrome

Successfully treating the "heavy hitters" of today's illnesses, such as chronic fatigue, AIDS, and cancer, is Dr. Stoff's specialty. He draws upon a wide range of alternative medicine therapies to accomplish this—nutrition, homeopathy, Chinese herbs, Anthroposophic medicines, relaxation techniques, guided imagery, and massage, among others. Health is restored to the whole patient, not just the body, says Dr. Stoff.

Misdiagnosis of chronic fatigue syndrome is common and creates additional pain and frustration, which could likely have been avoided by an *individualized* approach to the patient.

The goal is to help each person achieve a working balance between physical healing and emotional, mental, even spiritual aspects of their life. "We assist and encourage the patient to take an active role in the healing process," says Dr. Stoff, explaining the holistic approach of his integrated medicine clinic, Solstice Clinical Associates.

The first step before designing a treatment plan is extensive testing. Dr. Stoff believes in evaluations of a patient's blood, urine, and stool, consultations with staff physicians and specialists, followed by an assessment of a client's innate healing resources and state of mind. The new patient will spend an hour with Dr. Stoff, who specializes in homeopathy and is a world-acknowledged expert in holistic protocols for chronic fatigue syndrome. His 1988 book, *Chronic Fatigue Syndrome: The Hidden Epidemic*, mentioned earlier, is recognized as a standard work in the field of alternative medicine solutions for this illness.[12]

For more information about **urine tests and stool analyses**, see Chapter 2: Testing, pp. 34-72. For more about **psychological factors in CFS**, see Chapter 11: Healing Psychological and Emotional Factors, pp. 292-317.

QUICK DEFINITION

A **lymphocyte** is a form of white blood cell, representing 25% of the total count, whose numbers increase during infection. Lymphocytes, produced in the bone marrow, come in two forms; B cells, which produce antibodies to neutralize foreign matter in the blood, and T cells, matured in the thymus gland (behind the breastbone) and having many functions in the body's immune response.

Next, the patient meets with George B. Olson, Ph.D., an immunologist and expert in guided imagery. Dr. Olson often prepares instructional tapes for clients, taking them through the stages of generating mental images of healing. Lance J. Morris, N.M.D., a naturopathic physician trained in acupuncture, herbs, homeopathy, and structural/energy work, then provides a nutritional assessment and some counseling.

Finally, the new patient talks with one of several staff psychologists who assesses the patient's self-image and attitude about the illness. There may be psychological or unconscious factors, such as secondary gain or codependency, that make it advantageous for the patient to remain sick. As Dr. Stoff puts it, "Most importantly, what we want to know is this: what are this person's perceived roadblocks to healing? Through close collaboration among our staff members, we provide an individualized and comprehensive treatment program based on an in-depth understanding of each of our patients."

Quite often, Dr. Stoff's team gets a patient who has received the "proverbial million-dollar workup" from conventional medicine, but still has no clear diagnosis. The tests Dr. Stoff runs are targeted at discovering the level of function of the various systems in a patient's body. The results of a test for levels of T and B immune cells, called lymphocytes (SEE QUICK DEFINITION), for example, tell Dr. Stoff if the person's immune system is fighting a chronic viral infection and, if so, which type. The more details Dr. Stoff has about a patient's immune system and the status of its different cells, the better he is able to design treatment.

Dr. Stoff checks the patient's organic acid levels (found in the urine) as a gauge of how well their system can detoxify itself. "Our extensive laboratory tests show us where the patient's problems lie. That way I can tell, for example, if the person has an underlying autoimmune problem." (An autoimmune disorder is one in which the immune system attacks the body's own tissues; examples include multiple sclerosis, rheumatoid arthritis, lupus, diabetes mellitus, and chronic thyroiditis.) Some physicians, including Dr. Stoff, put CFS in this category as well.

Not infrequently—at the rate of about two patients per month—Dr. Stoff discovers that a patient actually has cancer, misdiagnosed as chronic fatigue syndrome. Often, conventional doctors fail to do a complete series of tests and come up with a chronic fatigue syndrome diagnosis because it seems to fit the variety of symptoms, says Dr. Stoff. But this can be misleading and sometimes simply wrong, not to mention fatal. "As much as possible, we try to approach the patient without any blinders on. I don't just rubber-stamp another doctor's diagnosis."

Nor is the final prescription out of a therapeutic cookbook: "We may see 100 women with breast cancer, but the treatment protocol will be different for each. We don't have any canned protocols that we take off the shelf just because a person has a *presumed* diagnosis." The clinic's staff meets to discuss their findings and together come up with an overall treatment plan. "We don't miss a trick," says Dr. Stoff. "That's how we consistently get good results." Customarily, a patient stays in Tucson for two days for a complete evaluation and initial treatment prescription. If the patient has cancer or a serious autoimmune problem, it may require staying in town for a month to receive daily intravenous treatments.

> **"We don't have any canned protocols that we take off the shelf just because a person has a presumed diagnosis. The treatment protocol is different for each person," says Jesse Stoff, M.D.**

Paul's Case: Down and Out with Chronic Fatigue

Paul came to Dr. Stoff's clinic suffering from chronic fatigue syndrome. The 39-year-old former missionary was so exhausted that some days he even lacked the energy to get out of bed. Paul had a constant sore throat, swollen glands, recurrent low-grade fever, muscle and joint aches, headaches, chronic indigestion, sleeping disorders, depression, and problems with memory, concentration, and focus. He was tired all the time, took frequent naps, and often could not keep his eyes open in the mornings.

During his time as a missionary, Paul had often skipped meals even though he was performing strenuous physical work. His body had become undernourished and continual stress regarding money problems further depleted his system, Dr. Stoff learned. "Paul crashed and burned from this lifestyle and, as a result, he was down for the count by the time I met him." Although Paul's work had been in the back country of South America, Dr. Stoff's blood, urine, and stool tests did not reveal the presence of any exotic tropical or parasitic infections. But Paul did have high levels of Epstein-Barr virus (SEE QUICK DEFI-

Epstein-Barr virus (EBV) is a herpes-like virus thought to be the cause of infectious mononucleosis and Burkitt's lymphoma. It is contracted through the cells in the lining of the mouth and throat, and can therefore be spread by sharing utensils, kissing, and unsanitary habits. EBV symptoms, frequently duplicated in other conditions, include debilitating fatigue, fever, swollen glands, arthritic symptoms, multiple allergies, and difficulties in concentrating. People with chronic fatigue syndrome often have a high level of EBV antibodies in their blood, but EBV is no longer regarded (as it was in the 1980s) as the sole or even necessarily a contributing cause for chronic fatigue.

DHEA (dehydroepiandrosterone)is naturally produced by the human adrenal glands and gonads with optimal levels occurring around age 20 for women and age 25 for men. After those ages, DHEA levels gradually decline so that a person 80 years old produces only a fraction of the DHEA they did when they were 20. As an antioxidant, hormone regulator, and the building block from which estrogen and testosterone are produced, DHEA is vital to health. Low DHEA levels have been associated with cancer, diabetes, multiple sclerosis, hypertension, obesity, AIDS, heart disease, Alzheimer's, and immune dysfunction illnesses. Test subjects using supplemental DHEA reported improved sleeping patterns, better memory, an improved ability to cope with stress, decreased joint pain, increases in lean muscle, and decreases in body fat. No serious side effects have been reported to date, although acne, oily skin, facial hair growth on women, deepening of the voice, irritability, insomnia, and fatigue have been reported with high DHEA doses.

NITION), commonly associated with chronic fatigue syndrome. His inadequate diet, high physical demands, and stress had left his system seriously deficient in many amino acids and essential fatty acids, says Dr. Stoff.

Even more serious, Paul's basic biological rhythms and hormonal cycles were out of balance. For example, his levels of ACTH (adreno-cortico-tropic hormone, secreted by the pituitary gland, vital for adrenal gland health) were undetectable; his DHEA (SEE QUICK DEFINITION) was almost negligible; his cortisol (SEE QUICK DEFINITION) levels were way too high; and he had multiple enzyme (SEE QUICK DEFINITION) failures based in his pancreas, which made his system unable to absorb nutrients from foods or supplements. "Paul's immune system wasn't working properly because his body could no longer regulate these natural, deep-set cycles," explains Dr. Stoff.

Dr. Stoff's treatment program had many facets. First, he gave Paul a series of Anthroposophic (SEE QUICK DEFINITION) remedies (*Echinacea Argentum*, to stimulate the immune system; *Apis Belladonna*, to work against inflammations; and *Cardus Marianus*, to detoxify the liver) through a single injection every day for ten days. Next, Dr. Stoff put Paul on a multivitamin and an acidophilus supplement. To help regulate his biological cycles and promote sleep, he recommended melatonin (a brain hormone from the pineal gland) at the initial dose of 9 mg at bedtime, then gradually lowering it to 3 mg daily. Dr. Stoff also started Paul on a commercial amino acid formula called Amino-virox™ (2 capsules, 3 times daily, taken 30 minutes before meals) and a multi-nutrient supplement called Immune Boosters (3 capsules daily, with meals).

To counter Paul's depression, promote sleep, and increase levels of serotonin, a key brain chemical, Dr. Stoff gave him 5-hydroxy-tryptophan, a form of the amino acid L-tryptophan (100 mg at bedtime). To restore depleted levels of dopamine, another important brain chemical, Dr. Stoff prescribed Catemine, a form of the amino acid L-tyrosine, and activated vitamin B6 (peridoxal-s-phosphate). The goal was to balance the relationship between two vital brain chemicals, the neurotransmitters (SEE QUICK

DEFINITION) serotonin and dopamine, which, in turn, would reset Paul's biocycles. To address Paul's enzyme deficiencies and to increase his nutrient absorption, Dr. Stoff prescribed an enzyme formula called Absorbaid.

After three days on this program, Paul began to feel much better; his energy levels were markedly improved. This was evidence that his body was resetting its biological clock. A month later, Dr. Stoff added a natural form of the adrenal hormone DHEA (100 mg, taken at dinner) to Paul's regimen. In all, it took about 18 months before Paul was fully recovered. Normally, chronic fatigue syndrome patients recover faster, "but Paul was so nutritionally depleted that it took much longer."

Dr. Stoff has successfully treated at least 1,500 cases of chronic fatigue syndrome. Based on his experience, the return to health involves three stages. First, you put the viruses involved into remission. Second, you have to repair the cellular and systemic damage. Third, the patient must "learn the lessons of the disease" so that the same lifestyle and emotional patterns are not repeated in the future. Paul had to learn how to pace himself, maintain his priorities, and "gain insight into the deeper significance" of his illness. To further this, the clinic staff taught Paul guided visualization techniques and gave him stress reduction counseling.

The goal, says Dr. Stoff, "is to get the person feeling 110% improved without taking any supplements, but this third stage, when they're fully functional, feeling great, and without symptoms, is the longest. Then things slowly, but progressively improve." In general, most of Dr. Stoff's chronic fatigue patients "do well fairly quickly if they follow our directions." As for Paul, he recently left for Russia to do missionary work. ∎

Cortisol is a hormone secreted by the adrenal glands which are located atop the kidneys. Cortisol secretion (as well as the adrenal gland's other hormones, DHEA, adrenaline, and aldosterone) occurs in daily cycles, peaking in the morning and having the lowest values at night. Cortisol promotes protein building, regulates insulin and glycogen synthesis, and helps produce prostaglandins. Under conditions of stress, high amounts of cortisol are released; chronic excess secretion is associated with obesity and suppressed thyroid function. Imbalances in cortisol secretion are linked with low energy, muscle dysfunction, impaired bone repair, thyroid dysfunction, immune system depression, sleep disorders, poor skin regeneration, and decreased growth hormone uptake.

Enzymes are specialized living proteins fundamental to all living processes in the body, necessary for every chemical reaction and the normal activity of our organs, tissues, fluids, and cells. There are hundreds of thousands of these Nature's "workers." Enzymes enable the body to digest and assimilate food. There are special enzymes for digesting proteins, carbohydrates, fats, and plant fibers. Specifically, protease digests proteins, amylase digests carbohydrates, lipase digests fats, cellulase digests fiber, and disaccharidase digests sugars.

Anthroposophic medicine is an extension of conventional Western medicine developed by Austrian scientist Rudolf Steiner, in conjunction with European physicians, in the 1920s. It is based on a spiritual model of the human being and its medicines as extensions of homeopathic remedies. In the U.S., there are about 60 practitioners, all M.D.s, plus hundreds of nurses, but in German-speaking countries, there are thousands of practitioners. In addition, there are several major hospitals in Germany and Switzerland devoted exclusively to this medical approach.

A **neurotransmitter** is a brain chemical with the specific function of enabling communications to happen between brain cells. Chief among the 100 identified to date are acetylcholine, gamma-aminobutyric acid (GABA), serotonin, dopamine, and norepinephrine. Acetylcholine is required for short-term memory and all muscle contractions. GABA works to stop excess nerve signals and thus keeps brain firings from getting out of control; serotonin does the same and helps produce sleep, regulate pain, and influence mood, although too much serotonin can produce depression. Norepinephrine is an excitatory neurotransmitter.

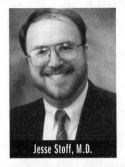

Jesse Stoff, M.D.

Based on Dr. Stoff's experience, the return to health involves three stages. First, you put the viruses involved into remission. Second, you have to repair the cellular and systemic damage. Third, the patient must "learn the lessons of the disease" so that the same lifestyle and emotional patterns are not repeated in the future.

Mapping the Multiple Causes of CFS

Paul's case illustrates the complexity of chronic fatigue syndrome and the need to address that complexity if treatment is going to be successful. As with many other illnesses, the conventional medical establishment searches for a single cause of CFS. It should be obvious that this limited focus does apply to the picture of Paul and the majority of CFS patients for whom illness was the result of the convergence of numerous factors.

Dr. Stoff and many other alternative physicians regard the idea of seeking a single cause as misguided. "There has been a search for bacterial, viral, or fungal activity," says Dr. Leon Chaitow, N.D., D.O., of London, England. "Since many of these (Epstein-Barr virus, herpes simplex, candidiasis) are commonly found to be present (active or dormant) in people with CFS, whatever was found was considered to be 'the cause' of the entire syndrome." Paul's case (and others discussed in this book) makes it clear that a complex illness such as chronic fatigue results from the convergence of many layers of imbalance and dysfunction. To expect to find a single cause is medically foolish.

Like Dr. Stoff, Dr. Chaitow believes strongly that CFS is and must be treated as a multisymptomatic condition, a condition he describes as "similar to an onion in which each peeled layer reveals another layer, or symptomatic factor, underneath. Focus on immune function would be more beneficial than focus on the virus, which is simply taking advantage of the situation," he observes.

EDITOR'S NOTE

Jesse Stoff, M.D., is medical director of Solstice Clinical Associates. From 1985-1991, Dr. Stoff was editor of the *Journal of Anthroposophic Medicine* and, from 1986-1991, he was vice president of the Physicians' Association for Anthroposophic Medicine. Dr. Stoff is coauthor of the best-selling *Chronic Fatigue Syndrome: The Hidden Epidemic* (Harper Collins, 2nd Edition, 1992). To contact Jesse Stoff, M.D.: Solstice Clinical Associates, Southwest Professional Plaza, 2122 North Craycroft Road, #112, Tuscon, AZ 85712; tel: 520-290-4516; fax: 520-290-6403.

Undoing Chronic Fatigue in Stages—
The Scope of This Book

Testing—Before a physician can design an effective treatment plan, it is necessary to determine precisely what is happening in the patient's body. In order to repair the damaged body systems, as Dr. Stoff says, you must first knock out the viruses and infections and eliminate the other factors that are weakening these systems.

Chapter 2 covers the range of testing that is useful to pinpoint the imbalances, deficiencies, infectious agents, and specific immune system weaknesses which are contributing to your CFS. This includes testing for: viral and bacterial infection, candidiasis, and parasites; immune system function; hormonal levels; heavy metal toxicity; enzyme deficiencies; allergies; and nutritional deficiencies. Most of the testing involves simple blood, urine, and stool analyses, but your conventional doctor may not be aware of the specific parameters to investigate.

Viruses, Infections, Candidiasis, and Parasites—Research and clinical evidence has shown that parasites, candidiasis, viruses, and other infections are often present in patients with chronic fatigue syndrome. After testing to determine exactly which of these invaders are present, treatment then begins with eliminating them, as a first step toward restoring the body's natural healing abilities. Chapter 3 explains how these infections can contribute to CFS and discusses an array of techniques used by leading alternative medicine practitioners to successfully rid their patients of the infectious burden on their immune systems.

Restoring Immune Vitality—A depleted immune system is a central feature in CFS. The immune system is the body's basic defensive system with which it resists infection and disease formation—it keeps the body immune from illness. For someone with CFS, the immune system has been operating at a constant, heightened level of activity for a prolonged period. Ironically, this seemingly heightened level of activity is marked by diminished competency; it seems to work harder, but it is actually incapacitated. Chapter 4 describes options for fortifying your depleted immunity.

For **Immune Boosters** (with different formulations of vitamins, minerals, and botanicals: breakfast, lunch, dinner; available without prescription), **Catemine**, and **Absorbaid**, contact: Solstice Vitamin Company, 982 Stuyvesant Avenue, Union, NJ 07083; tel: 800-765-7842 or 908-810-0909. For **Amino-Virox**, contact: Tyson and Associates, 12832 South Chadron Avenue, Hawthorne, CA 90250; tel: 800-318-9766; fax: 310-675-4187. For **Anthroposophic medicines** (available to physicians; some may be obtained without a prescription), contact: Weleda, Inc., 175 North, Route 9 West, P.O. Box 249, Congers, NY 10920; tel: 914-268-8572; fax: 914-268-8574. Raphael Pharmacy, 7957 California Avenue, Fair Oaks, CA 95628; tel: 916-962-1099.

"Focus on immune function would be more beneficial than focus on the virus, which is simply taking advantage of the situation," says Leon Chaitow, N.D., D.O.

Detoxifying the Body—The accumulation of toxins in the body is often another feature of CFS and creates a further burden on the immune system. Whether from stress, poor diet, or chemicals in food and the environment, these toxins need to be removed from the body if the immune system is to be restored to health. Chapter 5 presents methods for removing toxins from the body, especially from the intestines.

An Underactive Thyroid Gland—Although an underactive thyroid was not one of the elements contributing to Paul's chronic fatigue, Dr. Stoff and other physicians have encountered this condition, known as hypothyroidism, in numerous patients diagnosed with CFS. While hypothyroidism is technically considered a separate illness and not a cause of CFS, many CFS patients have not been properly tested for thyroid problems and distinct categorization of the two illnesses is not necessarily of benefit to the patient. Hypothyroidism may be one of the many factors contributing to a person's CFS.

In Chapter 6, you will learn how the thyroid gland and the hormones it produces are integral to the maintenance of your energy levels and to the health of all of your body systems. Stephen Langer, M.D., and Raphael Kellman, M.D., two alternative medicine practitioners who specialize in treating the thyroid, detail cases from their patient files illustrating their successful reversal of hypothyroidism and the associated chronic fatigue.

Mercury in the Mouth Can Lead to CFS—Another hidden factor which often contributes to CFS is mercury toxicity from dental fillings. Again, though Paul's illness did not involve this particular element, it is often a component in CFS. The mercury that most people in the U.S. have in their teeth is actually classified by the Environmental Protection Agency as a hazardous waste. In Chapter 7, biological dentists and other alternative physicians explain the effects of mercury on the body and relate case histories of chronic fatigue patients whose illnesses were turned around after mercury-amalgam filling removal.

Enzyme Deficiency—As Dr. Stoff discovered in the tests he ran on Paul, enzyme deficiencies were interfering with Paul's absorption of nutrients from food and supplements. Enzymes are needed to digest food; when they are deficient, numerous problems develop in the gastrointestinal system and eventually in the immune system. Without the necessary fuel, his already weakened body was further depleted. In Chapter 8, enzyme experts Maile Pouls, Ph.D., and Lita Lee, Ph.D., describe the far-reaching effects of enzyme deficiencies and their vital role in intestinal health, and how a precise program of enzyme and other nutrient supplementation can help reverse serious health problems such as chronic fatigue syndrome.

Underlying Allergies—One of the symptoms shared by CFS, fibromyalgia, and environmental illness is allergies; in the case of the latter, the allergies are so severe as to be debilitating. In Chapter 9, Milton Hammerly, M.D., describes how hidden allergies and related intestinal imbalance can perpetuate CFS. Devi Nambudripad, D.C., L.Ac., R.N., Ph.D., presents cases in which chronic fatigue was reversed by getting rid of allergies using her Nambudripad Allergy Elimination Technique. Finally, Susan Lange, O.M.D., L.Ac., recounts the story of her own recovery from environmental illness—the ultimate allergy—and explains the "sick building syndrome."

Other Factors That Can Generate Fatigue

Fatigue can result from a variety of conditions other than chronic fatigue syndrome, according to Leon Chaitow, N.D., D.O. These include:

- Adrenal insufficiency caused by excessive stress and/or the overuse of stimulants (tea, coffee, chocolate, cola, alcohol, tobacco, drugs)
- Anemia (low levels of iron or vitamin B12 in the blood result in anemia; a blood test can verify this diagnosis)
- Candidiasis (often misdiagnosed as CFS in women)
- Cardiovascular causes (if breathlessness and/or chest pain on exertion accompanies fatigue, the heart may be involved)
- Chronic ill-health (many chronic diseases have fatigue as a symptom)
- Depression
- Diabetes
- Headaches
- Hypoglycemia (low blood sugar)
- Obesity
- Premenstrual syndrome (the connection will be obvious if fatigue occurs at the same time in the monthly cycle)
- Sleep disturbance or inadequate sleep
- Stress

You may note that a number of the causes listed are also symptoms of chronic fatigue syndrome. This highlights the circularity of symptoms and illness. Depression is both a symptom and a cause of fatigue, as are headaches, candidiasis, PMS, poor stress-coping skills, and sleep disorders. The presence of these factors can produce a downward spiral of illness and it becomes difficult to tell which came first, the fatigue or the other exhibited symptoms.

Nutritional Deficiencies Weaken the Immune System—Like most CFS patients, Paul had numerous nutritional deficiencies; in his case, they were the result of an inadequate diet, enzyme deficiencies, the heavy physical demands of his work, and stress. Once the underlying factors which are producing the deficiencies are identified and treated, it is necessary, according to Dr. Stoff and other alternative physicians, to replenish the body's supply of vitamins, minerals, amino acids, and other essential nutrients. This will help bolster the immune system and give the body the strength to begin healing itself. Chapter 10 details the nutrients that are commonly deficient in chronic fatigue conditions and those useful in fortifying the immune system.

Healing the Psychological Side of CFS—Dr. Stoff referred to the need for people with CFS to "learn the lessons of the disease" in order not to repeat the emotional, psychological, and lifestyle patterns which contributed to their illness. He provided Paul with the tools of guided visualization and stress reduction counseling to gain these insights. In Chapter 11, clinical cases from alternative medicine physicians illustrate how lifestyle choices, psychological factors, and suppressed emotions can contribute to CFS. You will learn how homeopathy, traditional Chinese medicine, flower remedies, and color therapy can assist in resolving the psychological and emotional aspects of illness. You will also learn more about the relationship between CFS and depression, the main psychological/emotional symptom of the syndrome.

Herbal Medicine Can Help Treat Causes and Symptoms—There are a variety of herbs which can be of assistance in the treatment of CFS by both addressing underlying causes and providing symptomatic relief. An example of the former are herbs which support and strengthen the immune system or adrenal glands. In the latter category, herbs can offer relief from the array of CFS symptoms ranging from fatigue to muscle aches. They have the advantage over conventional medications of doing so without side effects. Chapter 12 offers a compendium of herbs with research presenting evidence of their efficacy in particular applications.

By the time you have finished these chapters, you will have a comprehensive view of CFS and many practical recommendations for putting an end to your chronic fatigue, including a list of helpful physicians and substances.

From The Vapors to Soldier's Heart to Tahoe Flu: A Brief History of Chronic Fatigue

The first cases of chronic fatigue syndrome may have occurred in the 19th century in the form of "the vapors," followed in the early 20th century by a malady of World War I veterans called "soldier's heart." It wasn't until the mid-1980s, however, that the disorder received widespread attention as the result of a virtual epidemic in the small Lake Tahoe resort town of Incline Village, Nevada.

Beginning early in 1984, Daniel Peterson, M.D., and Paul Cheney, M.D., were baffled by the several patients a day who came to their office suffering from persistent extreme fatigue and whole-body muscle aches. Later it was learned that doctors across the country were treating patients for similar symptoms, but nowhere was the disease as prevalent in a population as in Incline Village.

By June of 1985, the number of afflicted patients consulting Drs. Peterson and Cheney was 90; by July, 120; and by the end of the summer, 150. The U.S. Centers for Disease Control (CDC) ignored the situation until the doctors sent them 12 samples of the Tahoe patients' blood, all of which tested abnormally high for the Epstein-Barr virus (EBV) antibodies, as had samples from other sources. These results prompted the CDC to launch an investigation which did not lead to the discovery of why the disorder was so concentrated in Incline Village, but did eventually result in its classification as a recognized illness. In addition, the CDC investigators came to the conclusion that Epstein-Barr was not necessarily the source. The patients involved also had high antibody levels for cytomegalovirus and herpes simplex. Later, other viruses were pinpointed in connection to the disease as well. Meanwhile, the numbers of those affected in Incline Village had risen to nearly 200 out of the town's population of 20,000.

Variously labeled Tahoe flu, chronic Epstein-Barr, or chronic mononucleosis, in 1987, the CDC gave the elusive illness the official name of chronic fatigue syndrome (CFS) and, in 1988, released guidelines for diagnosis (see "Required Symptoms for a Diagnosis of Chronic Fatigue, According to the U.S. Centers for Disease Control, p. 14). A glib reporter dubbed CFS "Yuppie flu" as a result of the published demographics. At that time, those who were seeking medical help for CFS were predominantly white and upper middle-class. While CFS still tends to be an adult disease and affects more women than men, the epidemic has since become "democratic," leaving no one exempt.

As a footnote, Drs. Cheney and Peterson were repaid for bringing the epidemic to official and public attention by being labeled quacks in their own community. Many people preferred to believe this was an imaginary illness and blamed the doctors for perpetuating patients' fantasies and hypochondria and, in the process, scaring away the tourist trade which was the economic backbone of the town. Dr. Cheney moved his practice to North Carolina, where patients from all over the country came to consult with him. [13]

Drugs Whose Side Effects Resemble Symptoms of Chronic Fatigue

A ccording to the *Physicians' Desk Reference*, the following drugs can produce side effects similar or identical to symptoms associated with chronic fatigue syndrome. If you are taking any of these drugs, they may be compounding or even producing your symptoms. For example, with a drug such as Centrax Capsules (a brand name version of diazepam, a tranquilizer), common side effects include mild drowsiness, weakness, and confusion, while less common side effects include depression, lethargy, headache, stupor, dizziness, and numerous others. It should be obvious that many of these symptoms are identical to problems experienced by patients with CFS. (Percentages refer to the number of individuals affected.)

Accutane Capsules
  (approximately 1 in 20)

Actimmune (14%)

Alferon N Injection (6% to 14%)

Anafranil Capsules (35% to 39%)

Aredia for Injection (up to 12%)

Atrofen Tablets (2% to 4%)

Blocadren Tablets (3.4% to 5%)

BuSpar (4%)

Cardura Tablets (12%)

Cartrol Tablets (7.1%)

Catapres to TTS (4% to 6%)

Centrax Capsules (11.6%)

CHEMET (succimer) Capsules
  (5.2% to 15.7%)

Combipres Tablets (about 4%)

Cordarone Tablets (4% to 9%)

Dantrium Capsules (among the
  most frequent)

Depo to Provera Contraceptive
  Injection (more than 5%)

Desyrel and Desyrel Dividose
  (5.7% to 11.3%)

DynaCirc Capsules (0.4% to 3.9%)

Engerix to B Unit to Dose Vials (14%)

Epogen for Injection (9% to 25%)

Ergamisol Tablets (6%)

Ethmozine Tablets (3.1% to 5.9%)

Fludara for Injection (10% to 38%)

Foscavir Injection (More than 5%)

Hismanal Tablets (4.2%)

Hivid Tablets (less than 1% to 34%)

Hylorel Tablets (25.7% to 63.6%)

Hytrin Tablets (11.3%)

Intron A (18% to 84%)

Kerlone Tablets (2.9% to 9.7%)

Lariam Tablets (among the most frequent)

Leucovorin Calcium for Injection
  (2% to 13%)

Levatol (4.4%)

Lopid Tablets (3.8%)

Lopressor Ampuls, Tablets (10%),

HCT Tablets (10 in 100 patients)

Lozol Tablets (greater than
  or equal to 5%)

Ludiomil Tablets (4%)

Marplan Tablets
(among the most frequent)

Mesnex Injection (33%)

Mexitil Capsules (1.9% to 3.8%)

Mykrox Tablets (4.4%)

NebuPent for Inhalation Solution
(53% to 72%)

Neupogen for Injection (11%)

Nipent for Injection (29%)

Nolvadex Tablets (3.8%)

Normodyne Injection, Tablets
(2% to 10%)

Norpace Capsules, CR Capsules
(3% to 9%)

Norvasc Tablets (4.5%)

Parlodel Capsules, SnapTabs
(1% to 7%)

Polygam, Immune Globulin Intravenous
(Human) (3% to 6%)

Prinivil Tablets (3.3%)

Prinzide Tablets (3.7%)

Procardia XL Extended Release Tablets
(5.9%)

Procrit for Injection (9% to 13%)

Proleukin for Injection (53%)

Prozac Pulvules & Liquid,
Oral Solution (4.2%)

Reglan Injectable, Syrup,

Tablets (10%)

Roferon to A Injection (89% to 95%)

Rowasa Rectal Suppositories,
Rectal Suspension Enema (3.4%)

Rythmol Tablets (1.8% to 6%)

Sectral Capsules (11%)

Seldane Tablets (2.9% to 4.5%)

Supprelin Injection (1% to 10%)

Tambocor Tablets (7.7%)

Tegison Capsules (50% to 75%)

Tenex Tablets (3% to 12%)

Tenoretic Tablets (0.6% to 26%)

Tenormin Tablets and I.V. Injection
(0.6% to 26%)

Toprol XL Tablets
(about 10 of 100 patients)

Trandate Injection (1% to 10%),
Tablets (2% to 11%)

Valrelease Capsules
(among the most common)

Vaseretic Tablets (3.9%)

Visken Tablets (8%)

Wellbutrin Tablets (5%)

Xanax Tablets (48.6%)

Zebeta Tablets (6.6% to 8.2%)

Zestoretic (3.7%)

Zestril Tablets (3.3%)

Zoloft Tablets (10.6%)

Testing

THE KEY TO UNDERSTANDING
THE CAUSES OF YOUR
CHRONIC FATIGUE

AS CHRONIC FATIGUE syndrome expert Jesse Stoff, M.D., explained in Chapter 1, using a variety of medical tests to find out the interlinking causes of a patient's CFS is the first order of business. Unfortunately, no single standard medical test exists to detect chronic fatigue syndrome in all its complexity, so diagnosis depends on a history of illness which fits the pattern of CFS, along with ruling out all other conditions with similar symptoms. These include multiple sclerosis, systemic lupus erythematosus, cancer, unresolved hepatitis B or C, sleep apnea, narcolepsy, alcohol or substance abuse, side effects of medication, severe

> A careful medical history, a physical examination, and laboratory tests can pinpoint specific infections often associated with CFS and provide an inventory of the pattern of symptoms, which may be the surest way to diagnose the illness.

obesity, and such psychiatric illnesses as major depressive disorder, schizophrenia, bipolar disorder, dementia, and eating disorders (anorexia and bulimia).[1]

Getting a clear symptom picture is often difficult due to the tendency of CFS symptoms to fluctuate in degree and severity, not only over a period of weeks or months, but even from day to day. A cyclical pattern of illness and reasonable health is the result. Frequently, after a severe bout of CFS, a patient resumes normal activity and exercise, only to relapse into extreme fatigue after a period of time. But if a number of CFS symptoms persist for six months (see sidebar:

"Required Symptoms for a Diagnosis of Chronic Fatigue, According to the U.S. Centers for Disease Control," p. 14) and other causes have been eliminated, it is considered likely that the person has CFS.[2]

A careful medical history, a physical examination, and selected laboratory tests (highlighted in this chapter) can pinpoint specific infections often associated with CFS and provide the physician with an inventory of the pattern of symptoms. This may be the surest way to diagnose the illness, says Leon Chaitow, N.D., D.O., of London, England.

In addition to the well-known symptoms of CFS, Murray R. Susser, M.D., of Santa Monica, California, notes that, unlike in healthy people, brain circulation in CFS patients gets worse after exercise. Therefore, as part of getting a complete symptomatic picture, he tests patients after exercise for decreased blood circulation in the brain. He also tests the cortisol level in the blood which (unlike in healthy people) decreases in CFS patients after exercise. Low levels of this hormone (vital for dealing with stress) suggests the likelihood of CFS.[3]

Tests Covered in This Chapter

- **Electrodermal Screening**
- **Anti-Candida Antibodies Panel**
- **Stool Analysis**
- **Urine Analysis**
- **CBC Blood Test Report**
- **Immune System Testing**
  -T and B Cell Panel
  -Natural Killer Cell Function
  -Nitrogen Balance
  -Biological Terrain Assessment
- **Hormone Testing**
  -Saliva Assay Report
  -TRH Test (thyroid)
  -Adrenal Stress Index
  -DHEA Challenge Test
- **Heavy Metal Toxicity Screening**
  -ToxMet Screen
- **Testing for Enzyme Deficiencies**
  -Loomis Urinalysis
- **Allergy Testing**
  -NAET
  -Skin Testing
  -IgG ELISA Test
- **Testing for Nutritional Deficiencies**
  -Individualized Optimal Nutrition
  -Functional Intracellular Analysis
  -Pantox Antioxidant Profile
  -Oxidative Protection Screen

Testing for the Underlying Causes

As discussed in Chapter 1, alternative medicine physicians are less focused on getting a definitive diagnosis of CFS, aside from eliminating other disorders, than they are in gathering as much information as possible on the underlying causes that are producing the patient's symptoms. Without this information, any treatment program is guesswork. For this reason and depending on the individual's symptoms, according to the physicians presented in this book, it may be

Alternative medicine physicians are less focused on getting a definitive diagnosis of CFS than they are in gathering as much information as possible on the underlying causes that are producing the patient's symptoms.

wise to test for the following: candidiasis, parasites, and bacterial and viral infections; immune system abnormalities; hormonal imbalances and deficiences; heavy metal toxicity; enzyme deficiencies; allergies; and nutritional deficiencies.

Electrodermal Screening: Versatile Energy Testing

Electrodermal screening (EDS) is a quick method to identify most of these conditions, especially ones involving toxic or allergic substances. A blunt, noninvasive electric probe is placed at specific points on the patient's hands, face, or feet, corresponding to acupuncture points at the beginning or end of energy meridians. Minute electrical discharges from these points serve as information signals about the condition of the body's organs and systems, useful for the physician in evaluation and in developing a treatment plan.

The normal waiting period of laboratory analysis is avoided through the immediate feedback provided by this computerized testing of the body's organs and systems via acupuncture points. As a cross-reference, specific blood, urine, and stool analyses can then be ordered to serve as confirmation of electrodermal results. By quickly pinpointing problems, EDS can prevent unnecessary, guesswork testing. For example, if EDS indicates that a person has a specific type of parasite, running a stool analysis for that parasite eliminates the trial and error of the often long process of testing to see if parasites, in general, are a problem. EDS can also be helpful in determining the body's tolerance to medications or remedies which may be prescribed.

The key idea with EDS is that it is a "data acquisition process" in which the trained practitioner conducts an "interview" with the patient's organs and tissues, gathering information about the basic functional status of those systems and their energy pathways, says James Hoyt Clark of Orem, Utah, an EDS inventor and educator. As such, EDS

For more information about the **LISTEN System and EDS seminars**, contact: James Hoyt Clark, Biosource, Inc., 1388 West Center Street, Orem, UT 84057; tel: 801-226-1117. For more information about the **Omega Acubase system and seminars**, contact: Vaughn Cook, L.Ac., Digital Health, Inc., 1770 East Fort Union Blvd., #101, Salt Lake City, UT 84121; tel: 801-944-4070; fax: 801-944-4067. For **Acupro**, contact: Doug Lieber, Computronix Electro-Medical Systems, 145 Canyon Oaks Drive, Argyle, TX 76226; tel: 817-241-2768; fax: 817-455-2605. For more information about **electrodermal screening, energy medicine, and devices**, contact: Occidental Institute Research Foundation, P.O. Box 100 Penticton, British Columbia, Canada V2A 6J9; tel: 604-497-6020; fax: 604-497-6030.

is an investigational, not diagnostic, device because it requires the physician's knowledge of acupuncture, physiology, and therapeutic substances to interpret the energy imbalances, establish their precise focus, and select the most appropriate therapeutic response.

EDS can indicate the degree of stress that is affecting an organ and can monitor the progress of therapy, avoiding trial and error and general guesswork. According to the way EDS devices are calibrated, initial readings above 60 can indicate an inflammation somewhere in the body, while readings below 45 can often indicate physiological changes brought about by a degenerative process. The physician's task is to find a single substance or combination of substances that will balance the point, which means bringing its EDS reading back close to

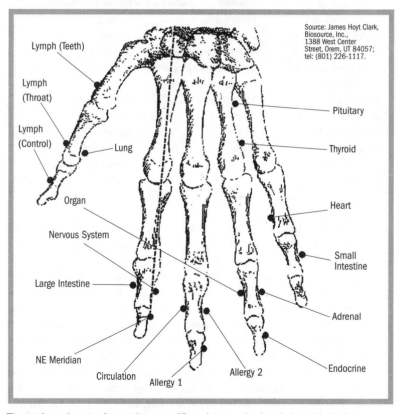

Electrodermal screening probes specific points on the hands (see black dots above) to gather information about the health function or possible toxicity of organs and body systems. These points are part of acupuncture meridians.

Substances Whose Effect on the Body Can Be Pinpointed with Electrodermal Screening

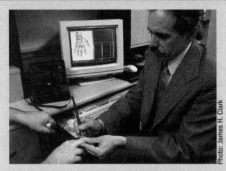

alcohol products
amino acids
animal danders
Ayurvedic herbs
blossoming flowers
cacti and succulents
chemicals
Chinese/Japanese herbs
cleaners
colors and dyes
dental products
digestive enzymes
endocrines
environmentals
essential oils
flower essences
food
gems/minerals
geopathic agents
grasses, weeds
habit-forming drugs

homeopathics-
   combinations
homeopathics-drainage
homeopathics-polychrest
homeopathics-singles
hormones
insects
metals
miasms
minerals
molds/fungi

nosodes
parasites
pesticides
phenolics
sarcodes
shrubs
snakes
spiders
tree pollens
veterinary viruses
vitamins

50. For example, the pancreas readings for a person with diabetes will become balanced when the correct and appropriate dose of insulin is placed within the EDS circuit.

The more sophisticated EDS devices, such as the LISTEN system from Biosource (developed by James Hoyt Clark), Omega Acubase from Digital Health, Inc., and Acupro from Computronix, contain an inventory of energy signals corresponding to several thousand different substances. This inventory is called the Product Library; the LISTEN system is programmed with information for about 4,000 substances. These include most of the homeopathic remedies, grass, weed, and tree pollens, foods, toxic chemicals, dental materials, molds, bacteria, healthy and diseased organ states, and conventional drugs.

"The LISTEN system is not diagnostic; it doesn't pick the remedy," explains Bruce Shelton, M.D., M.D.(H), Di.Hom., founder and director of the Allergy Center in Phoenix, Arizona. Dr. Shelton rou-

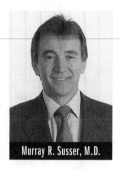

Murray R. Susser, M.D.

"The most common infections we find are yeast and parasites," reports Dr. Susser. "We also find hidden bacterial infections such as Lyme disease and abscesses in the teeth and sometimes chronic prostatitis, chronic sinusitis, and chronic gastritis."

tinely uses EDS as a front-line testing procedure to identify multiple toxins and allergens in his patients. "I use the device as a yes/no meter for what I'm thinking about the patient." EDS only indicates, based on the operator's skillful input, whether a given substance will balance a condition. "When a substance balances the symptoms highlighted by EDS, it means you need it as a remedy," says Dr. Shelton.

For more about **allergies**, see Chapter 9: Addressing the Allergy Connection, pp. 232-258.

Testing for Candidiasis, Parasites, and Bacterial and Viral Infections

While the presence of multiple infections often associated with CFS may not provide definitive proof that a person has the illness, knowing what the body is contending with is the first step in treatment design.

"The most common infections we find are yeast [*Candida albicans*] and parasites," reports Dr. Susser. "We also find hidden bacterial infections such as Lyme disease [*Borrelia burgdorferi*] and abscesses in the teeth and sometimes chronic prostatitis, chronic sinusitis, and chronic gastritis." Elevated antibody levels (activated immune proteins) to certain viruses are frequently found in the blood of CFS patients. These include Epstein-Barr, cytomegalovirus, human herpes virus–6, herpes simplex, rubella, and enteroviruses such as Coxsackie.

The Anti-Candida Antibodies Panel—As mentioned above, electrodermal screening can identify the presence of most of these infectious agents. Follow-up blood tests or other laboratory workups can quantify the presence of these agents. Candidiasis, an overgrowth of the yeastlike fungus *Candida albicans* (a normal flora of the skin, mouth, intestinal tract, and vagina), can be determined by stool or blood analyses. One blood test, called the Anti-Candida Antibodies Panel, measures the levels of the IgG and IgM antibodies (SEE QUICK DEFINITION) against *Candida*; the IgG levels indicate both past and ongoing infection, while the IgM may be a truer reflection of present infection.

Parasites—Another factor that may be weakening the CFS patient's immune system from the inside is parasites. The human body may have unwelcome residents that are harmful to health, literally eating us from the inside, using our nutrients and often plugging up our lymphatic vessels. The possible presence of parasites in the body, mostly in the intestines, is a little-appreciated but major health problem, according to nutrition educator Ann Louise Gittleman.[4] People assume they are vulnerable to parasites only if they travel in tropical areas, but this is a dangerous misconception, says Gittleman. Anyone can get them (and many probably already have) from merely staying at home.

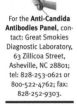

For the **Anti-Candida Antibodies Panel**, contact: Great Smokies Diagnostic Laboratory, 63 Zillicoa Street, Asheville, NC 28801; tel: 828-253-0621 or 800-522-4762; fax: 828-252-9303.

Undiagnosed parasitic infections (from microscopic protozoa to various species of worms) may account for a great deal of the otherwise unexplained diseases currently besetting America. One estimate contends that 25% of New York City residents have a parasitic infection and that, by the year 2025, 50% of the projected 8.3 billion world population will have them. Parasites tend to reside in the intestines, but they can also migrate to the blood, lymph, heart, liver, gallbladder, pancreas, spleen, eyes, and brain. While in place, they can produce numerous symptoms: constipation, diarrhea, gas, bloating,

Antibodies	Normal	Abnormal	Reference Range
IgG	500.0		(REF. RANGE 500-8000)
IgM	50.0		(REF. RANGE 50-3000)
IgA	50.0		(REF. RANGE 50-8000)
Candida Antigen	2.0		(REF. RANGE 0-10)
Immune Complex	1200.0		(REF. RANGE 0 - 7000)

The Anti-Candida Antibodies Panel measures the levels of key immune defense proteins or antibodies (the immunoglobulins IgG and IgM) against the yeast *Candida albicans*.

irritable bowel syndrome, joint and muscle aches, allergies, anemia, skin problems, sleep disturbances, chronic fatigue, and gradual immune dysfunction.

According to Gittleman's research, parasite damage can be extensive. Parasites can destroy cells faster than they can be regenerated; they can release toxins that damage tissues, resulting in pain and inflammation; and, over time, they can depress, even exhaust, the immune system. Of the dozens of specific parasites of concern to human health, the major groupings include microscopic protozoa, roundworms, pinworms, hookworms (Nematoda), tapeworms (Cestoda), and flukes (Trematoda).

Parasitic infection, however, is as difficult to diagnose as chronic fatigue syndrome itself. One of the main problems related to the study of parasitic infections and their link to systemic illness is the fact that "most parasitology laboratories fail to find the majority of intestinal parasites in stool specimens submitted to them," according to the *Journal of Advancement in Medicine*.[5] David Casemore, M.D., of the Public Health Laboratories in Bodewuddan, Rhyh, England, adds that parasitic infection "is almost certainly underdetected, possibly by a factor of ten or more."[6] Steven Bailey, N.D., of Portland, Oregon, reports that one patient with AIDS required examination of 12 stool samples before giardiasis (infection with the protozoan *Giardia lambia*) was diagnosed.[7] Unfortunately, this is not an unusual occurrence.

According to Martin Lee, Ph.D., director of Great Smokies Diagnostic Laboratory in Asheville, North Carolina, many doctors, hospitals, and laboratories fail to diagnose parasitic infection because they rarely allow the time for careful analysis or multiple procedures using stool specimens collected over several days. Dr. Lee suggests that if you suspect you may have an intestinal parasite, or just want to be tested as a preventative measure, make sure your physician, hospital, or lab follows the guidelines set by the U.S. Centers for Disease Control and the *Manual of Clinical Microbiology*.

The Comprehensive Digestive Stool Analysis (described below) provides useful indications of general parasitic activity. Immunofluores-cent staining may be another method to detect your parasites. This technique uses antibodies against parasites tagged with fluorescent dyes which make them highly visible under the microscope.

A Dental Marker of Chronic Fatigue?

One of the primary setbacks to treating chronic fatigue syndrome has been the lack of a specific medical "marker" that would indicate a clinical way to diagnose the syndrome. Burke A. Cunha, M.D., chief of the Infectious Disease Division of Winthrop-University Hospital in Mineola, New York, has discovered arch-shaped, bright red membrane tissue in the back of CFS patients' mouths. Located on both inner sides of the mouth next to the back molars, these "crimson crescents," as Dr. Cunha calls them, intensify in color as the patient's condition worsens, and fade as the patient improves.

Dr. Cunha states that the crescents appear in 80% of CFS patients but show up in less than 5% of non-CFS patients with sore throats, and not at all in patients with mononucleosis or strep throat. He states, "If your patient has crimson crescents, you now can say his condition is probably chronic fatigue syndrome."[8] Although Dr. Cunha's findings are recent and have not been confirmed by other health practitioners, the existence of such a marker for CFS bears further investigation.

As they attack specific parasites, the antibodies will show up only where there is a parasitic presence.

What a Stool Analysis Can Indicate: A Glossary of Terms

In addition to parasites, there are many other intestinal factors which may be playing a role in your illness. A healthy digestive system is central to the maintenance of overall health. Problems that begin in the intestines have far-reaching effects on the body and can contribute to the development of serious illnesses. Digestive problems, such as diarrhea, constipation, irritable bowel syndrome, bloating, gas, or indigestion, are usually part of the symptom picture in CFS, fibromyalgia, and environmental illness.

Understanding how well, or poorly, food is digested and measuring other parameters of intestinal health in a patient with one of these disorders can provide therapeutic insights and point the way to healing. A stool analysis can serve as this "window" into digestive inadequacies. The following is a glossary of terms used in this type of analysis along with an explanation of what each of the values can tell you:

Dysbiosis Index—Intestinal dysbiosis refers to an imbalance of intestinal flora. Specifically, these flora include friendly, beneficial bacteria called probiotics (for example, *Lactobacillus acidophilus* and *Bifidobacterium bifidum*) and unfriendly or harmful bacteria (for example, *Pseudomonas aeruginosa*). In dysbiosis, the unfriendly bacteria predominate; they begin fermentation, producing toxic by-products which interfere with the normal elimination cycle. The dysbiosis index reflects the balance of friendly and pathogenic bacteria, and those markers related to the flora, such as pH and SCFAs.

Colonic Environment

Lactobacillus and **Bifidobacteria**–These bacteria are involved in vitamin synthesis, the detoxification of procarcinogens (substances that become carcinogenic or cancer-causing), and they support the immune system. Deficiencies of *Lactobacillus* have been linked with a higher risk for various chronic diseases.

For information about the **Comprehensive Digestive Stool Analysis,** contact: Great Smokies Diagnostic Laboratory, 63 Zillicoa Street, Asheville, NC 28801; tel: 828-253-0621 or 800-522-4762; fax: 828-252-9303.

gamma Streptococcus–This is a bacteria normal to the intestines; its presence in the analysis is not an indication of digestive imbalance.

Candida albicans–The intestinal tract normally contains small amounts of this yeast. In some cases, however, wide use of antibiotics or birth control pills and a high-carbohy-

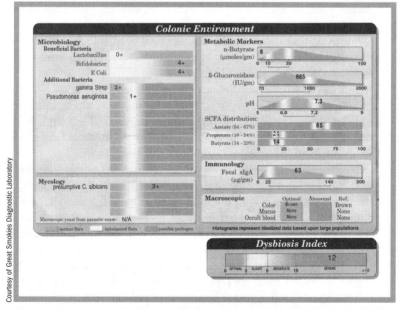

Courtesy of Great Smokies Diagnostic Laboratory

The stool analysis provides important information about the health status of the intestines and their function, especially regarding the population of numerous bacteria, both helpful and pathogenic. This relationship, when it is imbalanced, is called dysbiosis, as indicated in the chart above.

A healthy digestive system is central to the maintenance of overall health. Problems that begin in the intestines have far-reaching effects on the body and can contribute to the development of serious illnesses.

drate diet may cause an overgrowth of the *Candida* yeast, causing a condition called candidiasis. Overgrowth of *Candida albicans* and other intestinal yeasts has been linked to food allergies, migraines, vaginitis, irritable bowel syndrome, indigestion, and asthma.

Pseudomonas aeruginosa—Associated with wound infections, infected burn lesions, and urinary tract infections, this bacterium produces a characteristic blue pus and causes infections in the context of a weakened immune system. These problems do not normally occur in the colon; however, *P. aeruginosa* in the colon may or may not be symptomatic. If symptomatic, it may contribute to diarrhea and inflammation.

Macroscopic (appearance)—Yellow to green stools may indicate diarrhea and a bowel sterilized by antibiotics; black or red may reflect bleeding in the gastrointestinal tract; tan or grey can indicate a blockage of the common bile duct; mucus or pus can point to irritable bowel syndrome, polyps, diverticulitis, or intestinal wall inflammation; and occult blood might result from eating too much red meat, from hemorrhoids, or possibly from colon cancer.

pH—pH is a reflection of the acid/alkaline balance in the colon. The preferred range is 6.0 (mildly acidic) to 7.2 (mildly alkaline). Fecal pH reflects the status of colonic digestive processes, SCFAs (see below), beneficial bacteria, and bacterial metabolism. An elevated fecal pH is associated with a higher risk of colitis and colon cancer.

N-butyrate—This is a form of butyric acid, a primary energy source for the colon cells; it must be present in adequate amounts for healthy metabolism (energy, nutrient, and water release from foods) in the colon. Butyric acid is needed to digest short-chain fatty acids (SCFAs). Low levels of N-butyrate are associated with a higher risk of colon cancer.

Total SCFA—Short-chain fatty acids, such as acetate, propionate, N-butyrate, and valerate, are produced when the colon ferments soluble fibers. SCFAs are important because they provide 70% of the energy needed by the cells lining the colon.

SCFA distribution—Elevated levels of any of the four SCFAs can indicate poor nutrient absorption in the colon or bacterial overgrowth, while decreased levels suggest lack of dietary fiber, unbalanced metabolic processes, or dysbiosis. The key factor here is the ratio among the four SCFAs, which usually remains relatively constant in healthy individuals but can shift noticeably when metabolism becomes disordered.

Beta-glucuronidase—This is an enzyme produced by various bacteria in the colon. Elevated levels may result from bacterial overgrowth, an abnormal intestinal pH, too much dietary fat (especially from meat), or low levels of beneficial bacteria. Elevated levels can increase bioactivation of carcinogens in the bowel, thus increasing the risk of colon cancer.

Fecal sIgA—Fecal secretory IgA is a specialized immunoglobulin, which is one of a class of five specially designed antibody proteins produced in the spleen, bone marrow, or lymph tissue. They are involved in the immune system's defense response to foreign substances. Fecal sIgA serves as the first line of defense against invading pathogens, toxins, and food allergens in the intestines. Low levels mean an increased susceptibility to infection and food allergies.

Measures of Digestive Dysfunction

Triglycerides—Most dietary fats are triglycerides, a term that denotes their chemical structure. During digestion, lipase, a pancreatic enzyme, breaks triglycerides down into glycerol and free fatty acids. Elevated fecal triglyceride levels indicate incomplete fat metabolism and possible problems in the pancreas.

Chymotrypsin—Relative levels of this digestive enzyme, produced in the

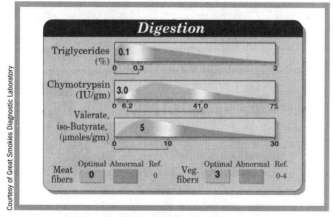

The degree of digestive dysfunction can be indicated by studying the levels of numerous biochemicals and fibers, shown above.

intestines, can indicate the patient's enzyme status and activity. Decreased levels mean the pancreas is not releasing enough enzymes and/or that the stomach is low on digestive acids, which are needed to activate chymotrypsin. Elevated levels suggest a rapid transit time (the speed at which fecal matter moves through the intestines).

Valerate and iso-butyrate—Valerate and iso-butyrate are short-chain fatty acids produced when intestinal bacteria ferment protein. Elevated levels indicate that the protein was not digested properly in the stomach and intestines.

Meat and vegetable fibers—These are crude microscopic markers for digestive function. Elevated levels may indicate inadequate chewing, stomach acid, or digestive enzymes.

Measures of Absorption

LCFAs—Long-chain fatty acids are normally absorbed directly by intestinal mucosa. Elevated levels reflect malabsorption of fats, a result of maldigestion or inflammation of the lining of the small intestine.

Cholesterol—Cholesterol in the feces comes from either dietary fats or the breakdown of the cells lining the intestines. Generally, fecal cholesterol levels remain stable, despite dietary intake; elevated fecal levels suggest malabsorption or irritation of the mucosal lining.

Total fecal fat—This represents the sum of all fats or lipids, except for SCFAs, and can indicate either maldigestion or malabsorption.

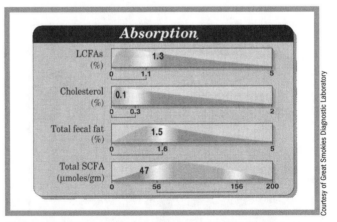

Food consumption does not equal absorption. That's why it's necessary to pinpoint the levels of the four substances shown above as they are critical indicators of how well nutrients are being absorbed.

What a Urine Analysis Reveals:
A Glossary of Terms

A urine analysis provides another window into what precisely is happening in a CFS patient's body. Again, chronic digestive problems are often associated with CFS and a 24-hour urine analysis can pinpoint what is going wrong in digestion. Then the appropriate therapies can be implemented to help break the cycle of CFS in which imbalances in one system of the body feed imbalances in another.

For the test, a patient's total urine output is collected over a 24-hour period, then analyzed in a laboratory for the status of key biochemical factors. These can include kidney function, levels of bowel toxicity, pH, vitamin C, calcium, and other essential nutrients, and how the body is handling proteins, fats, and carbohydrates. The following are specific values measured in urine analysis:

Volume–The total urine output, either excessive (polyuria) or minimal (oliguria), in relationship to the specific gravity indicates how well the kidneys are functioning.

Indican–This indicates the degree of toxicity, putrefaction, gas, and fermentation in the intestines. Indican comes from putrefying proteins in the large intestine which are kicked back into the blood and excreted through the kidneys. Indican is extremely toxic and causes many symptoms; the higher the level, the greater the intestinal toxemia or inflammation in the digestive tract. Readings as close to zero as possible are desirable.

pH–Based on hydrogen ion concentration, this value indicates the degree of

For information about receiving a **urine analysis**, contact: Dr. Lita Lee, P.O. Box 516, Lowell, OR 97452; tel: 541-937-1123; fax: 541-963-1132. Also contact: Dr. Maile Pouls, Health Enhancement Center, 517 Liberty Street, Santa Cruz, CA 95060; tel: 408-423-7538; fax: 408-425-2222.

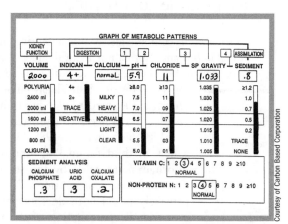

Urine analysis results. A patient's total urine output is collected over a 24-hour period, then analyzed in a laboratory for the status of key biochemical factors (shown above).

urine acidity versus alkalinity on a scale of zero to 14, with urine pH usually ranging from 4.5 to 8.0 and with 7.0 being neutral.

Chlorides–These are salt residues in the urine and the values here give information on salt intake and assimilation.

Specific gravity–This value measures the weight of total dissolved substances (solutes) in the urine against an equal amount of water, such that a normal reading of 1.020 means the urine is 20% heavier than water. Specific gravity shows the general water content (hydration) of the body. Values can typically range from 1.005 to 1.030; a high reading indicates solute concentration and kidney stress.

Total sediment analysis–This indicates the amount of dissolved organic and mineral substances remaining in the urine after digestion; an optimal total reading for the three sediment categories is 0.5.

Calcium phosphate–A reading here indicates the status of carbohydrate digestion; a level of 0.5 signifies normal carbohydrate digestion.

Uric acid–Levels of uric acid signify the status of protein digestion; optimal digestion yields a reading of zero.

Calcium oxalate–This value indicates the status of fat digestion; a reading of zero signifies optimal fat digestion.

Vitamin C–Levels of vitamin C indicate body reserves of this key nutrient; a reading of 1 is high, 2 to 5 normal, and 6 to 10 deficient.

Using the Complete Blood Count as a Guide to Therapy

In addition to comprehensive stool and urine analyses, blood tests can reveal important information about the biochemical status of a person and, as with the other tests, serve as an invaluable guide to developing the most effective, individually tailored treatment program. However, the standard blood tests of conventional medical practice do not necessarily provide a complete picture.

For more information about the **CBC Blood Test Report**, contact: Carbon Based Corporation, 153 Country Club Drive, Incline Village, NV 894451; tel: 702-832-8485; fax: 702-832-8488. **Patricia Kane, Ph.D.**, may be contacted at: Carbon Based East, Five Osprey, Millville, NJ 08332; tel: 609-825-2200 or 609-825-8333; fax: 609-825-2143.

With this in mind, in 1985, Mark A. Schauss developed a new method for making optimum, practical use of information revealed by the standard blood test. His Carbon Based Corporation's Blood Test Report inexpensively offers both doctors and patients a five-part user-friendly formulation of the information, opening "a therapeutic window" to one's unique biochemistry, says Schauss. The test also empowers users to take more control of their health care by allowing them to make more informed decisions.

The Blood Test's Basic Status Report alphabetically lists the amounts detected of about 44 substances normally found in the blood. But it also ranks these items, such as cholesterol, lymphocytes, sodium, and bilirubin, according to their relative deviation from the mean value. Schauss calls this ranking "% Status," which demonstrates by what percentage the client's readings are higher or lower than a statistical norm. For example, normal sodium levels range from 135 to 145, so a one-point deviation is substantial as there are only ten points for normalcy, Schauss explains. On the other hand, normal triglycerides range from zero to 250, so a one-point change here is not significant. The idea is to provide a statistical context and normative comparison for the test results as measured against agreed-upon standards of what is normal, Schauss says.

The Blood Test's Panel Report groups the results according to 14 biochemical considerations, such as electrolytes, kidney function, acid or alkaline pH, nitrogen, and protein. "You can review each of the panels at a glance for unbalanced patterns in your patient's blood chemistry," says Schauss. The Disease Indicators Report compares the total blood status to indicators of any of 140 diseases. Here, known disease patterns, as revealed in a blood analysis, are correlated with the individual's results. For example, the test might indicate a 62.5% match for myasthenia gravis, a 40% match for folic acid deficiency, and a 33.3% match for angina pectoris.

According to CBC medical director Patricia Kane, Ph.D., the CBC Blood Test Report can "depict a patient's potential disease patterns, that is, whether abnormalities in their blood indicate a predisposition toward a certain disease."

According to Carbon Based Corporation (CBC) medical director Patricia Kane, Ph.D., the CBC Blood Test Report can "depict a patient's potential disease patterns, that is, whether abnormalities in their blood indicate a predisposition toward a certain disease. On the lookout for that disease, a physician can investigate further, perhaps stopping the disease before it strikes. By predicting these patterns, the test offers a new outlook toward preventive medicine."

The Drug Interactions Report identifies potential aggravating effects if the patient were to use any of hundreds of conventional drugs. For example, if one's total bilirubin is out of balance, the use of aspirin, penicillin, niacin, or streptomycin is contraindicated because

P.O. Box 829
Millville, NJ 08332
609-825-2200

The % Status is the weighted deviation of the laboratory result.

Low Results

Test	% Status		Result
B.U.N.	-64.29	L	6.00
Creatinine	-61.11	L	0.40
Hematocrit	-58.00	L	36.20
Basophil Count	-50.00	L	0.00
Basophils	-50.00	L	0.00
MCV	-47.33	L	79.56
GGT	-45.45	L	9.00
CO2	-42.31	L	21.00
Iron, Total	-42.14	L	41.00
Uric Acid	-41.23	L	3.00
Sodium	-40.00	L	136.00
Lymphocytes	-37.50	L	25.00
Sodium/Potassium Ratio	-35.37	L	27.76
Eosinophil Count	-30.00	L	140.00
Hemoglobin	-27.50	L	12.90
MCH	-27.47	L	28.35
Triglycerides	-26.80	L	58.00
Lymphocyte Count	-26.25	L	1750.00

High Results

Test	% Status		Result
Anion Gap	89.00	H	17.90
Monocytes	83.33	H	12.00
LDH	70.00	H	242.00
Calcium	66.67	H	10.50
SGOT	53.03	H	46.00
Phosphorus	43.33	H	5.80
MCHC	40.88	H	35.64
Albumin	28.57	H	4.50

Basic Status Report for a patient with depression. Based on the results of a standard blood test, this report arranges the data according to the highs and lows, or % Status. This shows by what percentage the client's readings are higher or lower than a statistical norm.

these would further the imbalance. Finally, the Biochemical Pharmacology Report suggests which supplements are indicated for the given abnormal blood chemistry; the exact dosages are left to a physician to determine. Carbon Based Corporation delivers the five-part report to clients within 48 hours for a cost of about $100, including blood test fees.

Testing the Immune System

Measuring the activity of the immune system is a vital component in determining the level and kind of disease involved and thus the type of support needed to restore immune strength. As mentioned in Chapter 1, certain levels of T and B immune cells (lymphocytes) can indicate a chronic virus and identify the strain. According to Charles W. Lapp,

M.D., of Raleigh, North Carolina, immune testing of CFS patients often reveals, in addition to increased T-cell activity, abnormal levels and impaired function of natural killer cells (foreign protein destroyers) and the presence of autoantibodies (an antibody which attacks the body's own cells) such as antithryroid antibody.

Highly elevated levels of lymphokines or cytokines (interleukin 1, 2, and 3) may also be in evidence. Lymphokines are released by lymphocytes and cytokines by lymphocytes and other cells in response to specific antigens (foreign disease-producing substances). Lymphokines assist cellular immunity by stimulating macrophages (the immune system's vacuum cleaners). Cytokines combat local and systemic inflammation. Dr. Lapp reports that extremely high levels of interleukin 1 and 2 are usually only seen in CFS, AIDS, and blood-related malignancies.[9]

Jesse Stoff, M.D., of Tucson, Arizona, relies on standard blood tests to establish the state of a patient's biochemistry and immune function and provide the information needed to design an individualized treatment program targeting the specific deficiencies or areas of weakness. The tests he runs most frequently are a T and B Cell Panel, natural killer (NK) cell function, and nitrogen balance.

The T and B Cell Panel—This test, Dr. Stoff says, gives information about 25 immune system components and the structural status of an individual's immune system. Some viruses and other infections are also detected by this test. The T and B Cell Panel and the blood test for NK cell function are relatively inexpensive standard laboratory tests that any physician can order. Through these tests, the clinician can see where the hole exists in the person's immune system defense and whether the deficiency is in T, B, or NK cells. Then you can determine which immunomodulators (substances that can regulate, or modulate, the activities of the immune system) will work best to plug the hole.

Testing nitrogen balance reveals the ratios between amino acids (protein building blocks). "Having amino acids in the correct ratios is akin to giving the NK cells the biochemical "teeth" they need to perform their work," Dr. Stoff explains. "It's important to note that if the natural killer cells lack the biochemical support (from nutrients) they need to work appropriately, stimulating them will get you nowhere."

The principles of immunomodulation can also be useful for individuals who may not be sick but want to keep their immune system in top working order. All you need is one simple blood test

The Major Players in Your Immune System

The immune system guards the body against foreign, disease-producing substances. Its "workers" are various white blood cells.

A **lymphocyte** is a specialized form of white blood cell, representing 25% to 40% of the total blood count, whose numbers increase during viral infection and when a person is fighting cancer. Lymphocytes are produced in the bone marrow and come in two basic forms: B cells and T cells.

B cells mature in the bone marrow and produce antibodies to neutralize foreign cells (this is known as humoral immunity). B cells account for 10% to 15% of all lymphocytes.

T cells mature in the thymus gland and react to and destroy specific invading antigens (this is known as cell-mediated immunity); 75% to 80% of lymphocytes are T cells. T cells are predisposed to respond to specific foreign substances (antigens) or infections.

Helper T cells (also known as T4 or CD4 cells) secrete immune proteins (particularly the interleukins and interferon) to stimulate B cells and macrophages, and activate Killer T cells; they account for 60% to 75% of T cells.

Killer T cells (T8 or CD8 cells) bind to the specific invader and secrete enzymes to destroy it; they account for 25% to 30% of T cells.

Suppressor T cells prevent excessive immune reactions by suppressing antibody activity.

Natural Killer (NK) cells are a type of nonspecific, free-ranging lymphocyte that is neither a B nor T cell. Unlike other lymphocytes, NK cells are not activated by a specific antigen—they can recognize and quickly destroy any antigen on first contact. They have potent cell-killing activity, being "armed" with an estimated 100 different biochemical poisons for destroying foreign cells. As with antibodies, their role is surveillance, to rid the body of aberrant or foreign cells before they can grow and produce cancer or infection. NK cells account for

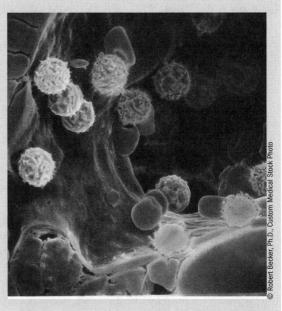

5% to 10% of all lymphocytes. An estimated 65% of normal healthy individuals have NK cell function between 30 and 160, 20% between 20 and 29, 10% between 161 and 250, and 5% have less than 20.

Macrophages are a form of white blood cell (originally produced in the bone marrow and called monocytes) that can literally swallow germs and foreign proteins, then release an enzyme that chemically either damages or kills the substance. The name means "big" (macro) "swallower" or "eater" (phage). Macrophages are the vacuum cleaners and filter feeders of the immune system, ingesting everything that is not normal healthy tissue, even old body cells.

An **antibody** is a protein molecule containing about 20,000 atoms, made from amino acids by B lymphocyte cells in the lymph tissue and set in motion by the immune system against a specific foreign protein, or antigen.

to measure natural killer cell function; an NK cell function test typically costs about $200. If your NK values are normal, don't worry about it; if they're subnormal, you will now have valuable diagnostic information that a physician can use to help restore your immune system to an optimal level.

For more on **immunomodulators** for strengthening the immune system, see Chapter 4: Restoring Immune Vitality, pp. 108-131.

If your results are below normal, further testing is advisable—a T and B Cell Panel will tell you if there is a viral trigger—to determine where the problems originate. Then, immunomodulating supplementation can help reverse the underlying weakness before it becomes a full-blown illness. This kind of early monitoring could likely have prevented many people's chronic fatigue syndrome because it tests for precisely the factors involved in CFS; namely, multiple infections, impaired NK function, and a variety of other immune deficiencies.

Biological Terrain Assessment: Analysis at the Cellular Level

The Biological Terrain Assessment (BTA) analysis is carried out in only ten minutes by a computerized device called a BTA S-1000. The device uses a pen-shaped microelectrode to determine pH, resistivity, and redox values in blood, saliva, and urine. A sample of blood (0.5 ml), saliva (0.5 ml), and first morning urine is obtained following a 12-14 hour fast. If a person eats an acid-producing, alkaline-producing, salty, or antioxidant (SEE QUICK DEFINITION) food just before the BTA, the testing reflects more about the ingested food than the body's baseline condition.

Here's the medical thinking behind the test. French biologist

An Immunological Test to Indicate Chronic Fatigue

Jay Levy, M.D., of the Division of Hematology and Oncology at the University of California at San Francisco, has developed an immunological test which distinguishes patients with CFS from healthy people and from those with other disorders having similar symptoms, such as systemic lupus erythematosus, documented depression, acute viral-like illness, and prolonged fatigue without other CFS criteria.[10]

Dr. Levy emphasizes that the test is not yet diagnostic, but is used as a kind of prescreening to identify possible CFS candidates for further study. Dr. Levy and his colleagues have found that the immune systems of people with CFS, unlike those of healthy people, are in a constant overactive state and never return to a normal operating level. This overactivity is what is behind the deep fatigue; paradoxically, this heightened activity overlays a condition of dysfunction and immune incompetency.

In this test, CFS patients with the most severe symptoms (based on a study sample of 147 patients) tend to have increased activation markers on CD8 cells and with reduced numbers of CD8 suppressor cells. Here you see the immune imbalance: one aspect is inappropriately activated, the other exists in insufficient numbers. The test involves monitoring CD8 cells (the proteins on killer T cells which are attacked by viruses). "Most noteworthy is the statistical evidence that an individual with two or more of the CD8 cell subset alterations has a high probability (90%) of having active CFS," says Dr. Levy.[11]

Louis Claude Vincent, Ph.D., discovered that the key to healing was not the use of powerful drugs but, rather, knowing the patient's biochemistry and the optimal conditions. He called these the "terrain" of body function.

Biological terrain is a phrase used to describe the conditions, general health, and activity level of cells. This includes the status of microorganisms at the cellular level: some are beneficial to life and health, others are not. Each type of bacteria, fungus or virus thrives in a precise biochemical medium. Viruses require a fairly alkaline environment to function, whereas fungi favor a more acidic environment; bacteria can thrive under various conditions, but their growth is best stimulated by a high-sugar environment. An excess of toxins in one's diet and environment tends to increase the production of acid within cells, forcing the body to compensate by producing a strong alkaline chemical reaction in the blood which, in turn, tends to favor the growth of fungi.

Dr. Vincent concluded that the components of the blood, urine, and saliva afford insight into the way the body functions. By monitoring biochemical changes in these fluids and by making appropriate changes in diet, lifestyle, and medical treatment, health can be reestablished and disease processes retarded or possibly reversed. In the pioneering tradition of Dr. Vincent, naturopathic physician and chiropractor Robert Greenberg, D.C., N.M.D., D.C., of the Whole Health Centre in Chesterfield, Missouri, developed an approach to assessing health known as Biological Terrain Assessment, or BTA. This test enables him to determine the optimal conditions for a specific patient's internal environment.

According to Dr. Greenberg, the healthy body must satisfy three criteria to function at the highest level: 1) optimal pH (acid-base balance); 2) optimal oxidation-reduction potential; and 3) resistivity (the opposite of electrical conductivity). Through BTA, these factors are measured in blood, urine, and saliva to yield a total of nine measures.

Before we learn how BTA does this, let's examine these three factors in more detail. "The pH reading tells us whether enzymatic activity in the body is occurring properly and if digestion and absorption of vitamins and other nutrients is ade-

QUICK DEFINITION

An **antioxidant** (meaning "against oxidation") is a natural biochemical substance that protects living cells against damage from harmful free radicals. Antioxidants work against the process of oxidation—the robbing of electrons from substances. If unblocked or left uncontrolled, oxidation can lead to cellular aging, degeneration, arthritis, heart disease, cancer, and other illnesses. Antioxidants in the body react readily with oxygen breakdown products and free radicals, and neutralize them before they can damage the body. Antioxidant nutrients include vitamins A, C, and E, beta carotene, selenium, coenzyme Q10, pycnogenol (grape seed extract), L-glutathione, superoxide dismutase, and bioflavonoids. Plant antioxidants include *Ginkgo biloba* and garlic. When antioxidants are taken in combination, the effect is stronger than when they are used individually.

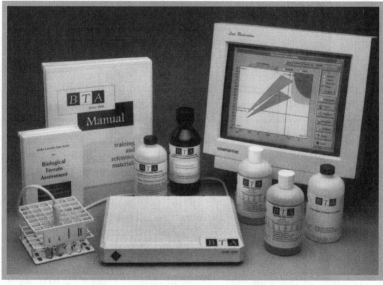

The Biological Terrain Assessment unit analyzes blood, urine, and saliva samples and displays information about an individual's cellular health on its monitor.

"Blood is a good indicator of toxicity and oxygen balance, while saliva offers insight into a person's digestive capacities," says Dr. Greenberg. Taken together and analyzed by means of the BTA S-1000, these measures provide a benchmark for determining whether or not someone is getting healthier.

For information about **BTA S-1000**, contact: Biological Technologies International, P.O. Box 560, Payson, AZ 85547; tel: 520-474-4181; fax: 520-474-1501. The approximate cost of the equipment is $10,550.

For more on **cellular terrain**, see Chapter 4: Restoring Immune Vitality, pp. 108-131.

quate," says Dr. Greenberg. "It can also alert us to the potential presence of environmental or industrial contaminants, substances that prove very damaging to the body's delicate chemistry." In general, the urine is a better indicator of pH changes than the blood because the blood's pH level is very tightly controlled; however, both measures together, along with salivary pH, give a more complete picture of the body's chemical balance.

Oxidation-reduction potential (abbreviated as redox) refers to the degree of "oxidative stress" on the body, or how much free-radical burden (oxidation of tissues) the body is exposed to. "Because of the effects of stress, poor air, poor food quality, and lack of aerobic exercise typical of most Americans, these values are generally much lower than they should be to sustain a healthy body," says Dr. Greenberg. "If the values remain low for extended periods of time, the person will be more susceptible to cancer and other illnesses."

The third factor, resistivity, is a measure of a tissue's resistance to the flow of electrical current, as opposed to conductivity which indicates the ability to transmit or conduct electrical current through a cell, nerve, or muscle. With low resistivity (high conductivity), there is typically a congestion or buildup of mineral salts. High resistivity (low conductivity) means a lack of minerals, which indicates the need to further evaluate the individual for specific deficiencies of these vital elements.

"Urine is a good indicator of the body's secretory ability and toxic load on cells," says Dr. Greenberg. "Blood is a good indicator of toxicity and oxygen balance, while saliva offers insight into a person's digestive capacities." Taken together and analyzed by means of the BTA S-1000, these measures provide a benchmark for determining whether or not someone is getting healthier. "The goal is to move the body toward the optimal benchmark, which is the same regardless of age, weight, and sex," Dr. Greenberg explains. "We find that people

A Primer on Cellular Terrain

The term **pH**, which means "potential hydrogen," represents a scale for the relative acidity or alkalinity of a solution. Acidity is measured as a pH of 0.1 to 6.9, alkalinity is 7.1 to 14, and neutral pH is 7.0. The numbers refer to how many hydrogen atoms are present compared to an ideal or standard solution. Normally, blood is slightly alkaline, at 7.35 to 7.45; urine pH can range from 4.8 to 7.5, although normal is closer to 7.0.

Acid-base metabolism refers to the metabolic processes that maintain the balance of acids and bases (alkalines) in body fluids. Acids release hydrogen ions, while bases accept them. The total number of these hydrogen ions present determines the pH of a fluid. Too many hydrogen ions (a pH below 7.0) produce an acidic state called acidosis, while too few hydrogen ions (a pH above 7.0) cause an alkaline excess called alkalosis; both can lead to illness.

Oxidation-reduction is the basic chemical mechanism in the cell by which energy is produced from foods. Electrons (negatively charged particles in an atom) are removed from one atom, resulting in "oxidation" of this first atom, and then are added or transferred to another atom, resulting in "reduction" of this second atom. This continual process of energy metabolism is actually a flow of electrons, or a minute electrical current, within the cell.

---

who attain these benchmarks seem capable of maintaining sound health indefinitely."

The therapeutic approach indicated by BTA findings will vary greatly from one patient to the next. "The BTA may uncover inadequate enzymatic secretions in one person and chronic and degenerative stress in another. As a result, they are placed on different nutritional and lifestyle modification programs and require unique nutritional support or therapies. When the patient's body chemistry is balanced and maintained with a healthy diet, proper vitamin and mineral supplementation, and adequate amounts of exercise and rest, the body can remain healthy and nourish a vibrant immune system to protect and sustain it."

Many patients who undergo a BTA came into their doctor's offices with reports of "normal" laboratory values, based on a blood test and other standard tests. Yet these same individuals display illness both objectively and subjectively, even though their standard blood results do not show it. "Often potent influences exist within the patient's system which can include pollutants, environmental poisons, parasites, viruses, fungi, invasive microbes, lack of adequate vitamins and minerals, lack of oxygen, and excessive carbon dioxide," says Dr. Greenberg. Most standard laboratory tests are incapable of detecting these elements and, as a result, many patients remain sick; meanwhile, their doctors contend that nothing more can be done.

For example, Dr. Greenberg evaluated Susan, 36, who had frequent outbreaks of debilitating herpes sores in her mouth. During an episode, they would become so numerous that Susan had trouble eating and drinking. She had consulted many physicians and tried all the drugs they prescribed, but nothing helped her. "We did a biological Terrain Assessment and discovered a cellular picture that looked very much like a heavy metal profile," says Dr. Greenberg. On this basis, he ordered a hair analysis and 24-hour urine test, both of which revealed that Susan had high concentrations of mercury, probably leached into her tissues from her dental amalgams. She had all her mercury amalgams replaced and in the last 18 months has not had a single herpes sore, says Dr. Greenberg.

Testing Hormone Levels

Hormone (SEE QUICK DEFINITION) imbalances are common in CFS. As was the case with Paul in Chapter 1, the adrenal hormones DHEA (SEE QUICK DEFINITION) and cortisol and the hormone ACTH (adreno-cortico-tropic hormone, secreted by the pituitary gland and essential for adrenal health) are frequently implicated in the disorder. Since the adrenal glands play a central role in maintaining the body's energy levels, when these glands are functioning poorly, the result is fatigue. Low amounts of melatonin, the pineal gland hormone which regulates the body's sleep cycle, may also be contributing to the overall symptom picture of CFS.

An underactive thyroid, a condition called hypothyroidism, is another important component to consider when investigating the causes of your chronic fatigue. As you will learn in Chapter 6, thyroid problems often go undiagnosed and, for someone with CFS, eliminating or confirming the thyroid as a factor should be a first step.

Initial testing and subsequent monitoring of hormone

levels in the blood provide specific guidelines for supplementation in order to restore hormonal balance in the body, one component in reversing chronic fatigue. In addition to standard blood testing, the Aeron LifeCycles Saliva Assay Report, TRH test for thyroid function, Adrenal Stress Index, and DHEA Challenge Test can provide further useful information.

Aeron LifeCycles Saliva Assay Report

"The concept of hormone replacement therapy is the first long-term concept related to anti-aging medicine," states John Kells, president of Aeron LifeCycles in San Leandro, California, a laboratory that offers a saliva-based test for measuring levels of eight different hormones. Most of the key hormones in a man's or woman's body—estrogen, testosterone, DHEA—decline as we age, leaving us more susceptible to reduced physiological functioning and possibly disease. The goal of hormone replacement is to prevent illness and enhance the quality of life, says Kells, but he notes that "there is a fair bit about this that is not yet known."

There is no evidence, he says, "that people will necessarily live longer if they replace hormones in decline, but experts in this field are hopeful that they will live disease-free longer and will not succumb to the early onset of disease that many now believe is associated with decline in body function and hormone levels." If you maintain these levels, you will probably slow down the aging process, says Kells. There are age-associated optimal levels of progesterone, estradiol, estriol, estrogen, and cortisol. Aeron LifeCycles uses these as a reference point in their saliva assay, Kells explains. These target values can then be used as a dosage guideline for supplementation. "The goal is to try to bring the hormone levels back up to a level that existed in our physiological youth," he says.

The Aeron LifeCycles Saliva Assay Report, which can be ordered by both laypeople and physicians, provides graphs of individual hormone levels. Changing levels can be plotted over time on the same graph if supplementation or subsequent testing is done. Although hormones are present in saliva only in fractional amounts compared to the blood, "clinically relevant and highly accurate levels of hormones can be determined in saliva," says Kells. "Saliva testing provides a means to establish whether or not your hormone levels are within the expected normal range for your age."

The saliva assay has several advantages over traditional

For more information about the **Aeron LifeCycles Saliva Assay Report**, contact: Aeron LifeCycles, 1933 Davis Street, Suite 310, San Leandro, CA 94577; tel: 510-729-0375 or 800-631-7900; fax: 510-729-0383.

blood testing for hormones. It is painless and noninvasive, and tests can be performed simply, at any time or place. As DHEA, cortisol, estrogen, progesterone, and testosterone levels are highest in the morning, it is far more convenient to be able to test them at home (and then immediately ship the saliva sample to Aeron's laboratory) than to drive to a physician's office possibly at a later time when levels have naturally fallen off a little.

As the test is less expensive than blood testing, you can do frequent testing to monitor changes (brought on by interventions such as diet, exercise, herbs, stress reduction, or acupuncture) and to adjust dosages of over-the-counter hormones such as DHEA or melatonin, Kells says. In general, Kells explains that it is best to establish a baseline level of saliva hormones first, then after intervention (which can include hormone supplementation), test a second time to measure the changes.

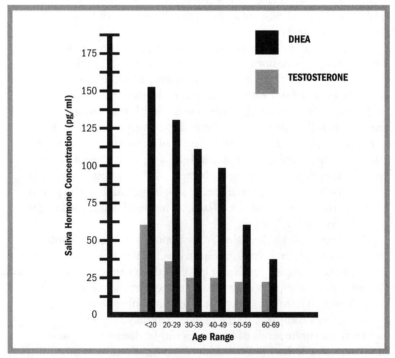

The Aeron LifeCycles Saliva Assay Report provides graphs of individual hormone levels. This chart shows the age-dependent range of testosterone and DHEA in females. The graph clearly shows how DHEA and testosterone levels decline with age.

TRH: The Gold Standard of Thyroid Tests

A major contributing factor to the development of chronic fatigue is often an underactive thyroid gland, an endocrine gland located in the neck. Here the CFS patient is confronted with two obstacles: first, many doctors pay little or no attention to the thyroid; and second, standard tests for thyroid function are often misleading.

Many patients fall through the cracks of medicine's obliviousness to thyroid function or, if they're fortunate enough to have a thyroid test, they may get "normal" results because most standard tests are not sensitive enough to identify hypothyroidism. The result is erroneous diagnoses. Patients with depression get a Prozac prescription; those with unchecked weight gain get a weight loss drug; those who are tired all the time get a label of "chronic fatigue syndrome" but no treatment.

The TRH (thyrotrophin-releasing hormone) test is a far more sensitive laboratory measure than routine thyroid blood tests and can show conclusively that a patient is suffering from an underactive thyroid, explains Raphael Kellman, M.D., a New York City physician who specializes in thyroid-related cases and uses the test regularly in his clinical practice. "Our center has seen hundreds of patients whose routine thyroid tests revealed nothing, but who then failed the TRH stimulation test, allowing us to make the appropriate diagnosis. In patients I've seen with three or more typical symptoms of hypothyroidism, 35% to 40% have tested "normal" in standard tests, while TRH tests show they have an underactive thyroid."

"The TRH test reveals a deeper physiological level by looking at the function of the thyroid and by measuring abnormal function levels, as compared to standard blood tests and the TSH test which measures only pathology," says Raphael Kellman, M.D.

The TRH is an inexpensive test, costing about $100, says Dr. Kellman. First, through a simple blood test, the physician measures the patient's level of TSH (thyroid-stimulating hormone), then gives an injection of TRH (a completely harmless synthetic hormone modelled after the TRH secreted by the hypothalamus gland in the brain), and finally draws blood 25 minutes later to remeasure the TSH. The TRH injection stimulates the pituitary gland

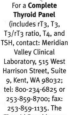

For a **Complete Thyroid Panel** (includes rT3, T3, T3/rT3 ratio, T4, and TSH, contact: Meridian Valley Clinical Laboratory, 515 West Harrison Street, Suite 9, Kent, WA 98032; tel: 800-234-6825 or 253-859-8700; fax: 253-859-1135. The Thyroid Panel has an average price of $85 and must be ordered by a physician.

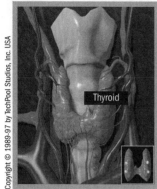

Thyroid

Many patients fall through the cracks of medicine's obliviousness to thyroid function or, if they're fortunate enough to have a thyroid test, they may get "normal" results because most standard tests are not sensitive enough to identify hypothyroidism.

which produces thyroid-stimulating hormone; if the thyroid is underfunctioning, the pituitary gland will secrete excess TSH upon stimulation. If the second TSH blood test measures are high (above 10), it tells us the patient's thyroid is underactive. A TSH reading of 15 is suspicious, while 20 strongly points to hypothyroidism.

"Routine testing assumes that if TSH is high, then thyroid hormone must be low, but in these tests a high TSH is only detectable in cases of extreme abnormalities," Dr. Kellman explains. "The TRH test reveals a deeper physiological level by looking at the *function* of the thyroid and by measuring abnormal function levels, as compared to standard blood tests and the TSH test which measures only pathology." The TRH test was once widely used by American physicians, but was replaced by the quicker, easier TSH. "In the age of assembly-line medicine, doctors jettisoned the TRH because it is cumbersome and time-consuming, and opted for the easy route," comments Dr. Kellman. "But this is a grave mistake of modern medicine, causing needless suffering for many people. The standard blood tests measuring thyroid levels are ineffectual."

Understanding the utility of the TRH test has implications for several of today's leading health problems, says Dr. Kellman. For example, he estimates that 50% of people reporting chronic fatigue actually have an *undiagnosed* underactive thyroid. Depression, a common symptom of CFS, is also linked with abnormal TRH results and an underactive thyroid, says Dr. Kellman. For those who have received a diagnosis of hypothyroidism, the TRH can be used to monitor medication dosage. "If you are currently on thyroid medication yet still complain of fatigue, the TRH test can tell us if you are being medicated properly," explains Dr. Kellman. "Many lives have been changed—and healed—from this one test."

Adrenal Stress Index (Saliva Test)

Symptoms commonly associated with chronic fatigue syndrome such as lack of energy, headaches, sleep disturbances, low body temperature, and muscle and joint pain can be caused by an imbalance in the adrenal glands. The adrenal glands, one above each kidney, secrete key stress hormones such as cortisol, DHEA, and adrenaline. Levels of these hormones are often abnormal in people with CFS, which could also be defined as a continual stress response. The Adrenal Stress Index (ASI), a simple, noninvasive test, can pinpoint whether an imbalance in the adrenal glands might be contributing to CFS.

For more about the **thyroid gland, its hormones, and its role in chronic fatigue,** see Chapter 6: Reversing Hidden Thyroid Problems, pp. 164-189.

The adrenal glands do not secrete their hormones at a constant level throughout the day; instead, hormones are released in a cycle, with the highest volume in the morning and the lowest at night. This 24-hour cycle, known as the circadian rhythm, can influence a variety of body functions, from immune response to quality of sleep. If the adrenal glands secrete hormones improperly (due to an abnormal adrenal rhythm), fatigue and muscle pain may result.

The ASI saliva test evaluates how well one's adrenal glands are functioning by tracking the 24-hour cycle. Four saliva samples taken at intervals throughout the day are used to reconstruct the adrenal rhythm in the laboratory and determine whether the three main stress hormones are being secreted in proper proportion to each other, and at the right times. Based on the results, a physician can prescribe the appropriate treatment to restore the balance of hormones and correct the circadian rhythm.

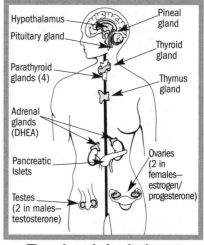

Hypothalamus
Pituitary gland
Parathyroid glands (4)
Adrenal glands (DHEA)
Pancreatic Islets
Testes (2 in males—testosterone)
Pineal gland
Thyroid gland
Thymus gland
Ovaries (2 in females—estrogen/progesterone)

The adrenal glands do not secrete their hormones at a constant level throughout the day; instead, hormones are released in a cycle, with the highest volume in the morning and the lowest at night.

For information on the **Adrenal Stress Index saliva test** and **DHEA Challenge Test**, contact: Diagnos-Tech, Inc., 6620 South 192nd Place, J-104, Kent, WA 98032; tel: 800-878-3787 or 425-251-0596; fax: 206-251-0637. fax: 425-251-0637.

DHEA Challenge Test (Saliva Test)

As was the case with Paul in Chapter 1, the hormone DHEA is often deficient in people with CFS, and taking a DHEA supplement to raise the levels is relatively easy. However, while many people taking DHEA report significant improvement in sleeping patterns, energy level, and ability to cope with stress, some people actually experience the opposite effect.

Depending upon a person's genetic makeup, a certain amount of DHEA from a supplement may be converted by the body into the hormones testosterone and estradiol (a type of estrogen). If you are genetically predisposed to convert DHEA, you may experience unwanted side effects with supplementation as a result of increased amounts of testosterone and estradiol. These side effects can include fatigue, insomnia, irritability, acne, oily skin, deepening of the voice, and an increase in body hair.

Through a simple saliva sample, the DHEA Challenge Test determines whether, in your particular case, DHEA supplements will improve or worsen your health. The test works by measuring levels of the two hormones (testosterone and estradiol) in the saliva both before and after a five- to seven-day treatment with the DHEA hormone (15 mg for women, 25 mg for men). If your testosterone and estradiol levels are too high following the "challenge" to the system, continuing to take DHEA supplements is probably not advisable.

Testing for Heavy Metal Toxicity

Increasingly, practitioners of alternative medicine find that chronic low-level exposure to a variety of toxic heavy metals poses serious health dangers if the toxins are allowed to stay in the body. These toxins are commonly found in our food, water, and air, as well as in cooking utensils, cosmetics, auto exhaust, tobacco smoke, many of the building materials and fabrics in our work and living environments, and dental materials in our teeth (mercury fillings).

Typical symptoms of heavy metal toxicity can include nervous system disorders, depression, fatigue, skin rashes, high blood pressure, hyperactivity, nausea, irritability, headaches, and more serious conditions including autism, intelligence deficits, and cancer. Testing for heavy metal toxicity can identify which metals are present and in what amounts. On the basis of this information, a physician is able to develop an individualized detoxification and nutritional prescription program both to eliminate the toxic metals from the system and to restore depleted essential nutrients.

The following test for heavy metal toxicity can give you the information you need from only a blood and/or urine sample.

ToxMet Screen

The ToxMet Screen, from MetaMetrix Medical Laboratory, provides an inexpensive but detailed analysis of the levels of specific heavy metals in a patient's system, based on a urine sample. The test typically costs about $100 and is ordered by a physician.

ToxMet tests for levels of four highly toxic heavy metals (arsenic, cadmium, lead, and mercury); it also reports on levels for ten potentially toxic elements, such as aluminum, bismuth, boron, nickel, and strontium. Finally, information is gathered on a patient's status regarding 14 essential metals and minerals, such as copper, calcium, chromium, molybdenum, selenium, and vanadium. When test results exceed limits believed to be safe, the report indicates a "high" concentration.

For example, one patient was high in arsenic (65 units compared to a high limit of 40) and cadmium (3.7 compared to the limit of 2). ToxMet also indicated that this patient had high levels of calcium, magnesium, manganese, and zinc.

Typical symptoms of heavy metal toxicity can include nervous system disorders, depression, fatigue, skin rashes, high blood pressure, hyperactivity, nausea, irritability, headaches, and more serious conditions.

Testing for Enzyme Deficiencies

For information on the **ToxMet Screen**, contact: MetaMetrix Medical Laboratory, 5000 Peachtree Industrial Boulevard, Suite 110, Norcross, GA 30071; tel: 770-446-5483 or 800-221-4640; fax: 770-441-2237.

If you recall from Chapter 1, Paul had depleted enzyme levels which meant he was unable to absorb the nutrients from food and supplements properly. Enzymes (SEE QUICK DEFINITION), essential in the breakdown of nutrients and the clearing of toxins in the blood, come from two sources: they are manufactured in the pancreas and we get them from our food.

If our food doesn't contain the necessary enzymes, which is often the case in the highly processed standard American diet, then the pancreas must work overtime to produce more enzymes. This taxes the pancreas and also depletes the number of enzymes available to circulate in the blood and clear toxins. When this state of affairs is prolonged, digestive and absorption problems develop and toxins accumulate beyond the body's ability to eliminate them. Therefore, before implementing dietary changes and a regimen of nutritional supplements as part of a total treatment program, it is advisable to determine if enzyme deficiencies are present. Without investigating this possibility, the most careful diet and highest quality supplements will have little or no effect.

A 24-hour urine analysis is all it takes. Specific parameters of the test reveal the status of digestive function in three food groups: protein, carbohydrates, and fats. Abnormal values in uric acid indicate a deficiency of protease, the enzyme which digests protein. If calcium phosphate values are abnormal, it means there is a deficiency of amylase, the enzyme which digests carbohydrates. Lastly, the calcium oxalate component is linked to lipase, the enzyme which digests fats. (See "What a Urine Analysis Reveals," pp. 47-48.)

Loomis Urinalysis

In her work as an an enzyme therapist, Lita Lee, Ph.D., of Lowell, Oregon, relies on the urinalysis developed by Charles Loomis, D.C., founder and president of 21st Century Nutrition in Madison, Wisconsin. She emphasizes that a 24-hour urine sample is the only way to pinpoint enzyme deficiencies. In addition to enzyme deficiencies, the Loomis test isolates digestive disorders and nutrient deficiencies.

For the test, Dr. Lee asks clients to avoid taking vitamins, minerals, enzymes, herbs, or other supplements during the 24-hour testing period and for at least a day before the test. No dietary changes are necessary, she says. The client collects urine in a sterile container, noting the total urine volume eliminated (in cups, or other units of measure) each time, along with any symptoms experienced while urinating. The sample is then analyzed by someone who specializes in Loomis urinalysis.

Allergy Testing

For information on **Loomis urinalysis**, contact: 21st Century Nutrition, 6421 Enterprise Lane, Madison, WI 53719; tel: 800-662-2630.

Allergies are a characteristic component of CFS, fibromyalgia, and environmental illness. Identifying and taking steps to eliminate these allergies or avoiding exposure to the offending substances is a vital part of reducing the burden on the immune system. In the case of environmental illness, the extent of the allergies presents a daunting prospect, but the level of disability created by the constant allergic reaction makes the process of identification all the more necessary.

There are numerous tests to identify allergens, or allergy-causing substances, but two of the most effective are the Nambudripad Allergy Elimination Technique and electrodermal screening, mentioned previously but discussed here in regard to allergies. Other, more conventional tests include skin testing and the IgG ELISA test.

Nambudripad Allergy Elimination Technique (NAET)

Developed by Devi Nambudripad, D.C., L.Ac., R.N., Ph.D., this method of both detecting and permanently eliminating allergies and sensitivities combines applied kinesiology's (SEE QUICK DEFINITION) muscle response testing with acupuncture and chiropractic. To identify an allergen, the patient holds a vial containing the suspected allergy-causing substance in one hand while the practitioner tests the muscle strength of the patient's arm or leg. A weak muscle response indicates an allergy or sensitivity to that substance. Treatment involves the patient again holding the substance while the NAET practitioner uses acupuncture or acupressure to reprogram the way the body responds to the substance, thereby removing the allergic charge.

Electrodermal Screening

This form of testing (described above, see pp. 36-39) is widely used in Europe, and to an increasing extent in the U.S., to screen for both food and environmental allergies, and to determine what remedy to use to properly neutralize the allergic reaction.

"A small [painless] current of electricity is introduced at specific acupuncture points on the patient," explains Fuller Royal, M.D., of Las Vegas, Nevada. "Various allergens are then introduced into the circuitry, enabling the physician to determine any change in the way the patient reacts to the current." Dr. Royal states that using electrodermal screening allows him to accurately test for a full spectrum of allergens, and that the entire battery of tests can be done in an hour. According to Dr. Royal, a reading of 50 is normal on a scale of 100 and "a reading of over 50 means allergens are present," he says. "As they are found, various treatment

Applied kinesiology, first developed by George Goodheart, D.C., of Detroit, Michigan, is the study of the relationship between muscle dysfunction (weak muscles) and related organ or gland dysfunction. Applied kinesiology employs a simple strength resistance test on a specific indicator muscle that is related to the organ or part of the body that is being tested. If the muscle tests strong, maintaining its resistance, it indicates health. If it tests weak, it can mean infection or dysfunction. For example, the deltoid muscle in the shoulder shares a relationship to the lungs and therefore is a good indicator of any problems there.

For more on **NAET treatment,** see Chapter 9: Addressing the Allergy Connection, pp. 232-258.

doses are also added into the circuit and the correct treatment will bring the reading back down to 50."

Skin testing

"Skin testing is one of the most consistent methods of testing people for pollen, mold, dust, chemical, and other environmental allergies," says Richard Wilkinson, M.D., who practices environmental medicine in Yakima, Washington. He recommends Serial Endpoint Titration or SET testing, which is far more accurate than the commonly used scratch test. The scratch test consists of lightly scratching the skin and placing a dilution of a suspected allergen in that spot. If it raises a wheal (bump) within 15 minutes, allergy is confirmed. Needless to say, identifying one's full range of allergies using this method is potentially a long and uncomfortable process.

During a SET test, a diluted form of a potential allergen is injected just below the skin. The body immediately reacts to the introduction of this foreign substance by forming a wheal of about 4 mm in diameter. In the next 10 minutes, the wheal will grow according to the severity of the immune reaction. Ten minutes after the injection, the wheal is measured again. A 5 mm diameter wheal indicates a non-allergic reaction, while a wheal 7 mm or larger indicates that you have an allergy.

If the test shows a positive result (meaning you are allergic to the substance), the process can then be repeated with increasingly diluted forms of the allergen. These new tests show how severely the body reacts to varying amounts of the substance. SET is one of the few tests (NAET is another) that can evaluate your degree of sensitivity to a known allergen.

The IgG ELISA Test

Most allergy tests only measure the presence of IgE (immunoglobulin E [SEE QUICK DEFINITION]) antibodies, while most food allergies are dealt with in the body by the IgG (immunoglobulin G) antibodies. The IgG ELISA (enzyme-linked immunoabsorbent assay) test offers new hope for food allergy sufferers. It is currently the only commercially available test of its kind for delayed food allergies.

"We know that one of the fundamental causes behind food allergies is the penetration of undigested or partially digested food from the digestive tract into the bloodstream," explains James Braly, M.D., medical director of Immuno Laboratories in Fort Lauderdale, Florida. "With the IgG ELISA test, we can measure the actual presence of specific foods and their specific IgG antibodies in the blood to precisely determine which foods a person is allergic to." Convenient and automated, the IgG ELISA test involves computer analysis of a blood sample for the presence of IgG antibodies against over 100 foods. The test can be done through the mail, as long as samples reach testing labs within 72 hours after the blood is drawn.

To contact **James Braly, M.D.:** Immuno Laboratories, 1620 West Oakland Park Boulevard, Fort Lauderdale, FL 33311; tel: 800-231-9197 or 954-486-4500; fax: 954-739-8583.

Tests to Identify Nutritional Deficiencies

Nutritional deficiencies are usually a feature of chronic fatigue syndrome, whether due to impaired digestion (as a result of the multiple infections involved), poor diet, stress, environmental toxins, or a combination of these factors. Specific nutritional deficiencies can contribute to certain CFS symptoms. For example, a lack of amino acids (SEE QUICK DEFINITION), the protein building blocks of neurotransmitters (SEE QUICK DEFINITION), can lead to depleted levels of those essential chemical messengers in the brain. Such a deficiency has been linked to depression, anxiety, and other mood disorders.

As with other aspects of treatment, in order to design an effective program of nutritional supplementation, it is necessary to identify all deficiencies. Thorough testing can avoid prescribing the wrong supplement and save time and expense in the long term. Among the laboratory tests for nutrient status, the four discussed below are relatively inexpensive and provide detailed, practical information.

An **immunoglobulin** is one of a class of five specially designed antibody proteins produced in the spleen, bone marrow, or lymph tissue and involved in the immune system's defense response to foreign substances. The main types of immunoglobulins, grouped according to their concentration in the blood, are: IgG (80%), IgA (10% to 15%), IgM (5% to 10%), IgD (less than 0.1%), IgE (less than 0.01%). Technically, all antibodies are immunoglobulins.

Individualized Optimal Nutrition (ION)
Using a blood and a urine sample, the ION (Individualized Optimal Nutrition) Panel from MetaMetrix measures 150 biochemical components. The test is highly useful for physicians who need detailed biochemical assessment of patients who have chronic fatigue or other immune disorders, multiple chemical sensitivities, cancer, heart disease, learning difficulties, or obesity. Specifically, ION checks for nutritional status in categories including vitamins, minerals, amino acids, fatty and organic acids, lipid peroxides, general blood chemistries (cholesterol, thyroid hormone, glucose), and antioxidants. In each category, a patient's levels are compared with predetermined limits.

Nutritional deficiencies are usually a feature of chronic fatigue syndrome, whether due to impaired digestion (as a result of the multiple infections involved), poor diet, stress, environmental toxins, or a combination of these factors.

Based on the individual's test results, ION can provide supplement recommendations. For the antioxidant panel, for example, ION provides a precisely tailored blend of 16 substances from coenzyme Q10 and copper citrate to beta carotene and vitamin C. Finally, ION summarizes the test results into nine categories according to disease risk, such as cardiovascular, liver function, intestinal balance, energy, digestive disorders, and thyroid status. In each case, an individual's biochemical status is contrasted against a healthy norm. The total ION test of seven panels typically costs between $600 and $1,000, although individual panels may be ordered.

FIA™ (Functional Intracellular Analysis)

These tests (as Comprehensive Profile 3000, B-Complex Profile 1100, Primary Profile 1500, Cardiovascular Profile 1600, or Antioxidants Profile 1400) measure the function of key vitamins, minerals, antioxidants, amino acids, fatty acids, and metabolites (choline, inositol) at the cellular level. They also assess the status of carbohydrate metabolism in terms of insulin function and fructose intolerance. The FIA measures how these micronutrients are actually functioning within the activities of living white blood cells rather than simply measuring the micronutrient levels in the blood (which may or may not provide useful information about cell metabolism). More specifically, FIA assesses the amount of cell growth for metabolically active lymphocytes (a type of white blood cell) as a way of identifying micronutrient deficiencies that are known to interfere with growth or immune function in the cells. These tests typically cost $300 or less.

Pantox Antioxidant Profile™

Using a small blood sample, this diagnostic screen measures the status of more than 20 nutritional factors as a way of determining the body's antioxidant defense system. It then compares the results against a database of 7,000 normal and healthy profiles. Specifically, the screen reports on lipoproteins (cholesterol, triglycerides), fat-soluble antioxidants (vitamins A and E, carotenoids, coenzyme Q10), water-soluble antioxidants (vitamin C, uric acid, bilirubin), and iron balance. The test helps answer the question: are you getting the right antioxidants in the correct amounts? The Pantox Profile is displayed in bar graphs with accompanying explanatory medical text, telling you if your levels of a specific nutrient are low and pose a health risk. The test cost to patients is about $300 and is often covered by health insurance, including Medicare.

It is important to realize that just because you consume a nutrient does not mean that your body has assimiliated it or that it is present and active in your bloodstream. Stress produced by the heightened activity of free radicals can seriously deplete your reserves of antioxidants, despite a healthy diet and nutritional supplementation (delivered imprecisely), explains Pantox Laboratories director Charles A. Thomas, Jr., Ph.D. The practical goal, he says, is for "an individual to take steps to change one's levels so as to join others who are experiencing a lower rate of degenerative diseases."

Oxidative Protection Screen

Introduced in November 1995, the Oxidative Protection Screen from Antibody Assay Laboratories of Santa Ana, California, can provide your physician with an actual biochemical analysis of how well your body is handling free radicals. This information, in turn, is valuable for a physician in assessing a patient's overall health, the degree of antioxidant "protection" one has, and the possible need for further nutrient supplementation.

When lipids (fatty acids and other oily organic compounds) are damaged by free radicals, they form lipid peroxides which circulate in the blood. Using a drawn blood sample from a patient, the lab test determines the amount of lipid peroxides in the plasma; these numbers vary with age and gender.

For a 20-year-old woman, for example, the normal range is 1.28-1.69 micromole/liter, but for a 60-year-old

For more information about **ION,** contact: MetaMetrix Medical Laboratory, 5000 Peachtree Industrial Boulevard, Suite 110, Norcross, GA 30071; tel: 770-446-5483 or 800-221-4640; fax: 770-441-2237. For **Functional Intracellular Analysis™,** contact: SpectraCell Laboratories, Inc., 515 Post Oak Boulevard, Suite 830, Houston, TX 77027; tel: 713-621-3101 or 800-227-5227; fax: 713-621-3234; website: http://www.spectra-cell.com. The **Pantox Antioxidant Profile** must be ordered by a licensed health-care practitioner. Contact: Pantox Laboratories, 4622 Santa Fe Street, San Diego, CA 92109; tel: 888-726-8698, 619-272-3885 or 800-726-8696; fax: 619-272-1621. **Oxidative Protection Screen** must also be ordered by a licensed health-care practitioner. Contact: Antibody Assay Laboratories, 1715 East Wilshire, #715, Santa Ana, CA 92705; tel: 714-972-9979 or 800-522-2611; fax: 714-543-2034.

female, it is 2.15-2.82 micromole/liter. An elevated amount, beyond this range, indicates a high production of free radicals, while the lower the amount of lipid peroxides, the stronger the antioxidant protection. The TOPI™ (Total Oxidative Protection Index) will indicate your system's overall ability to withstand the "attack" of free radicals and thus your individual degree of oxidative protection. The normal range here is 45% to 63%; ranges above 63% indicate a high degree of antioxidant protection and health. The test cost to patients is about $100.

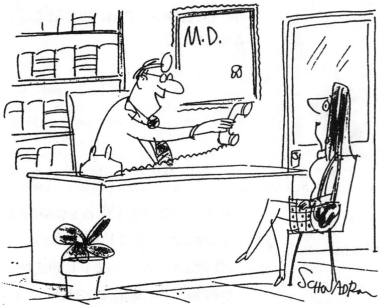

" I NOW OFFER NUTRITIONAL COUNSELING. HERE'S A RECORDING OF MY MOM'S RECIPE FOR CHICKEN SOUP. "

3

Eliminating Viruses,

INFECTIONS, CANDIDIASIS, AND PARASITES

PARASITES, CANDIDIASIS, viruses, and other infections are often present in patients with chronic fatigue syndrome. Whether these infections in combination are the cause of CFS or opportunistic invaders of a weakened immune system has not been conclusively demonstrated, but in either case, compromised immunity is a central feature of the syndrome and the infections involved perpetuate and

deepen immune dysfunction by further taxing an already overloaded system. As a result, an immune-strengthening protocol is integral to the CFS treatment programs of many alternative medicine physicians.

Some reseachers and doctors still hold

To focus on *only* EBV is a mistaken approach. One of the hallmarks of alternative medicine thinking and practice is that there is rarely, or never, a single cause of any illness; diseases are developed out of multiple converging imbalances and deficiencies.

stubbornly to the view that a single virus is behind CFS. The conventional medical profession has tended to focus on the herpes family of viruses which includes Epstein-Barr and oral and genital herpes. The Epstein-Barr virus (EBV; SEE QUICK DEFINITION) has received the most attention since its symptoms are duplicated in CFS sufferers, who usually test high for EBV antibody levels as well. These are immune proteins mobilized to defend the body against EBV molecules. In the early days of the CFS epidemic (the 1980s), conventional doctors assumed—and some insisted—that EBV was the cause of chronic fatigue syndrome. When patients with CFS started turning up without elevated levels of EBV, conventional physicians eventually reorganized their thinking on causality.

Even the National Institutes of Health (NIH) admits that there is no clear-cut evidence that the Epstein-Barr virus, or any other virus, is the primary cause of CFS. The NIH reports that recent studies found that acyclovir, a drug which blocks multiplication of the Epstein-Barr virus, is ineffective in CFS patients.[1] So to focus on *only* EBV is a mistaken approach. One of the hallmarks of alternative medicine thinking and practice is that there is rarely, or never, a single cause of any illness; diseases are developed out of multiple converging imbalances and deficiencies.

Infectious Agents: The Chicken or the Egg?

The wide-ranging, complex symptomology of CFS patients seems to indicate that the disorder includes more than EBV alone. Murray R. Susser, M.D., of Santa Monica, California, concedes that EBV may indeed be a major factor in CFS cases, but poses the possibility that EBV (dormant or suppressed) might be *reactivated* due to other weaknesses in immune function.[2]

"CFS can start with ordinary viral infections, such as those that cause respiratory infections like the common cold and flus," he explains. "There are 2,300 viruses which can cause a cold or flu and if one of those hits you and your body isn't able to get rid of it, then you have a chronic infection. In CFS, we often get hidden viral, parasite, and yeast infections which are results of a weakened immune system. One infection puts demand on the immune system which can't kick it, and another infection may join in, leading from one to another in a domino effect. With this constant infection, CFS behaves like the flu that never got better. I sometimes call it, 'the flu that became always.'"

Some of the infections in this domino effect may be retroviruses, a group which includes the leukemia and AIDS viruses, and which recent research has linked to CFS, reports Dr. Susser.[3] Sinusitis, inflammation of the sinuses which may be caused by a virus, bacteria,

QUICK DEFINITION

Epstein-Barr virus (EBV) is a herpes-like virus thought to be the cause of infectious mononucleosis and Burkitt's lymphoma. It is contracted through the cells in the lining of the mouth and throat, and can therefore be spread by sharing utensils, kissing, and unsanitary habits. EBV symptoms, frequently duplicated in other conditions, include debilitating fatigue, fever, swollen glands, arthritic symptoms, multiple allergies, and difficulties in concentrating. People with chronic fatigue syndrome often have a high level of EBV antibodies in their blood, but EBV is no longer regarded (as it was in the 1980s) as the sole or even necessarily a contributing cause for chronic fatigue.

"In CFS, we often get hidden parasite, yeast, and viral infections which are results of a weakened immune system. One infection puts demand on the immune system which can't kick it, and another infection may join in, leading from one to another in a domino effect," says Murray Susser, M.D.

Parasites are any organism that lives off another organism (called a host), and draws nourishment from it. Specifically, parasites are the protozoa (single-cell organisms), arthropods (insects), and worms that infect the body and cause major damage to tissues and organs. Common forms of the protozoan parasites are *Giardia lamblia* which causes giardiasis, *Entamoeba histolytica* which produces dysentery, and *Cryptosporidium*, a cause of diarrhea particularly in people with immunologic diseases such as AIDS. The most common arthropod parasites are lice, mites, ticks, and fleas. Worm parasites include pinworms, roundworms, tapeworms, whipworms, *Trichinella spiralis* (worms usually acquired from eating tainted pork), hookworms, Guinea worms, and filaria (threadlike worms that inhabit the blood and tissues).

or allergies, is also common in cases of CFS.

Other factors may leave the body vulnerable to infections, parasites (SEE QUICK DEFINITION) or an overgrowth of *Candida albicans* (a yeast-like fungus). For example, poor digestion is a contributing cause of parasitic infection. "Someone who has a low acid level (a measure of the pH, or general chemical balance) in his stomach won't digest food properly, so whatever parasites come through in the food won't get sterilized out," says Maoshing Ni, D.O.M., Ph.D., L.Ac., president of Yo San University in Santa Monica, California. "That's what hydrochloric acid [digestive acid in the stomach] does, it sterilizes the food and kills off all the germs. When it's not effective at doing that, the parasites get passed along into the intestines." A complicating factor of parasitic infection is that most people who have parasites don't know it.

Parasitic infection, in turn, can lead to candidiasis. This overgrowth of *Candida albicans* in the intestinal tract is often found as a complication of giardiasis (infection with the protozoan *Giardia lamblia*, a highly contagious and virulent unicellular organism found mostly in the contaminated waters of lakes, streams, and oceans). Like CFS itself, candidiasis is reaching epidemic proportions in the United States.

Considered an opportunistic infection (one that develops when the body is compromised by other infections), candidiasis has serious consequences since it increases gut permeability to undigested foods and bowel toxins. These can then enter the bloodstream where they induce an immune response, as well as promote intolerance or sensitivities to common foods. The reverse can also occur—continual allergic reactions in the body and the circulation of allergens create an ideal environment for candidiasis.

Both candidiasis and parasites are often the result of an excessive

The Insider's View of Stomach pH

An effective way to determine the pH (the ratio of acidity to alkalinity) in the stomach is the Heidelberg pH capsule system. This "tubeless gastric analysis" is a way of showing abnormal conditions of acidity or alkalinity in the stomach or small intestines, according to its manufacturer.

The term pH, which means "potential hydrogen," represents a scale for the relative acidity or alkalinity of a solution. Acidity is measured as a pH of 0.1 to 6.9, alkalinity is 7.1 to 14, and neutral pH is 7.0. The numbers refer to how many hydrogen atoms are present compared to an ideal or standard solution. Normally, blood is slightly alkaline, at 7.35 to 7.45; urine pH can range from 4.8 to 7.5, although normal is closer to 7.0.

A miniature electronic transmitter is put inside a small capsule made of polyacrylate (inert and indigestible) which the patient swallows; once in the stomach, the capsule transmits, by radio signals, continuous and/or changing values for the pH of that area. The capsule is active for about 22 hours after ingestion. These results (fluctuations of pH) are displayed in graph form, called a gastrogram. The stomach's pH can be challenged by introducing an alkalinizing drink such as sodium bicarbonate; the gastrointestinal system's response to this challenge is itself valuable information about its health.

The technique was developed in the 1950s by German researcher Hans G. Nöller, M.D., professor of pediatrics at the University of Heidelberg. Dr. Nöller sought an alternative to the invasive, uncomfortable stomach tube procedure commonly used by gastroenterologists to assess stomach and small intestine function. Since its invention, over 200 scientific studies have reported on the Heidelberg pH capsule's application for a variety of gastrointestinal conditions.

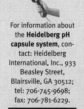

For information about the **Heidelberg pH capsule system**, contact: Heidelberg International, Inc., 933 Beasley Street, Blairsville, GA 30512; tel: 706-745-9698; fax: 706-781-6229.

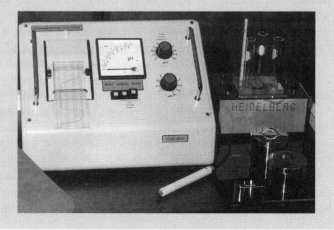

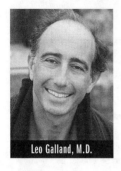

Leo Galland, M.D.

Any person with unexplained fatigue, multiple allergies (especially to food), chronic gastrointestinal complaints, such as bloating, diarrhea, abdominal pain, flatulence, or chronic constipation, should be screened for intestinal parasites, according to Leo Galland, M.D.

For more about **candidiasis and allergies**, see Chapter 9: Addressing The Allergy Connection, pp. 232-258.

use of antibiotics, which kill much of our body's important intestinal flora, thereby inviting opportunistic infections. Leon Chaitow, N.D., D.O., of London, England, describes the likely candidate for *Candida* overgrowth as someone whose medical history includes: steroid hormone medication (such as cortisone or corticosteroids), often prescribed for skin conditions such as rashes, eczema, or psoriasis; prolonged or repeated use of antibiotics which are frequently given for urinary and ear infections, sinusitis, bronchitis, and other infections; ulcer medications (such as Tagamet and Zantac); or oral contraceptives.

While candidiasis is more commonly linked to CFS, parasites are frequently overlooked as a contributing factor and even when testing is ordered, it often fails to detect them (see Chapter 2: Testing, pp. 34-73). As evidence of parasite involvement in CFS, Leo Galland, M.D., of New York City, reports that 82% of those who suffered from chronic fatigue syndrome were cured of their symptoms when treated for parasitic infection. In one study, over one-third of the CFS patients tested were found to be infected with *Giardia lamblia*.[4]

The clinical profile of parasitic infection resembles that of CFS: chronic fatigue, joint and muscle pain, immune dysfunction, allergies, skin conditions such as rashes and hives, nervousness, and digestive problems. Dr. Galland's research indicates that major health problems can be caused by even mild parasitic infection. Consequently, his view is that any person with unexplained fatigue, multiple allergies (especially to food), and chronic gastrointestinal complaints, such as bloating, diarrhea, abdominal pain, flatulence, or chronic constipation, should be screened for intestinal parasites.

Prolonged viral or bacterial infection, candidiasis, and parasites tax the immune system and contribute to malabsorption of nutrients which results in nutritional deficiencies. Obviously, eliminating this drain on the body is a treatment priority. To accomplish this, many alternative medical doctors employ a two-pronged approach: targeting the infectious agents and bolstering the immune system so it can fulfill its purpose of fighting off such agents.

Detoxification therapy to rid the body of an accumulation of toxins from a variety of sources may be a component of both. Chapter 4 discusses detoxification methods along with alternative medicine techniques for rebuilding the immune system in general. In this chapter, we focus on treating the specific infections, candidiasis, and parasites using the two-pronged approach.

Is Chronic Fatigue the New Face of Polio?

Just as tuberculosis, once believed to have been eradicated by modern medicine, has now returned in more virulent, drug-resistant strains, so may polio be with us again in a disguised form. We may be mistakenly calling it chronic fatigue syndrome (U.S.) or myalgic encephalomyelitis (England). According to William Campbell Douglass, M.D., editor of the medical newsletter *Second Opinion*, polio is more common than ever and may actually be caused by the polio vaccination. This intriguing and potentially electrifying theory is based on information Dr. Douglass gleaned from several clinical studies.

Dr. Douglass argues that the Salk and Sabin vaccines, widely administered to children in the 1950s for poliomyelitis, did not eliminate polio at all but forced it to change its form. While the vaccines suppressed the polio virus, the virus was replaced by genetically similar ones, such as Coxsackie virus which is often found in elevated levels in CFS patients. The Coxsackie family of viruses, first isolated in 1948, consists of 29 different strains and is linked to numerous illnesses. When physicians first began identifying these viruses in the blood of CFS patients, they failed to discern their connection with polio.

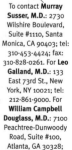

To contact **Murray Susser, M.D.:** 2730 Wilshire Boulevard, Suite #1110, Santa Monica, CA 90403; tel: 310-453-4424; fax: 310-828-0261. For **Leo Galland, M.D.:** 133 East 73rd St., New York, NY 10021; tel: 212-861-9000. For **William Campbell Douglass, M.D.:** 7100 Peachtree-Dunwoody Road, Suite #100, Atlanta, GA 30328; tel: 770-668-0432.

The sustained use of polio vaccines for over 40 years has resulted in "at least 72 viral strains that can cause polio-like diseases," says Dr. Douglass. Before the polio vaccines, there were only three polio viruses. He notes that he was not the first to point to evidence of "the changing of polio rather than the elimination of it." As early as 1934, cases of "atypical" polio were reported in Los Angeles; "abortive poliomyelitis" was reported in Switzerland in 1939.

Dr. Douglass suggests that the trend towards the emer-

"We now know that chronic fatigue syndrome is not a new disease, but simply an 'aborted form' of the more serious paralytic polio," states William Campbell Douglass, M.D.

gence of a new polio—its predominant symptom changing from infantile paralysis to adult muscle weakness—has rapidly increased since the polio vaccines were introduced. "We now know that chronic fatigue syndrome is not a new disease, but simply an 'aborted form' of the more serious paralytic polio," he states. If Dr. Douglass' speculations prove correct, the credibility of conventional medicine's mass vaccination program will be seriously undermined. It is hardly a public health benefit if a vaccine simply modifies an existing disease, forcing it to take another form in the next generation of patients. The indiscriminate use of vaccines may prove to be as counterproductive as has the overprescription of antibiotics.

Treating Viral and Bacterial Infections

Viruses do not respond to antibiotics, so these drugs are only prescribed for bacterial infections or to prevent a bacterial infection from developing in the immune-weakened environment created by a virus. Although alternative medicine physicians sometimes resort to an antibiotic, they generally try to avoid it because of the further problems it creates in the body, such as clearing out all the beneficial intestinal flora along with the infection-causing bacteria and thus creating a prime environment for candidiasis and parasites.

In addition to strengthening the immune system to bolster the body's own defense mechanisms against disease-producing microorganisms, alternative medicine employs antimicrobial herbs to reduce the viral and bacterial load on the body. These include echinacea, goldenseal, citrus seed extract, aloe vera, and tea tree oil, among others. Pau d'arco bark, obtained from a tropical tree native to Brazil, has particularly strong antiviral qualities. (See herbal medicine treatments for candidiasis and parasites, later in this chapter.)

According to Lita Lee, Ph.D., an enzyme therapist in Lowell, Oregon, coconut oil is an antiviral useful to chronic fatigue patients for several reasons. "Medical research on the use of coconut oil for chronic fatigue patients shows it to have an antiviral effect," she reports. In addition, it is antiallergenic and antiseptic, promotes thyroid function, regulates blood sugar, and protects mitochondria (the cells' energy "factories") against stress injuries, she says. "Coconut oil has gotten a bad rap," she adds. "It is actually one of the most healthy saturated fats."

See Chapter 4: Restoring Immune Vitality, pp. 108-131, and Chapter 12: Correcting Chronic Fatigue With Herbs, pp. 318-338.

Another strong antiviral botanical is an extract of shitake mushroom called LEM (for *Lentinus edodes mycelium*, the immature form of the fungus). Research at Yamaguchi University in Tokyo, Japan, demonstrated LEM's ability to inhibit viruses and stimulate the immune system.[5] It may stop the spread of a virus by blocking the virus' receptor sites. LEM appears to boost the immune system by stimulating macrophages and lymphocytes, both of which are "workers" in immune defense against toxins, viruses, and other invading microorganisms.

Thus far the research on LEM's antiviral qualities has taken place in a test tube, but *HealthWatch*, the newsletter of the CFIDS (chronic fatigue and immune dysfunction syndrome) Buyers Club, reports that LEM is the "all-time best-selling nutritional supplement used by CFIDS sufferers."[6]

An Antiviral Nutritional Program

Shari Lieberman, Ph.D., C.N.S., a nutrition scientist and certified nutrition specialist based in New York City, developed a multivitamin/mineral formula called Optimum Protection which she uses (at a dosage of four tablets daily) as the basis of an antiviral, antibacterial nutritional supplement program for CFS patients. Here are the components of her program, with typical dosages (the components and dosages will vary, depending upon the individual):

Kyolic Premium EPA—This product is a combination of garlic and fish oil (EPA or eicosapentaenoic acid, an omega-3 essential fatty acid). "I combine these because garlic is a broad spectrum antibiotic and fish oil is excellent for inflammation and any sort of autoimmune phenomenon," Dr. Lieberman says. "I classify CFS as an autoimmune disease." She recommends four capsules a day.

Quercetin—This bioflavonoid (vitamin C helper) is a substance with antihistamine, anti-inflammatory, and antiviral properties. "It's an antihistamine like vitamin C, it's great for patients who have allergies, rhinitis, sinusitis, even environmental allergies. It's also effectively antiviral. I use it with any viral syndrome, including CFS and HIV," she reports. She normally recommends 1,000-1,500 mg per day.

A Flu Virus May Contribute to Fibromyalgia

In a study of the possible connection between flu viruses and fibromyalgia (chronic muscle pain), nine out of ten fibromyalgia patients tested positive for antibodies to influenza type A, while three out of ten in an age- and sex-matched second group of people with fibromyalgia tested positive for influenza B.[7] Influenza A is a viral infection which mainly affects the respiratory and autonomic nervous systems.

The sympathetic branch of the autonomic nervous system is associated with arousal and stress, increasing heart rate, blood pressure, and muscle tension. Obviously, if this branch is affected by a flu virus, muscle tension would be affected as well. The researchers conclude that influenza A may be implicated in the development of fibromyalgia, the primary symptom of which is widespread muscle pain.

N-acetyl cysteine (NAC)–NAC is an amino acid precursor for the production of glutathione which reduces free radical damage to DNA and prevents the depletion of other antioxidants. N-acetyl cysteine is also an antiviral and is effective in breaking up mucus as well. "I'll use NAC if the person has some upper-respiratory symptoms or if they have environmental allergies," reports Dr. Lieberman. A typical dosage is 500 mg twice a day.

Glycyrrhizinate–An active component of licorice, glycyrrhizin is "probably the most studied antiviral compound on the planet," according to Dr. Lieberman. However, she often has difficulty obtaining it. The typical dosage for the capsules made by Jarrow Formulas is two or three daily. Glycgel (made by Thorne Research) is in gel form and the typical dosage is ½ teaspoon twice a day.

Echinacea–As mentioned above, echinacea is known for its antimicrobial qualities. Dr. Lieberman favors Echinaguard, a tincture form of echinacea. She normally recommends 30-50 drops once a day, in an ongoing cycle of four days on, four days off.

Coenzyme Q10–Coenzyme Q10 is a substance not made by the human body, but found naturally in sardines, salmon, mackerel, and beef heart. "Coenzyme Q10 is 100% for energy. It increases the oxygen consumption of your cells and is crucial for making ATP, which is our energy," states Dr. Lieberman. A typical dosage is 100 mg once or twice daily.

Maitake D-Fraction–The above supplements are the basics of the program. If the patient is experiencing predominantly viral symptoms,

Dr. Lieberman then adds maitake D-fraction to the regimen. This is an extract of the antiviral maitake mushroom, one of the medicinal mushrooms (shiitake and reishi are others) known to have powerful immune-enhancing effects. This tincture can be mixed with the Echinaguard at the same typical dosage, 30-50 drops once a day, four days on, four days off.

Acidophilus–*Acidophilus* is one of the beneficial bacteria, microbes that inhabit the human gastrointestinal tract where they are essential for proper nutrient assimilation. The human body contains several trillion beneficial bacteria comprising over 400 species, all necessary for health. Among the more well-known are *Lactobacillus acidophilus* and *Bifidobacterium bifidum*. Overly acidic bodily conditions, chronic constipation or diarrhea, dietary imbalances, consumption of highly processed foods, and the excessive use of antibiotics and hormonal drugs can interfere with probiotic function and even reduce the number of these microbes, setting up conditions for illness.

If a person has gastrointestinal problems, which is true of 50% of her CFS patients, then Dr. Lieberman includes the powdered, refrigerated variety of *acidophilus* to help restore intestinal balance, at a dosage of ½ teaspoon once or twice a day, mixed with water or juice or sprinkled on food.

Aloe Vera–This herb is also useful for gastrointestinal complaints. "Aloe vera is soothing, can ease inflammation, and has natural plant enzymes which help with digestion," says Dr. Lieberman. She recommends ¼ cup, twice daily.

For someone whose system is severely weakened by CFS and who has irritable bowel symptoms, Dr. Lieberman starts the program at low dosages and gradually builds to the full amount. "A patient's stomach may be so bad that they can't tolerate the full dose of vitamins until you clear the irritable bowel," she says.

One of her main approaches for healing the digestive problems is to take patients off dairy and gluten (a vegetable protein found in wheat, rye, oats, and barley). "I have found gluten to be extremely deleterious to immune function, certainly in patients with CFS and other autoimmune disorders," says Dr. Lieberman. In addition, "viruses love fat and sugar," she observes, so cutting them out of the diet is part of the antiviral program.

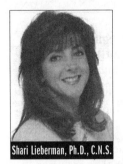

Shari Lieberman, Ph.D., C.N.S.

"I have found gluten to be extremely deleterious to immune function, certainly in patients with CFS and other autoimmune disorders," says Dr. Lieberman. In addition, "viruses love fat and sugar," she observes, so cutting them out of the diet is part of the antiviral program.

Shari Lieberman, Ph.D., C.N.S. is available by appointment only. To schedule an appointment, call: 212-929-3152. For **Glycyrrhizinate** and **Quercetin**, contact: Jarrow Formulas, Inc., 1824 South Robertson Boulevard, Los Angeles, CA 90035; tel: 800-726-0886 or 310-204-6936; fax: 310-890-8955. For **Glycgel**, contact: Thorne Research, P.O. Box 3200, Sandpoint, ID 83864; tel: 800-228-1966 or 208-263-1337; fax: 208-265-2488. For **Echinaguard**, contact: Nature's Way, 10 Mountain Springs Parkway, Springville, UT 84663; tel: 800-962-8873 or 801-489-1500; fax: 801-489-1640. **Optimum Protection, Kyolic Premium EPA**, and the other products mentioned by Dr. Lieberman are available from health food stores. These items may also be ordered by mail, contact: Hickey Chemists, 212-223-6333 (U.S. only).

A Homeopathic Antiviral Program for Chronic Fatigue Syndrome

New evidence suggests that chronic fatigue can be reversed using a homeopathic (SEE QUICK DEFINITION) approach to viral therapy. According to a study of 219 case histories, nearly all patients reported significant improvement after receiving homeopathic treatments which targeted the three main viruses—Epstein-Barr, Coxsackie, and cytomegalovirus—most commonly associated with chronic fatigue syndrome.

The study involved an unusually diverse group of participants. Among the 219 cases, ages ranged from 2 to 78 years, and length of symptoms extended anywhere from one month to 30 years. Significantly, more than half had unsuccessfully attempted treatment by another method before admission to the study. Despite this apparent diversity among participants, however, blood tests revealed that all were infected with one of these three viruses, and that many carried some combination of the three.

Researchers patterned their treatment plan on a fourfold approach previously used to successfully cure hepatitis. Participants received twice weekly injections of four different medicinal preparations: first, a highly diluted form (nosode—SEE QUICK DEFINITION) of the virus or viruses detected by the initial blood test, to stimulate the body's immune response against the infecting agent; second, a homeopathic preparation made from extracts of live organ tissues, to improve tissue regeneration and organ function (organ therapy); third, substances given to boost the immune system in general; and fourth, complex homeopathic remedies tailored both to the disease and to the patient, according to individual presentation of symptoms.

The homeopathic remedies included any combination of the following: Heel Coenzyme compositum and Wala Betula Arnica, Heel Echinacea compositum and Wala Meteoric Iron-Phosphorus-Quartz, Heel Engystol and Wala Pancreas Meteor, Galium-Heel and oral Wala Aurum Prunus, Heel Lymphomyosot and oral Wala Skorodit, and Heel Ubichinon compositum.

After an average of five to six weeks of treatment, nearly all participants noted a significant improvement in their physical function and overall health. Because most of the patients could not afford the expense of another blood test, reseachers had to rely on subjective self-reporting instead of clinical data; even so, their results are impressive. Complete recovery occured in 82% of the cases, while the remaining 18% resolved their symptoms after a second or third series of treatments. As one long-time sufferer of CFS described his recovery, "I have been dead for ten years and now I am alive again."

The study demonstrates that complex homeopathic remedies, when used in conjuction with nosodes, organ therapy, and immune system enhancement, can provide a treatment capable of reversing chronic fatigue syndrome. "This treatment is not open-ended," the study's authors point out. "Rather, it will most likely result in a cure in a specified time of five to six weeks." The prospect of a CFS cure should give hope to CFS sufferers, the authors conclude, because many are understandably frustrated by endless medical treatments which result in only marginal improvement.[8]

Olive Leaf Extract Can Kill Viruses

Olive leaf extract may be one of the most powerful natural medicines against viruses and bacterial infection. The active component of the olive leaf is oleuropein (the bitter element removed from olives when they are processed). Researchers at Upjohn, the pharmaceutical giant based in Kalamazoo, Michigan, found that the main component in oleuropein, a salt extract called calcium elenolate, is "virucidal (virus-killing) for all viruses against which it has been tested."

QUICK DEFINITION

Homeopathy was founded in the early 1800s by German physician Samuel Hahnemann. Today, an estimated 500 million people worldwide receive homeopathic treatment; in Britain, homeopathy enjoys royal patronage. Homeopathy is now practiced according to two differing concepts. In classical homeopathy, only one single-component remedy is prescribed at a time in a potency specifically adjusted to the patient; the physician waits to see the results before prescribing anything further. In complex homeopathy, typified by *Hepar compositum*, a prescription involves multiple substances given at the same time, usually in low potencies.

A **homeopathic nosode** is a super-diluted remedy made as an energy imprint from a disease product, such as tuberculosis, measles, bowel infection, influenza, and about 200 other substances. The nosode, which contains no physical trace of the disease, stimulates the body to remove all "taints" or residues it holds of a particular disease, whether it was inherited or contracted. Only qualified homeopaths may administer a nosode.

For more information about the **homeopathic remedies** cited, contact: Biomedical Homeopathic Industries, Inc., 11600 Cochiti SE, Albuquerque, NM 87123; tel: 800-621-7644 or 505-293-3843; fax: 505-275-1672.
For **olive leaf extract** (Alive and Well™ for consumers and Prolive™ for medical professionals), contact: Allergy Research Group, 400 Preda Street, San Leandro, CA 94577; tel: 510-639-4572 or 800-782-4274; fax: 510-635-6730; e-mail: info@nutricology.com.

The list of the viruses tested is impressive, including herpes, influenza A, Coxsackie, polio, encephalomyocarditis, and reovirus 3, among others. Upjohn researchers believe that calcium elenolate, interacting with the protein coat of the virus, managed to reduce the ability of these organisms to convey infections.

A study at the Volcani Institute of Agricultural Research in Rehovot, Israel, tested oleuropein's effect on a bacteria similar to *Streptococcus* and found that it effectively killed the organism. It did so by damaging the cell membrane of the bacterium, causing intracellular constituents such as phosphorus, potassium, and glutamate to leak out and impoverish the cell.[9] The olive leaf also contains natural vitamin C helpers (bioflavonoids) such as rutin, luteolin, and hesperidin, which are needed to protect against infection.

Arnold Takemoto, B.S., a biochemist who designs nutritional programs in Arizona, used olive leaf extract in his work with a rheumatologist for cases of fibromyalgia and chronic fatigue syndrome. He comments: "It's the missing link that functions as an antiviral and antiretroviral agent by slowing down the organism's reproductive cycle." Olive leaf extract, he adds, "allows the patient's immune system to go on the attack."

Donald Gay, D.C., N.D., H.M.D., based in Toronto, Canada, has also used olive leaf extract in treating chronic fatigue syndrome. "What's needed is something that rids the person of bacterial and viral infections, and now I've found the appropriate compound," states Dr. Gay. He used the extract to cure his own sinusitis from which he had suffered for over ten years.[10]

Treating Candidiasis

Before we discuss a range of alternative treatments for candidiasis, let's look at a case illustrating the relationship between yeast overgrowth and fibromyalgia, and how treating candidiasis and correcting the intestinal imbalance it creates can reverse this painful disorder.

Gary Kaplan, D.O., a family physician, chronic pain specialist, president of the Medical Acupuncture Research Foundation in Los Angeles, California, and associate professor at Georgetown University Medical School in Washington, D.C., explains how testing for these underlying conditions serves as a foundation for designing a therapeutic treatment program:

Fighting the Viruses of Severe CFS with Heat Therapy

Bruce Milliman, N.D., of Seattle, Washington, reports success using hyperthermia (heat therapy) as the central element in a treatment program for severe cases of CFS. Dr. Milliman's treatment involves artificially inducing fever in order to augment the body's ability to fight viral infections. Patients must commit to a three-week course of treatment during which they stay home, get total bed rest, and undergo the fever treatment three times daily.

To induce hyperthermia, the patient soaks in a bath (as hot as is tolerable) for a full five minutes, while drinking a 12-ounce glass of tepid water mixed with 2,000 mg of vitamin C. Emerging from the bath, the patient quickly dries off and gets into a bed prepared with flannel sheets and wool blankets, placing a hot water bottle under the breast (women) or over the liver (men), and remaining under the blankets for 20 minutes. This procedure stimulates a natural fever response and the body will sweat profusely in its attempt to return to normal body temperature.

According to Dr. Milliman, fever is one of the immune system's natural adaptive mechanisms, and "turning up the thermostat" enhances immune response. He reports a 70% to 75% success rate with his patients who follow this daily protocol for the full three weeks. Dr. Milliman reports that most failures in fever therapy occur in individuals unwilling or unable to address simultaneous disorders such as yeast infections, dental amalgam reaction (to mercury), and hypothyroidism.

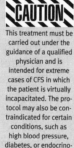

CAUTION

This treatment must be carried out under the guidance of a qualified physician and is intended for extreme cases of CFS in which the patient is virtually incapacitated. The protocol may also be contraindicated for certain conditions, such as high blood pressure, diabetes, or endocrinological problems.

Success Story: Reversing Fibromyalgia by Treating Candidiasis and Intestinal Imbalance

Lizzy, 42, came to my office with symptoms of fibromyalgia. She complained of generalized joint pain in her hands, hips, knees, and ankles, which had begun 12 months earlier. She also had sporadic but significant fatigue and sinus problems that never completely went away after each episode. For the frequent acne she had suffered from her whole adult life, she took a conventional drug called minocycline hydrochloride (a tetracycline antibiotic) to control the outbreaks.

At one point before seeing me, Lizzy had received a diagnosis of systemic lupus erythematosus, a dangerous autoimmune disease. However, blood work performed by another physician failed to confirm this diagnosis. Lizzy followed a healthy, mostly vegetarian diet, eating only a minimum of dairy products and meat and a great deal of whole grains. Despite her chronic pain, she exercised regularly by running and bicycling several times a week.

In the course of taking her health history, I learned that Lizzy's symptoms began shortly after a trip to Eastern Europe. In the months preceding this trip, Lizzy had been eating and sleeping poorly and was under constant stress regarding family matters. It is quite likely that in the course of her travels, Lizzy was exposed to something that set in motion an allergic reaction. In effect, you have a woman under stress who has experiences and exposures that push her over the immunological edge. The question is then, in what area will the immune resistance break down? In Lizzy's case, it broke down in the threefold area of colonic environment, digestion, and absorption.

My job as a physician is to figure out what steps to take to unload and de-stress her system, and to bring her intestinal microflora back into balance so that her digestion and absorption processes work well, and thereby restore her health. I help get things back into alignment and remove as many challenges to the body's functioning as I can so that its natural ability to heal itself is restored. Further, any significant psychological issues must be addressed as part of any comprehensive treatment program for a chronic condition.

Patients Report Onset of CFS After Hepatitis B Vaccine

Following the televised report in Canada of a nurse claiming that she acquired chronic fatigue syndrome following a vaccination for hepatitis B, 69 people called the television station to report the same experience. The U.S. Centers for Disease Control (CDC) investigated the claim of 60 of the callers. Although 53% met the CDC criteria for chronic fatigue syndrome, the CDC concluded that no scientific basis existed for their allegation, according to the *Canadian Medical Association Journal* (January 1, 1992).

Analyzing Her Colonic Environment—The relationship in time between Lizzy's travels abroad and the onset of symptoms suggested the possibility that she had picked up intestinal parasites. I requested that she send a stool sample to Great Smokies Diagnostic Laboratory for a comprehensive analysis of digestion, absorption, colonic environment, and yeast sensitivity. This test provides a great deal of information with regard to digestion of various foods, whether or not fats are being absorbed, what digestive enzymes are present, as well as whether intestinal bacteria are in balance or if yeasts are present in the stool. All of these factors may be contributing to a patient's symptoms.

I have found in a number of patients that parasite infestation can frequently produce an antigenic (SEE QUICK DEFINITION) reaction that leads towards generalized joint pain and sometimes asthma. The immune system judges antigens to be foreign, undesirable particles and mounts an immune response to their presence. For example, I had a male patient who developed

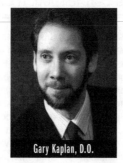

Gary Kaplan, D.O.

"My job as a physician is to figure out what steps to take to unload and de-stress my patient's system, and to bring their intestinal microflora back into balance so that their digestion and absorption processes work well, and thereby restore their health," says Gary Kaplan, D.O.

a *Giardia* infection followed by asthma symptoms, indicating an antigenic reaction; in other words, the antigenic reaction to the parasite manifested as asthma. When the *Giardia* was treated, the asthma symptoms disappeared.

As it turned out, Lizzy did not have a parasite problem, but her intestinal flora were out of balance, as indicated by a "severe" reaction on the Dysbiosis Index (see sidebar, "What a Stool Analysis Can Tell You," pp. 90-91). This high reading would certainly help account for her problems in digestion and absorption. Imbalances in bacterial microflora can also lead to skin problems, such as rashes and acne, joint pain, and digestive problems. On a macroscopic level the test revealed that Lizzy's stools were a normal brown color with no traces of blood or mucus, but their chemical nature, or pH (see sidebar), was slightly too alkaline at 7.3.

Among the beneficial bacteria we expect to find in the healthy colon, Lizzy was completely deficient of *Lactobacillus* varieties although she had an optimal level of *Bifidobacteria*. Among other bacteria, Lizzy's stool showed evidence of *gamma Streptococcus* in the normal range. Of nonbeneficial microbes, her stool measured *Pseudomonas aeruginosa* beyond the acceptable limit. As a result, she was growing some strains of bacteria in her colon that shouldn't be there. This data, however, should be interpreted carefully and the basic tenet of all alternative medicine is that you must look at the

An **antigen** is any biological substance (a toxin, virus, fungus, bacterium, amoeba, or other protein) that the body comes to regard as foreign and dangerous to itself. As such, an antigen induces a state of cellular sensitivity or immune reaction that seeks to neutralize, remove, or destroy the antigen by dispatching antibodies against it.

What Stool Analysis Can Tell You: A Glossary of Terms

Dysbiosis index—Intestinal dysbiosis refers to an imbalance of intestinal flora. Specifically, these flora include friendly, beneficial bacteria called probiotics (for example, *Lactobacillus acidophilus* and *Bifidobacterium bifidum*) and unfriendly or harmful bacteria (for example, *Pseudomonas aeruginosa*). In dysbiosis, the unfriendly bacteria predominate; they begin fermentation producing toxic by-products which interfere with the normal elimination cycle. The dysbiosis index reflects the balance of friendly and pathogenic bacteria, and those markers related to the flora, such as pH and SCFAs.

COLONIC ENVIRONMENT

Lactobacillus* and *Bifidobacteria—These bacteria are involved in vitamin synthesis, the detoxification of procarcinogens (substances that become carcinogenic, or cancer-causing), and they support the immune system. Deficiencies of *Lactobacillus* have been linked with a higher risk for various chronic diseases.

gamma Streptococcus—This is a bacteria normal to the intestines; its presence in the analysis is not an indication of digestive imbalance.

Pseudomonas aeruginosa—A bacterium associated with wound infections, infected burn lesions, and urinary tract infections, it produces a characteristic blue pus and causes infections in the context of a weakened immune system. These problems do not normally occur in the colon; however, *P. aeruginosa* in the colon may or may not be symptomatic. If symptomatic, it may contribute to diarrhea and inflammation.

Candida albicans—The intestinal tract normally contains small amounts of this yeast. In some cases, however, wide use of antibiotics, birth control pills and a high-carbohydrate diet may cause and overgrowth of the *Candida* yeast, causing a condition called candidiasis. Overgrowth of *Candida albicans* and other intestinal yeasts has been linked to food allergies, migraines, vaginitis, irritable bowel syndrome, indigestion, and asthma.

Macroscopic (appearance)—Yellow to green stools may indicate diarrhea and a bowel sterilized by antibiotics; black or red may reflect bleeding in the gastrointestinal tract; tan or grey can indicate a blockage of the common bile duct; mucus or pus can point to irritable bowel syndrome, polyps, diverticulitis, or intestinal wall inflammation; and occult blood might result from eating too much red meat, from hemorrhoids, or possibly from colon cancer.

pH—pH is a reflection of the acid/alkaline balance in the colon. The preferred range is 6.0 (mildly acidic) to 7.2 (mildly alkaline). Fecal pH reflects the status of colonic digestive processes, SCFAs (see below), beneficial bacteria, and bacterial metabolism. An elevated fecal pH is associated with a higher risk of colitis and colon cancer.

N-butyrate—This is a form of butyric acid, a primary energy source for the colon cells; it must be present in adequate amounts for healthy metabolism (energy, nutrient, and water release from foods) in the colon. Butyric acid is needed to digest short-chain fatty acids (SCFAs). Low levels of N-butyrate are associated with a higher risk of colon cancer.

Total SCFA—Short-chain fatty acids, such as acetate, propionate, N-butyrate, and valerate, are produced when the colon ferments soluble fibers. SCFAs are important because they provide 70% of the energy needed by the cells lining the colon.

SCFA distribution—Elevated levels of any of the four SCFAs can indicate poor nutrient absorption in the colon or bacterial overgrowth, while decreased levels suggest lack of dietary fiber, unbalanced metabolic processes, or dysbiosis. The key factor here is the ratio among the four SCFAs, which usually remains relatively constant in healthy individuals but can shift noticeably when metabolism becomes disordered.

For information about the **Comprehensive Digestive Stool Analysis**, contact: Great Smokies Diagnostic Laboratory, 63 Zillicoa Street, Asheville, NC 28801; tel: 704-253-0621 or 800-522-4762; fax: 704-252-9303.

Beta-glucuronidase—This is an enzyme produced by various bacteria in the colon. Elevated levels may result from bacterial overgrowth, an abnormal intestinal pH, too much dietary fat (especially from meat), or low levels of beneficial bacteria. Elevated levels can increase bioactivation of carcinogens in the bowel, thus increasing the risk of colon cancer.

Fecal sIgA—Fecal secretory IgA is a specialized immunoglobulin, which is one of a class of five specially designed antibody proteins produced in the spleen, bone marrow, or lymph tissue. They are involved in the immune system's defense response to foreign substances. Fecal sIgA serves as the first line of defense against invading pathogens, toxins, and food allergens in the intestines. Low levels mean an increased susceptibility to infection and food allergies.

MEASURES OF DIGESTIVE DYSFUNCTION

Triglycerides—Most dietary fats are triglycerides, a term that denotes their chemical structure. During digestion, lipase, a pancreatic enzyme, breaks triglycerides down into glycerol and free fatty acids. Elevated fecal triglyceride levels indicate incomplete fat metabolism and possible problems in the pancreas.

Chymotrypsin—A digestive enzyme produced in the intestines, its relative levels can indicate the patient's enzyme status and activity. Decreased levels mean the pancreas is not releasing enough enzymes and/or that the stomach is low on digestive acids, which are needed to activate chymotrypsin. Elevated levels suggest a rapid transit time (the speed at which fecal matter moves through the intestines).

Valerate and iso-butyrate—Valerate and iso-butyrate are short-chain fatty acids produced when intestinal bacteria ferment protein. Elevated levels indicate that the protein was not digested properly in the stomach and intestines.

Meat and vegetable fibers—These are crude microscopic markers for digestive function. Elevated levels may indicate inadequate chewing, stomach acid, or digestive enzymes.

MEASURES OF ABSORPTION

LCFAs—Long-chain fatty acids are normally absorbed directly by intestinal mucosa. Elevated levels reflect malabsorption of fats, a result of maldigestion or inflammation of the lining of the small intestine.

Cholesterol—Cholesterol in the feces comes from either dietary fats or the breakdown of the cells lining the intestines. Generally, fecal cholesterol levels remain stable, despite dietary intake; elevated fecal levels suggest malabsorption or irritation of the mucosal lining.

Total fecal fat—This represents the sum of all fats or lipids, except for SCFAs, and can indicate either maldigestion or malabsorption.

whole picture and not single out any one piece of information. When one element shifts, everything else changes accordingly.

The most glaring fact in Lizzy's stool analysis was the high level of yeast organisms (*Candida albicans*). Her levels approached the pathogenic. This overgrowth was behind the intestinal imbalance and many of her symptoms. To determine which prescription drugs and natural substances at what concentration would work best for her system in reducing the yeast overgrowth, I ran a second Great Smokies test called Sensitivity to Antifungal Agents. The test showed that the conventional antifungal drug Diflucan (fluconazole) was the "drug of choice."

Among the metabolic markers indicated in the stool analysis, Lizzy's levels of N-butyrate were somewhat depressed, under the preferred range of 10 to 30. This data told me that Lizzy was not metabolizing (SEE QUICK DEFINITION) her foods and extracting from them the fatty acids (such as from animal fats) her system needed. Many have observed a correlation between alkaline fecal pH and decreased levels of short-chain fatty acids (SCFAs). If you have low levels of N-butyrate, which is responsible for producing SCFAs from the metabolism of foods, then your SCFAs will be low as well. SCFAs result from the breakdown of carbohydrates and fiber; if SCFAs are in short

Sensitivity to Antifungal Agents

Minimum Inhibitory Concentration µg/ml
(lowest concentration required to inhibit growth of organism)
presumptive C. albicans

Prescriptive Agents		Typical*	Typical*	Typical*
Fluconazole	<0.5	2	2	2
Itraconazole	<0.5	2	2	2
Ketoconazole	<0.5	2	2	2
Nystatin	<2	10	10	10
Natural Substances				
Berberine	160	160	160	160
Caprylic Acid	500	500	500	500
Garlic	<125	500	500	500
Sanguinaria	<8	160	160	160
Undecylenic	500	500	500	500
Plant Tanins	<0.5	8	8	8
Uva-ursi	<8	160	160	160

Sensitivity to Antifungal Agents test. This test indicates how the patient is likely to respond to each of a number of agents, both natural and drug-based, capable of producing effects against fungi.

supply, this can mean the proper microflora are missing from the intestines, there is too little fiber in the diet, or the stool takes too long to move through the colon.

In Lizzy's case, she had a normal distribution of SCFAs, but a deficiency in total SCFAs. While the optimal range is 56 to 156, Lizzy's levels were only 47. This means she was creating the right amount of SCFAs, but as a whole, she wasn't digesting or absorbing them well. Counterbalancing this, Lizzy's levels of beta-glucuronidase, an enzyme needed to digest fats and cholesterol, were solidly normal. Also, the level of her fecal sIgA was well within the normal range.

The Status of Lizzy's Digestion and Absorption—The quality of a patient's colonic environment is directly affected by what they eat and how well, or poorly, it is digested and absorbed. Within the category of digestion, the laboratory test provides values in three key areas: triglycerides, chymotrypsin, and valerate iso-butyrate.

Lizzy's levels were acceptable in the first and third categories, but her chymotrypsin levels were seriously low. In regard to meat and vegetable fibers, which provide another measure of digestive function, Lizzy had no traces in her stool. This was not surprising, considering her mostly vegetarian diet. In fact, if Lizzy had been eating a meat-centered diet, she would have been feeling much worse and all her stool markers would have been further imbalanced. Her system was not geared to handle meat; fortunately, she had regulated her diet on her own and kept her meat consumption to a minimum.

Within the four categories indicating absorption, Lizzy's values were mostly unacceptable. Her levels of long-chain fatty acids (LCFAs) were slightly elevated. While her fecal cholesterol levels were in the normal range, her levels of total fecal fat were at the borderline of imbalance. As mentioned earlier, her chymotrypsin levels (another measure of absorption) were low.

To complement the considerable data I gained from the stool analysis, I ordered a blood test for Lizzy, from which I learned that her DHEA (SEE QUICK DEFINITION) levels were low (less than 200 mg/dL). Studies have shown that restoring optimal levels of DHEA reduced joint pain in test subjects with lupus. I started Lizzy on 25 mg daily of DHEA using the Pure Encapsulations brand. I have looked at

> **QUICK DEFINITION**
>
> **Metabolism** is the biological process by which energy is extracted from the foods consumed, producing carbon dioxide and water as by-products for elimination. Biochemically, metabolism involves hundreds of different chemical reactions, necessitating the involvement of hundreds of different enzymes, each of which handles a specific reaction. There are two kinds of metabolism constantly underway in the cells: anabolic and catabolic. In anabolic metabolism, the upbuilding phase, larger molecules are constructed by joining smaller ones together; in catabolic metabolism, the deconstructing phase, larger molecules are broken down into smaller ones. The anabolic function produces substances for cell growth and repair, while the catabolic function controls digestion (called hydrolysis), disassembling food into forms the body can use for energy.

Three principal factors were responsible for throwing Lizzy's digestive system out of balance and creating her symptoms: a yeast overgrowth, a wheat sensitivity, and a DHEA deficiency.

DHEA (dehydroepiandrosterone) is naturally produced by the human adrenal glands and gonads with optimal levels occurring around age 20 for women and age 25 for men. After those ages, DHEA levels gradually decline so that a person 80 years old produces only a fraction of the DHEA they did when they were 20. As an antioxidant, hormone regulator, and the building block from which estrogen and testosterone are produced, DHEA is vital to health. Low DHEA levels have been associated with cancer, diabetes, multiple sclerosis, hypertension, obesity, AIDS, heart disease, Alzheimer's, and immune dysfunction illnesses. Test subjects using supplemental DHEA reported improved sleeping patterns, better memory, an improved ability to cope with stress, decreased joint pain, increases in lean muscle, and decreases in body fat. No serious side effects have been reported to date, although acne, oily skin, facial hair growth on women, deepening of the voice, irritability, insomnia, and fatigue have been reported with high DHEA doses.

Osteopathy is a treatment method based on the principle that the structure of the body (the musculoskeletal system) is interrelated with the function of its systems and organs, and that disruptions in one can cause problems in the other, making both subject to a wide range of disorders. After a thorough evaluation, an osteopath performs adjustments (manipulations) on the patient, which help the body to correct its structural problems. These manipulations include cranial manipulation, relax and release techniques for the muscles and soft tissues, and articulation (similar to chiropractic adjustments). Osteopathy provides relief for patients suffering from a variety of conditions including spinal and joint problems, arthritis, allergies, chronic fatigue syndrome, high blood pressure, and headaches.

a number of DHEA products and find them, for the most part, to be unreliable in their ability to raise DHEA levels in my patients. The Pure Encapsulations formula, on the other hand, has been consistently effective.

Finally, as part of Lizzy's initial treatment plan, I suggested she start receiving osteopathic (SEE QUICK DEFINITION) manipulations and acupuncture to address the joint pain and sinusitis. After four treatments of each and daily use of DHEA, Lizzy's energy levels were better but the joint pain, especially in her hands, remained significant. It was my impression that the candidiasis in her intestines was contributing to this symptom. I started her on Diflucan, as indicated by her Sensitivity test.

I also suggested some dietary restrictions; in particular, I suggested Lizzy stay away from any foods made with wheat or yeast. Her system was unable to handle wheat; the chronic malabsorption of wheat gluten created an allergic-type reaction in her system which then contributed to the chronic joint pain. Intolerance to wheat (called gluten enteropathy or celiac disease) is far more common than people realize. In addition, Lizzy completely eliminated meat from her diet, sensing that her system may have been reacting poorly to even the small amounts she ate. Fortunately, Lizzy had already altered her diet by the time I met her. She knew that with a digestive system out of balance, a standard meat-based American diet would make her much sicker.

After 16 days on the Diflucan, Lizzy began to show unpleasant side effects, notably an itchy rash, and I stopped the medication. Her joint pain had improved considerably, presumably as the *Candida* had been brought under control, and her energy level continued to grow. No longer taking the Diflucan, Lizzy's rash disappeared, and she began to have dramatic improvement in her joint pain, fatigue, and sinusitis. About one month later, when Lizzy ate some wheat and meat as a test to her system, the joint pain returned along with muscle pain and joint swelling. However, once she stopped eating wheat again and maintained the allergen-free diet, all of these symptoms disappeared.

"I help get things back into alignment and remove as many challenges to the body's functioning as I can so that its natural ability to heal itself is restored," says Dr. Kaplan.

Often, allergy sufferers find their symptoms are worsened by dairy products, which increase mucus production; wheat intolerance often shows up as rashes and joint pain (as we saw in Lizzy's case). Nasal congestion and symptoms of asthma often improve after wheat is eliminated from the diet. In the case of red meat, the antibiotics and steroids routinely given to animals and ingested by meat eaters can aggravate numerous symptoms. Eliminating meat from the diet often leads to a reduction of these symptoms.

In my estimation, three principal factors were responsible for throwing Lizzy's digestive system out of balance (producing the abnormal stool analysis values) and creating her symptoms: a yeast overgrowth, a wheat sensitivity, and a DHEA deficiency. By reversing these, her fibromyalgia was resolved. ■

To contact **Gary Kaplan, D.O.**: Kaplan Clinic, 5275 Lee Highway, Suite 200, Arlington, VA 22207; tel: 703-532-4892; fax: 703-237-3105. For more information about **DHEA**, contact: Pure Encapsulations, Inc., 490 Boston Post Road, Sudbury, MA 01776; tel: 508-443-1999 or 800-753-2277; fax: 888-783-2277. For **Sinusan**, contact: Bioforce of America, Ltd., P.O. Box 507, Kinderhook, NY 12106; tel: 518-758-6060; fax: 518-758-9500. For the **Comprehensive Digestive Stool Analysis and Sensitivity to Antifungal Agents**, contact: Great Smokies Diagnostic Laboratory, 63 Zillicoa Street, Asheville, NC 28801; tel: 828-253-0621 or 800-522-4762; fax: 828-252-9303.

Other Alternative Medicine Treatments for Candidiasis

Successful treatment of candidiasis first requires the reduction of factors which predispose a patient to *Candida* overgrowth. Secondly, the patient's immune function must be strengthened. Diet, nutritional supplements, herbal medicine, Ayurvedic medicine, acupuncture, and enzyme therapy are some of the choices alternative medicine physicians employ to accomplish these ends.

Recovery from chronic candidiasis seldom takes less than three months and is usually well advanced by six months, but it can take longer to recover completely. Medical studies show that until bowel

Candida is under control, local manifestations (such as vaginal thrush) will continue to appear. Local treatment alone (for thrush or other symptoms) is not sufficient.

Diet

Yeast thrives on sugar, so to overcome candidiasis, sugar must be avoided in all its various forms. These include: sucrose, dextrose, fructose, fruit juices, honey, maple syrup, molasses, milk products (which contain lactose), most fruit (except berries), and potatoes (their starch converts into sugar). Candidiasis patients should also stay away from all alcohol since it is composed of fermented and refined sugar. "In treating candidiasis, my basic dietary taboos are sweets, alcohol, and refined carbohydrates," reports Leyardia Black, N.D., of Lopez Island, Washington.

Meat, dairy, and poultry consumption can also foster *Candida* growth because of the large amount of antibiotics used on the animals. Traces of antibiotics given to dairy cows can later show up in milk. Organic (hormone- and antibiotic-free) meat and poultry should be consumed whenever possible. For candidiasis patients, seafood (free of mercury toxins) and vegetable protein are preferable, since they are not only antibiotic free, but lower in fat.

Many candidiasis sufferers have allergies or sensitivities to various foods. Although *Candida albicans* yeast is not the same as yeast in foods (such as bread) a cross-reaction between food and yeast frequently occurs. As a result, foods containing or promoting yeast, such as baked goods, alcohol, and vinegar, should be avoided until possible sensitivities are clearly diagnosed.

Molds are another aspect of *Candida* sensitivity, according to Dr. Murray Susser. These include food molds (found in cheeses, grapes, mushrooms, and fermented foods) and environmental molds (found in wet climates, in damp basements, in plants, and outdoors). Mold and yeast can also exchange forms. Therefore, the ingestible molds of cheeses and fermented foods should be avoided. Avoiding food yeast and mold does not attack the *Candida* yeast itself, but is an attempt to ease stress on the immune system caused by substances which can trigger allergies.[11] Even so, avoidance of food yeast and mold should be considered on an individual basis. As Dr. Susser says, "My personal opinion is that most anti-*Candida* diets are too strict. It is unnecessary to take *Candida* patients off vinegar and mushrooms unless they are allergic to these things."

Dr. Susser advises patients to avoid yogurt because of its high sugar content, despite its high concentration of *Lactobacilli* which suppress "bad" bacteria and keep other organisms under control. He finds that freeze-dried *acidophilus* supplements in capsule form are more effective in combating bacteria than even unsweetened raw yogurt.

Nutritional Supplements

A general nutritional support program is frequently needed to help build up immune function and digestive efficiency, which may have become severely compromised after months or years of chronic candidiasis, according to Dr. Leon Chaitow. Specific supplementation can be helpful in reversing nutritional deficiencies and rebuilding weakened immune function.

Recommended supplements include:

■ Individual B vitamins (increase antibody response and are used in nearly every body activity)

■ Vitamin C (stimulates adrenaline and is essential to immune processes)

■ Vitamin E (the lack of which depresses immune response)

■ Vitamin A (builds resistance to infection and increases immune response)

■ Beta carotene (a vitamin A precursor which increases T cells)

■ Antioxidants, such as selenium, calcium, and zinc (immune-boosters useful in combating candidiasis)

■ Chromium, magnesium, and adrenal glandular extracts (stimulate adrenal function)

■ Probiotic (SEE QUICK DEFINITION) supplements (repopulate the intestines with "friendly" bacteria and correct the imbalance of flora created by the *Candida* overgrowth)

■ Essential fatty acids (such as evening primrose oil) may be considered as well[12]

As routine supplementation for treatment of candidiasis, James Braly, M.D., of Fort Lauderdale, Florida, offers the following regimen:

■ Vitamin C (8-10 g daily)
■ Vitamin E (one 400-IU capsule daily)
■ Evening primrose oil (six to eight capsules daily)
■ Max EPA (six capsules daily)
■ Pantothenic acid (250 mg daily)
■ Taurine (500-1,000 mg daily)
■ Zinc chelate (25-50 mg daily)
■ Goldenseal root extract with no less than 5% hydrastine (250 mg twice a day)

■ *Lactobacillus acidophilus* (one dry teaspoon, three times daily; if allergic to milk, use nonlactose *acidophilus*)

■ Dr. Braly also recommends supplementation of hydrochloric acid (HCl). He notes that the aging process, alcohol abuse, food allergies, and nutrient deficiencies create a lack of HCl in the stomach, which prevents food from being digested and permits *Candida* overgrowth. Such supplementation, he says, helps restore the proper balance of intestinal flora. Dr. Braly recommends one capsule of HCl and pepsin (a digestive acid in the stomach) at the start of meals, increasing cautiously to two to four capsules with each meal if needed.

Herbal Medicine

Herbs are often used to kill harmful yeasts and shore up immune function. They are used in teas, dried in capsules or tablets, or taken in suppository form. Herbs which contain berberain (an alkaloid found in the berbercia family) have proven particularly useful as anti-*Candida* agents. These include goldenseal, Oregon grape, and barberry.

Berberain is a natural antibiotic which acts against *Candida* overgrowth, normalizes intestinal flora, helps digestive problems, has antidiarrheal properties, and stimulates the immune system by increasing blood supply to the spleen. Soothing to inflamed mucous membranes, berberain can be taken as a tea, or in other fluid and dry forms.[13] Other antifungal and antibacterial herbs include German chamomile, aloe vera, ginger, cinnamon, rosemary, licorice, and tea tree oil.[14] Fennel, anise, ginseng, alfalfa, and red clover are also effective.

Dr. Braly's first line of attack on candidiasis is caprylic acid, a fatty acid found in coconut oil and shown to be an effective antifungal agent. Only if there is no improvement will Dr. Braly use conventional medication. Since caprylic acid is readily absorbed into the system, it should be taken in an enteric coated (absorbed in the small intestines rather than the stomach) or sustained release form.

In one study, 16 patients were given 1,800 mg daily of caprylic acid (the commercial brand Capricin) for 16 days, three patients were given 2,700 mg daily, and six received 3,600 mg per day. The results were a 30% to 90% reduction in *Candida* levels among those with the 1,800 mg dosage; a 70% to 100% reduction in the three patients taking 2,700 mg; and complete elimination of *Candida* in two weeks in all of those taking 3,600 mg.[15]

Dr. Susser agrees with the use of caprylic acid, but cautions that it is far from a panacea. "It's most useful when you combine it with a good diet, allergy care, the right nutrients, *acidophilus*, and other treatments," he says.

As mentioned above, Dr. Braly also recommends goldenseal root extract, standardized to 5% or more of its active ingredient, hydrastine, at a dose of 250 milligrams twice daily. In a recent study, goldenseal seemed to work better in killing off *Candida* than other common anti-*Candida* therapies, adds Dr. Braly. Other fatty acids derived from olives (oleic acid) and castor beans have also been found to be useful.

Garlic, a well-known folk remedy now formulated in odorless dry powder capsules, is a particularly effective antifungal agent. It has been shown to be effective against some antibiotic-resistant organisms. In cases of vaginal candidiasis, it can used as a suppository or douche. Pau d'arco bark has long been used to treat infections and intestinal complaints and is reportedly an analgesic, antiviral, diuretic, and fungicide. However, many products claiming to contain pau d'arco have only trace amounts or use a part of the tree other than the bark.[16]

Dr. Braly's first line of attack on candidiasis is caprylic acid, a fatty acid found in coconut oil and shown to be an effective antifungal agent against *Candida* overgrowth.

Ayurvedic Medicine

Ayurvedic (SEE QUICK DEFINITION) medicine considers candidiasis to be a condition caused by *ama*, the improper digestion of foods, according to Virender Sodhi, M.D. (Ayurveda), N.D., of Bellevue, Washington. As do other alternative medicine physicians, Dr. Sodhi attributes this digestive malfunction, and thus candidiasis, to the widespread use of antibiotics, birth control pills, and hormones,

When purchasing pau d'arco, be sure that the product contains lapachol, an organic compound found in high concentrations in pau d'arco and known for its antibiotic action.

environmental stress, and society's addiction to sugar in the diet. "Ayurvedic medicine believes that these stresses on the system cause carbohydrates to be digested improperly," he says. "Furthermore, the immune system in the gut becomes worn down."

Dr. Sodhi's candidiasis protocol involves strengthening the immune system and improving digestion through stimulation of the secretory IgA, the immunoglobulin (SEE QUICK DEFINITION) found in the mucoid lining of the intestines and lungs which may help prevent invasion of those surfaces by disease-producing bacteria and viruses.

To address the *Candida* overgrowth and thus bolster immunity, Dr. Sodhi uses grapefruit seed oil and tannic acid which act as antifungals and antibiotics, while *acidophilus* helps restore the balance of friendly bacteria in the intestines. Long pepper, ginger, cayenne, and the Ayurvedic herbs trikatu and neem taken a half-hour before meals increase immunoglobulin and digestive functions. He further recommends that his patients cleanse toxins from their systems using the pancha karma program, which involves herbs and dietary modification. With Dr. Sodhi's approach, candidiasis can usually be eliminated in four to six months.

Acupuncture

William M. Cargile, B.S., D.C., F.I.A.C.A., former chairman of research for the American Association of Oriental Medicine, has successfully reversed candidiasis with acupuncture, dietary recommendations, and herbs or other supplements as needed.

"Acupuncture treatment begins with the meridians [subtle energy channels] which influence genital function, spleen, and stomach," he explains. "These are yin [passive, receptive, cool] meridians and they correspond to areas of immune system enhancement. The goal is to normalize the metabolism of the cells in these areas." But Dr. Cargile adds that treatment is "a waste of time" if the patient does not also pay attention to nutrition, which he calls "a significant solution." (See the section on Diet above.) The following case makes this point clear.

Elena, 41, was suffering from severe candidiasis when she consulted Dr. Cargile. A single mother of three children, she had chronic low-grade sore throats and was taking five antibiotic prescriptions. "This had been going on for at least three years," Dr. Cargile says. "She was constantly bloated, had colonic distension, and had such bad oral thrush it looked like she had cotton in her throat. She had clearly destroyed the balance of her intestinal flora."

Dr. Cargile gave her a gargle solution of tea tree oil (an essential oil used in aromatherapy for numerous topical applications) which reduced the *Candida* pathogens in her mouth and throat. He recommended anti-*Candida* dietary changes and a douche with liquid *acidophilus*. Acupuncture treatments addressed meridians that passed through the larynx and throat. "After three treatments over a period of three weeks, she was 90% better," he states. "She had no oral *Candida* and was well on the road to recovery."

Enzyme Therapy

Lita Lee, Ph.D., an enzyme therapist based in Lowell, Oregon, uses plant enzyme supplements to treat yeast overgrowth. Many of her candidiasis patients come to her after unsuccessfully trying Nystatin, probiotics, homeopathics, fatty acid supplementation, and various herbs. "Certain cellulose enzymes will digest the common kinds of yeast, whereas other yeasts sometimes yield to amylase enzymes," reports Dr. Lee.

"I use a potent probiotic that contains *L. acidophilus*, *L. bifidus*, and certain cellulose enzymes, which digests yeast and reestablishes 'friendly' bowel bacteria." Dr. Lee relies upon another formula (containing protease, calcium, and magnesium) to cleanse the blood of toxic debris. This program is the most effective and fastest treatment for candidiasis Dr. Lee has discovered. "It also works well in combination with homeopathic and herbal remedies. I don't hesitate to add them to the enzyme protocol when needed," she states.

Treating Parasitic Infections

Although antibiotics and other drugs are often used to treat parasitic infections, this approach can pose a threat to overall health by upsetting the immune system, according to Dr. Leo Galland. Those who are already immunosuppressed or chronically ill should be especially careful. Dr. Chaitow agrees and advises pursuing a comprehensive supplement approach rather than medication.

"In many cases, antiparasitic prescriptive drugs have not proved to be lastingly effective," he points out. "They may diminish symptoms for one or two months, but the symptoms later return with full force." Parasites can be fought with high-dosage probiotic substances such as *Lactobacillus acidophilus*,

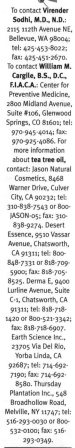

To contact **Virender Sodhi, M.D., N.D.**: 2115 112th Avenue NE, Bellevue, WA 98004; tel: 425-453-8022; fax: 425-451-2670. To contact **William M. Cargile, B.S., D.C., F.I.A.C.A.**: Center for Preventive Medicine, 2800 Midland Avenue, Suite #106, Glenwood Springs, CO 81601; tel: 970-945-4014; fax: 970-925-4086. For more information about **tea tree oil**, contact: Jason Natural Cosmetics, 8468 Warner Drive, Culver City, CA 90232; tel: 310-838-7543 or 800-JASON-05; fax: 310-838-9274. Desert Essence, 9510 Vassar Avenue, Chatsworth, CA 91311; tel: 800-848-7331 or 818-709-5900; fax: 818-705-8525. Derma E, 9400 Lurline Avenue, Suite C-1, Chatsworth, CA 91311; tel: 818-718-1420 or 800-521-3342; fax: 818-718-6907. Earth Science Inc., 23705 Via Del Rio, Yorba Linda, CA 92687; tel: 714-692-7190; fax: 714-692-8580. Thursday Plantation Inc., 548 Broadhollow Road, Melville, NY 11747; tel: 516-293-0030 or 800-532-0100; fax: 516-293-0349.

For more on **tea tree oil**, see "Tea Tree Oil—First Aid Kit in a Bottle," *Digest* #22, pp. 72-75.

How to Avoid Parasites

There are several precautions which will help you avoid parasites:

FOOD
- Do not eat raw beef—it can be loaded with tapeworms and other parasites.
- Do not eat raw fish or sushi—you are likely to get worms if you do.
- Wash your hands after handling raw meat or fish (including shrimp)—do not put your hands near your mouth without washing them first.
- Use a separate cutting board for meat and vegetables—spores from meat can seep into the board and contaminate vegetables or anything else you put on the board.
- Wash utensils thoroughly after cutting meat.
- Wash vegetables and fruit thoroughly—particularly salad items—as they often harbor parasites. Wash in one teaspoon Clorox per one gallon of water. Soak for 15-20 minutes. Then soak in fresh water for 20 minutes before refrigerating. Or, substitute a few drops of grapefruit seed extract.
- Do not drink from streams and rivers.

PETS
- Do not sleep near your pets—they harbor many worms and other parasites.
- De-worm your pets regularly and keep their sleeping areas clean.
- Do not let pets lick your face.
- Do not let pets eat off your dishes.

GENERAL
- Always wash your hands after using the toilet.
- Wash your hands after working in the garden—the soil can be contaminated with spores and parasites.

WHEN TRAVELING
- Do not drink the tap water.
- Start taking Chinese herbs or other preventive medications two weeks before traveling, and continue them while you travel.

CAUTION

"Antibiotics and other drugs are often used to treat parasitic infections, but this approach can pose a threat to one's overall health by upsetting the immune system. Those who are already immunosuppressed or chronically ill should be especially careful," says Leo Galland, M.D.

Bifidobacterium bifidum, and *Lactobacillus bulgaricus*. Treatment may last from eight to 12 weeks. Dr. Chaitow reports an 80% success rate in cases of seriously ill people afflicted with parasites and yeast overgrowth using this method.

Diet and Nutrition

If an intestinal parasitic infection is suspected, it is advisable to eliminate all uncooked foods from your diet and cook all meats until well done; soak both organic and inorganic vegetables in salted water (one tablespoon per five cups) for a minimum of 30 minutes before cooking. It is also suggested that you avoid coffee, all sugars including fruits and honey, and all milk and dairy products, with the possible exception of raw goat's milk. Raw goat's milk contains secretory IgA and IgG (immunoglobulins) which, as mentioned previously, help protect the intestinal lining from infectious agents. According to Steven Bailey, N.D., of Portland, Oregon, IgA and IgG have been found to be helpful in the treatment of parasites.

As with candidiasis, an intestinal parasitic infection may be only one element in the larger issue of suppressed immune function. A nutritional supplement program can address the restoration of both normal bowel and immune function. Nutritional supplements should include vitamin B12, vitamin A, calcium, magnesium, and the probiotics *Lactobacillus acidophilus*, *Bifidobacteria*, and *Lactobacillus bulgaricus*. Dr. Chaitow recommends beginning any antiparasitic protocol with high dosage probiotics to help rebuild intestinal flora ravaged by the parasitic infestation, as well as by other opportunistic infections, such as candidiasis. Probiotics are also imperative for fighting off any further infestation.

Herbal Medicine

The following herbal remedies have been reported to be safe and effective for the treatment of parasitic infections. Any of these remedies can also be used as a preventive measure against parasitic infection when water or food conditions are questionable. According to Dr. Galland, it is advisable to continue any treatment regimen until at least two parasitological tests, performed one month apart on "purged stool" specimens, are negative.

Citrus seed extract—Citrus seed extract is highly active against viruses, protozoa, bacteria, and yeast, and has long been used in the treatment of parasitic infections. It is not absorbed into the tissue, is nontoxic and generally hypoallergenic, and can be administered for up to several months, a length of time which may be required to eliminate *Giardia* and the candidiasis that often accompanies it.

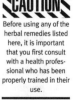

Before using any of the herbal remedies listed here, it is important that you first consult with a health professional who has been properly trained in their use.

Artemisia annua—This is an herbal remedy of Chinese origin. Its antiprotozoal activity is especially effective against *Giardia*, but some caution is advisable. It can initially cause a worsening of symptoms, allergic reactions, and some intestinal irritation. *Artemisia annua* is often prescribed by Dr. Galland, along with citrus seed extract. It may be used with additional herbs known for their antiparasitic activity and can also be used in conjunction with conventional drug therapy.

For more on **herbs**, see Chapter 12: Correcting Chronic Fatigue With Herbs, pp. 318-338.

Important Reminders During Any Parasite Treatment

Whatever treatment you employ to rid your body of parasites, the following recommendations can help ensure that the program is a success:

- If you have children and/or pets, they must be treated at the same time as the adults in the household to prevent reinfection.

- Drink more pure water (not from the tap) than usual to help the body flush out the dead parasites from your system; at least 64 ounces of water per day for a 150-pound adult.

- Sanitize your environment. When you have almost finished treatment, wash all pajamas, bed clothes, and sheets before using them again.

- Eat anti-parasitic foods. According to Ann Louise Gittleman, a nutrition educator in Bozeman, Montana, these include pineapple and papaya, either as fresh juice or in supplement form, in combination with pepsin and hydrochloric acid. Avoid all meats and dairy products for at least one week. You can also use pomegranate juice (four 8-ounce glasses daily), papaya seeds, finely-ground pumpkin seeds ($\frac{1}{4}$ to $\frac{1}{2}$ cup daily), and two cloves of raw garlic daily. Do not drink the pomegranate juice for more than four to five days.

- Modify your diet. For people with heavy parasitic infection, nutritionist Gittleman recommends a diet comprised of 25% fat, 25% protein, and 50% complex carbohydrates. You also need a regular intake of unprocessed flaxseed, safflower, sesame, or canola oils (two tablespoons daily), and higher than RDA amounts of vitamin A. Flaxseed oil is preferable because it has much higher levels of alpha linolenic acid (an omega-3 essential fatty acid commonly deficient in many people) than the other oils.

- Recolonize your intestines. You need to reintroduce beneficial, friendly bacteria (probiotics) into your intestinal system once you have flushed out the parasites, Gittleman advises. The bacterial strains most helpful here are *Lactobacillus plantarum, salvarius, acidophilus, bulgaris,* and *bifidus,* and *Streptococus faeceum,* which are available as nutritional supplements. *L. plantarum* is the most effective of these in combating parasite problems.

Artemisia absinthium—This is one of the oldest European medicinal plants. Known as "wormwood," it was highly prized by Hippocrates and used to expel worms (an application similar to that of *Artemisia annua* in the Chinese herbal tradition). *Artemisia absinthium* taken alone can be toxic, however, and therefore should be used in combination with other herbs to nullify its toxicity.

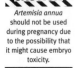

Artemisia annua should not be used during pregnancy due to the possibility that it might cause embryo toxicity.

Traditional Chinese Medicine

In traditional Chinese medicine (TCM—SEE QUICK DEFINITION), Chinese herbs are the primary treatment for parasites and the type used depends on the location of the parasites in the body, according to Dr. Maoshing Ni.

For intestinal parasites, the kind most often involved in chronic fatigue syndrome, purgative herbs are usually used. Pumpkin and quisqualis seeds are two common remedies. The pumpkin seeds are eaten raw, while the quisqualis seeds are usually roasted. Both are taken every morning on an empty stomach, approximately 10-12 seeds of either, for about two weeks. "Quisqualis and pumpkin seeds are mild and safe enough for adults and children to take daily as a preventative measure as well," says Dr. Ni.

Meliae seeds are much stronger than either pumpkin or quisqualis seeds, so they should only be taken in more severe cases. The meliae seeds paralyze the parasites for approximately eight hours, allowing the body to eliminate them through the bowels. Betel nut is another typical treatment for intestinal parasites. The nut is chewed raw like chewing tobacco.

"It can give a certain sense of euphoria, too, because it is slightly toxic," says Dr. Ni. "This is negligible, but some people might get diarrhea." Depending on the type of parasite, they may be able to get through the intestinal walls and into the bloodstream. "In situations like this you have to use some very strong antibiotic-like herbs," says Dr. Ni, "such as goldenseal and coptidis which are antiparasitic as well."

While eliminating the parasites with herbs, Dr. Ni also strengthens the immune system in order to get at the underlying cause of the parasitic infestation. Dr. Ni reports that nutrition and herbs such as ginseng, ligustri berries, and schisandra berries can accomplish this. He has good success with his three-month treatment program, which addresses both parasitic infection and immune suppression.

Dr. Ni recalls treating a woman previously diagnosed with chronic fatigue syndrome, candidiasis, yeast problems, and severe stomach difficulties. "We did a stool test and found that she also had parasites. This woman was extremely underweight. When she came to see me, she weighed 86 pounds—she was five feet, four inches tall. It took about three months for us to work on nourishing her body.

"Besides using herbs to kill off the parasites, I also used them to boost her immune system, and to deal with the yeast problem and her digestive weakness. In fact, this is the

QUICK DEFINITION

Traditional Chinese medicine (TCM) originated in China over 5,000 years ago and is a comprehensive system of medical practice that heals the body according to the principles of nature and balance. A Chinese medicine physician considers the flow of vital energy (*qi*) in a patient through close examination of the patient's pulses, tongue, body odor, voice tone and strength, and general demeanor, among other elements. Underlying imbalances and disharmony in the body are described in terminology analogous to the natural world (heat, cold, dryness, or dampness). The concept of balance, or the interrelationship of organs, is central to TCM. In TCM, imbalances are corrected through the use of acupuncture, moxibustion, herbal medicine, dietary therapy, massage, and therapeutic exercise.

To contact **Maoshing Ni, D.O.M., Ph.D., L.Ac.:** 1131 Wilshire Boulevard, Suite #300, Santa Monica, CA 90401; tel: 310-917-2200; fax: 310-917-2267

reason she got the parasites in the first place. After the three-month treatment, her stool tests were normal and remained that way. All her symptoms disappeared and her weight went back up to 108 pounds."

CAUTION

Although the Ayurvedic remedies mentioned here are safe and easy to self-administer, Dr. Sodhi recommends consultation with a doctor or qualified practitioner before beginning any treatment protocol in order to determine which of the various options will be best suited to one's individual needs and circumstances.

Ayurvedic Medicine

Ayurvedic medicine has many natural remedies which address specific parasitic infections, according to Virender Sodhi, M.D. The most effective herbs for *Giardia*, amoebas, *Cryptosporidium*, and other protozoal intestinal parasites are bilva, neem, and berberine, which can be taken in combination, he reports. He also recommends bitter melon, as well as such nutritional support as psyllium husk, turmeric, and *acidophilus* for the enhancement of the intestinal microflora. It may take several months to eliminate intestinal parasites.

"CFS can start with ordinary viral infections, such as those that cause respiratory infections like the common cold and flus," explains Murray R. Susser, M.D. "There are 2,300 viruses which can cause a cold or flu and if one of those hits you and your body isn't able to get rid of it, then you have a chronic infection. In CFS, we often get hidden viral, parasite, and yeast infections which are results of a weakened immune system."

Restoring Immune Vitality

ALONG WITH CLEARING all the opportunistic infections present in chronic fatigue syndrome, it is essential to rebuild the beleaguered immune system. Having been in an overactive and dysfunctional state for a prolonged period, often years, the immune system is in need of intensive support to return it to an optimal level of functioning and enable it to ward off current and future infection. Immunomodulation, using substances which target and adjust specific weaknesses in the immune system, and traditional Chinese medicine, a body of medical knowledge that includes acupuncture and Chinese herbal remedies, are two particularly effective alternative medicine methods for rebuilding immune strength.

Later in this chapter, you will learn about immunomodulators and other immune-building substances, as well as specific steps you can take to detoxify your body. First, let's look at how one alternative medicine physician rebuilds the immune system by focusing on detoxification of all the body's systems and by addressing both the physical and emotional aspects of the disease. A case of immune breakdown clearly illustrates the interrelationship of toxins and immunity.

For more information about **immune-building nutritional supplements and herbal medicine**, see Chapter 8: Replenishing Enzyme Deficiencies, pp. 212-231; Chapter 10: Ending Nutritional Deficiencies with Supplements, pp. 260-291. For more on the **immune system**, see Chapter 2: Testing, pp. 34-73.

Reversing Chronic Illness with Immune Support

Often the best medicine results after the healer is healed, an event fairly common among practitioners of alternative medicine. This was the case for

The Major Players in Your Immune System

Immune System: The immune system guards the body against foreign, disease-producing substances. Its "workers" are various white blood cells including 1 trillion lymphocytes and 100 million trillion antibodies produced and secreted by the lymphocytes. Lymphocytes are found in high numbers in the lymph nodes, bone marrow, spleen, and thymus gland.

Antibodies: An antibody is a protein molecule containing about 20,000 atoms, made from amino acids by B lymphocyte cells in the lymph tissue and set in motion by the immune system against a specific antigen (foreign and potentially dangerous protein). An antibody is also referred to as an immunoglobulin and may be found in the blood, lymph, colostrum, saliva, and the gastrointestinal and urinary tracts, usually within three days after the first encounter with an antigen. The antibody binds tightly with the antigen as a preliminary for removing it from the system or destroying it.

Lymph Nodes: Lymph nodes are clusters of immune tissue that work as filters or "inspection stations" for detecting foreign and potentially harmful substances in the lymph fluid. Acting like spongy filter bags, lymph nodes are part of the lymphatic system, which is the body's master drain. Cells inside the nodes examine the lymph fluid, as collected from body tissues, for foreign matter. While the body has many dozens of lymph nodes, they are, as noted previously, mostly clustered in the neck, armpits, chest, groin, and abdomen.

Lymph fluid flows in the lymphatic vessels throughout the body, helping to maintain the fluid level of cells and carrying various substances from the tissues to the blood. The human body has one to two quarts of lymph fluid, accounting for 1.5% to 3% of body weight.

Thymus and Spleen: The thymus, located behind the breastbone, secretes thymosin, a hormone that strengthens immune response. It also instructs certain lymphocytes to specialize their function. The spleen is like a large lymph node except that it filters blood rather than lymph fluid.

Lymphocyte: A lymphocyte is a form of white blood cell, representing 25% to 40% of the total count, whose numbers increase during infection. Lymphocytes, produced in the bone marrow and found in lymph nodes, come in two forms: T cells, which are matured in the thymus gland and have many functions in the body's immune response; and B cells, which produce antibodies to neutralize an antigen.

Immunoglobulin: Each lymphocyte produces a specific antibody or immunoglobulin. There are five main types of immunoglobulins, grouped according to their concentration in the blood: IgG, IgA, IgM, IgD, and IgE.

B cells: B cells mature in the bone marrow and produce antibodies to neutralize foreign cells (this is known as humoral immunity). B cells account for 10% to 15% of all lymphocytes.

T Cells: T cells specialize their immune function to become helper (CD4), suppressor (CD8), or natural killer (CD56) cells. Helper cells facilitate the production of antibodies by the B cells. Suppressor cells suppress B-cell activity.

Helper T cells: Also known as T4 or CD4 cells, helper T cells secrete immune proteins (particularly the interleukins and interferon) to stimulate B cells and macrophages, and activate Killer T cells; they account for 60% to 75% of T cells.

continued on next page

Natural Killer Cells: Natural killer (NK) cells are a type of nonspecific, free-ranging immune cell produced in the bone marrow and matured in the thymus gland. NK cells can recognize and quickly destroy virus and cancer cells on first contact. "Armed" with an estimated 100 different biochemical poisons for killing foreign proteins, they can kill target cells without having encountered them previously. As with antibodies, their role is surveillance, to rid the body of aberrant or foreign cells before they can grow and produce cancer. Decreased numbers of NK cells have been linked to the development and progression of cancer, as well as chronic and acute viral infections and other deficiencies of the immune system.

Macrophages: Macrophages are a form of white blood cell (originally produced in the bone marrow and called monocytes) that can literally swallow germs and foreign proteins, then release an enzyme that chemically damages, kills, or neutralizes whatever is ingested. The name means "big" *(macro)* "swallower" or "eater" *(phage)*. Macrophages are the vacuum cleaners and filter feeders of the immune system, ingesting everything that is not normal, healthy tissue, even old body cells or cancer cells.

Neutrophil: A neutrophil is a mature white blood cell formed in the bone marrow and released into the blood where it represents 54% to 65% of the total number of leuokocytes. Leukocytes are white blood cells divided into six types (neutrophils, basophils, eosinophils, monocytes, B lymphocytes, T lymphocytes) and two groups, according to the shape of the nucleus and the presence or absence of granules within the cells; one group includes primarily neutrophils, the other includes lymphocytes. The principal activity of the neutrophil is to ingest foreign particles, especially virulent bacteria and fungi.

Interferon: Interferon, familiar to many as a cancer treatment, is a natural protein produced by cells in response to a virus or other foreign substance. Vitamin C and certain herbs can also stimulate its production.

Interleukin: Interleukin is a class of proteins with various immune functions including T-cell activation.

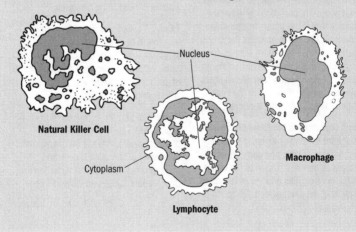

Natural Killer Cell

Nucleus

Cytoplasm

Lymphocyte

Macrophage

Constantine A. Kotsanis, M.D., medical director of MindBody Health Center International in Grapevine, Texas.

Dr. Kotsanis is a board certified specialist in nutrition, allergies, and ear, nose, and throat problems, but 12 years ago everything he knew about medicine from his conventional training failed to help him when he became unaccountably ill. Dr. Kotsanis, 38 years old at the time, was losing weight, unable to retain food in his stomach, and had diarrhea after each meal. He had consulted numerous physicians, but came back from these visits empty-handed. One physician insulted him by suggesting it was all in his head.

Dr. Kotsanis was dismayed at his declining health, his persistent allergies, and his inability to get better, even while using the best of what he knew from conventional allergy treatment. Things dragged on like this for two years, until he finally turned to his family for help. "I come from a family of health care practitioners from Greece," says Dr. Kotsanis, who attended medical school at the University of Athens. "While most of my relatives did conventional Western medicine and a few of my uncles were surgeons, some were herbalists who treated patients with plants, vitamins, and natural remedies." Dr. Kotsanis decided to seek healing from the knowledge held in that side of his family.

After considerable reading in the field of alternative medicine, Dr. Kotsanis went to Tijuana, Mexico, to seek treatment with Wolfram M. Kühnau, M.D., a German emigré and specialist in live cell therapy (SEE QUICK DEFINITION). As a child, Dr. Kotsanis had been exposed to a dangerously high level of the pesticide DDT; as an adult, his pancreas failed to produce enough digestive enzymes. The live cell injections stimulated his sluggish organs (pancreas, liver, and stomach).

After two days on live cell therapy injections, Dr. Kotsanis experienced a turnaround in his condition. His immune system was stimulated and his allergic symptoms were rapidly receding. Soon, "like magic," his symptoms were gone. Dr. Kotsanis left the Mexican clinic with a prescription for digestive enzymes and "friendly" bacteria (SEE QUICK

Cell therapy, as a means of promoting physical regeneration through injecting healthy cells into the body, was developed in the 1930s by the Swiss physician Paul Niehans, M.D. Since Dr. Niehans' work, cell therapy has come to mean the injection of cellular material from endocrine glands, organs, fetuses, or embryos of various animals (and sometimes humans) to stimulate healing and to treat numerous degenerative diseases, including cancer, arthritis, atherosclerosis, chronic fatigue, eczema, mental retardation, and others. More recently, shark embryo cells have been used as the source of live cells, collected before they have differentiated into specific immune- or organ-building cells.

Friendly bacteria, or probiotics, refer to beneficial microbes inhabiting the human gastrointestinal tract where they are essential for proper nutrient assimilation. The human body contains an estimated several trillion beneficial bacteria comprising over 400 species, all necessary for health. Among the more well known of these are *Lactobacillus acidophilus* and *Bifidobacterium bifidum*. Overly acidic bodily conditions, chronic constipation or diarrhea, dietary imbalances, consumption of highly processed foods, and the excessive use of antibiotics and hormonal drugs can interfere with probiotic function and even reduce the numbers of microbes, setting up conditions for illness.

"I realized that while conventional medicine may be good for acute problems, such as life threatening infections and trauma, as well as chronic irreversible problems requiring surgery, when it comes to chronic diseases, many conventional doctors have no idea what they are treating,"says Dr. Kotsanis.

DEFINITION), such as *L. acidophilus* and *L. bifidus*, to reconstitute the intestinal microflora which would facilitate better nutrient absorption.

"This experience changed my life and I started looking for more information," says Dr. Kotsanis. "I realized that while conventional medicine may be good for acute problems, such as life threatening infections and trauma, as well as chronic irreversible problems requiring surgery, when it comes to chronic diseases, many conventional doctors have no idea what they are treating. That is why we have an obligation to look on both sides of the fence. I don't think anyone has cornered the market in medicine. All disciplines have good things to offer. The knowledgeable physician will choose the appropriate treatment that fits the person and the disease."

Dr. Kotsanis calls this multimodal approach integrative medicine and it's the order of the day at his MindBody Health Center International, with its ten practitioners and six support staff who, together, treat about 2,500 patients each year. There is an optometrist, a clinical audiologist, an Ayurvedic counselor, and three psychotherapists and counselors. This unusual composition of medical staff reflects Dr. Kotsanis' ongoing pursuit of the best in integrative medicine.

Dr. Kotsanis adds expertise in allergy treatment, immunology, environmental medicine, orthomolecular medicine, acupuncture, homeopathy, neural kinesiology, neural therapy, and surgery. Other specialists, including osteopaths and chiropractors, consult at the Center on a rotating weekly basis, meeting with patients as needed, and imparting an "extended faculty" quality to the medical care the Center offers.

"As a rule, integrative medicine techniques tend to be more natural, with one of the fundamental principles being that treatments should actually augment the body's own abilities to heal itself," Dr. Kotsanis explains. "We have adopted the philosophy that supporting the body's own healing faculties is a wiser course for the best long-term results. This type of medicine is also called functional, because it addresses the body's natural functioning processes rather than addressing only the symptoms."

In Dr. Kotsanis' view, the approach benefits the patients by giving them far more choices in health care than that of conventional formats. "Sometimes you choose surgery, but sometimes you choose acupuncture," he observes. "You do whatever you need to do to alleviate the symptoms and improve the quality of life for that patient." Dr. Kotsanis' personal road to integrative medicine, including his firsthand experience with the miseries of chronic illness, has equipped him with both the compassion and medical insight to help many patients with long-term, seemingly immedicable conditions. The following case from his patient files makes this clear.

Success Story:
Reversing Immune System Breakdown

Millicent, 33, poses an all too common case of a person with entrenched, debilitating symptoms who consulted many doctors and ended up trusting none—that is, until she met Dr. Kotsanis. Millicent had a long history of chronic conditions, including fatigue, sinusitis, multiple infections, bronchitis, and pain, none of which were improved by repeated rounds of antibiotics or any other drugs or therapies offered.

At one point in her two years of "bouncing around" among physicians, Millicent went to a clinic specializing in environmental medicine. They tested her for allergies to multiple substances and determined that she was reactive to certain chemicals. Millicent received allergy desensitization injections, nutritional supplements, saunas, and dietary advice, but rather than experiencing improvement, her condition continued to deteriorate.

"We have adopted the philosophy that supporting the body's own healing faculties is a wiser course for the best long-term results," Dr. Kotsanis explains.

When Millicent first consulted Dr. Kotsanis, she was debilitated to the point that she could no longer maintain her former high-stress, demanding job. She couldn't sleep at night, but often fell asleep during the daylight hours. She was highly frustrated and a bit despondent about the seeming intractability of her condition, says Dr. Kotsanis.

"The core of her problem was a breakdown of her immune system," he says. "It had become hyperactive trying to deal with the multiple infections and allergies; then the antibiotics injured her digestive system and this contributed to her fatigue." A newlywed, Millicent

Electrodermal screening
is a form of computerized
information gathering,
based on physics, not
chemistry. A blunt, noninvasive electric probe is
placed at specific points
on the patient's hands,
face, or feet, corresponding to acupuncture points
at the beginning or end of
energy meridians. Minute
electrical discharges from
these points serve as
information signals about
the condition of the
body's organs and sys-
tems, useful for the
physician in evaluation
and developing a treat-
ment plan.

DMPS (2,3-dimercapto-
propane-1-sulfonate) is
the chelating (binding-
up) agent of choice for
the removal of elemental
mercury from the human
body. It can be given orally, intravenously, or intramuscularly and is useful
for people who have
been exposed to mercury
amalgam through their
dental fillings or for those
who show evidence or
suspicion of heavy metal
toxicity from other
sources.

Chelation therapy refers
to a method of binding
up ("chelating") toxins
(e.g. heavy metals) and
metabolic wastes and
removing them from the
body while at the same
time increasing blood
flow and removing arteri-
al plaque. One type of
chelation therapy
involves the chelating
agent disodium EDTA
given as an intravenous
infusion over a 3-¹/₂ hour
period. Usually 20 to 30
treatments are adminis-
tered at the rate of one to
three sessions per week.
Chelation therapy is
especially beneficial for
all forms of athero-
sclerotic cardiovascular
disease, including angina
pectoris and coronary
artery disease.

had lost all interest in sexuality as a consequence of her illness, and her marriage was at risk. "She was in a state of hopelessness—a young woman with no hope, no desire to do anything."

Initially, Millicent "tested" Dr. Kotsanis by agreeing to some acupuncture treatment. Millicent soon moved away, however, and did not return to the area for a year. Feeling only marginally better than when she left, Millicent again consulted Dr. Kotsanis.

Calling on the services of a consulting acupuncturist, Dr. Kotsanis had Millicent tested for heavy metal toxici-ty; he was concerned about the potential mercury leakage from her eight amalgam dental fillings. The acupunctur-ist, using electrodermal screening (SEE QUICK DEFINI-TION), determined that Millicent did have significant tox-icity in her body owing to mercury leakage. An analysis of Millicent's urine confirmed the mercury diagnosis.

Over the next six months, Millicent had her mercury fillings carefully removed. To assure the elimination of mercury residues from her body once the fillings were out, Millicent had infusions of a special nontoxic chemi-cal called DMPS (SEE QUICK DEFINITION) to chelate (SEE QUICK DEFINITION), or bind up, the heavy metal and pre-pare it for excretion from the body. After six DMPS infu-sions over a space of three months, Dr. Kotsanis assessed that the mercury had been removed from her body. Prior to the DMPS infusions, Millicent had worn a surgical mask all the time to filter out allergens and toxic materi-als from the air she breathed. She no longer required this mask once the mercury toxicity was eliminated, Dr. Kotsanis notes.

Concurrent with administering the DMPS, Dr. Kotsanis made nutritional and dietary recommendations for Millicent. These included flaxseed oil (two table-spoons daily); extra virgin olive oil (for cooking and in salads) to help the liver; raw flaxseeds (two teaspoons daily); organic foods; lean meats, such as organically raised chicken, venison, or lamb; and unusual grains such as quinoa, amaranth, and teff.

The more common grains, such as wheat and corn, as well as soybeans, have been far too genetically manipu-lated and, in Dr. Kotsanis' view, are best avoided by the chronically ill. Millicent was also instructed to avoid dairy products, red meats (for antibiotic and hormonal residues), and fish (for potential mercury contamination). Organic brown rice and oats were acceptable; the consumption of ¾ to one gallon of pure water every day was advised to help her system flush out toxins.

As a further aid in detoxifying, Dr. Kotsanis prescribed three products from Metagenics, taken in sequence: UltraClear-Plus®, UltraClear®, and Ultra-Clear Sustain®. These were taken in powder form, at the rate of two scoops daily, mixed with juice or water. To complement this daily regimen, Millicent took Metagenics' multivitamin (without iron) in a dosage of one tablet, two times daily. "Nutritional problems account for perhaps 50% of the problem in patients with chronic disease," says Dr. Kotsanis.

But Millicent still had discomfort and fatigue, and was subject to bouts of crying and serious depression. "Millicent was steadily getting better, but still dragging herself around. She was going through a lot of emotional distress," says Dr. Kotsanis. "I decided she should do some emotional detoxification because everyone who has a chronic disease needs this."

Emotional Detoxification—To Dr. Kotsanis, it is not only important to detoxify the internal organs, such as the liver, pancreas, and intestines, of toxic materials, but also to purge the often repressed emotions of pain, grief, and unresolved trauma, in order to achieve a lasting cure.

Dr. Kotsanis worked with psychologist Stephen Vasquez, Ph.D., of Bedford, Texas, who employs a combination of skillful psychological questioning and a form of strobic light therapy to elicit buried emotions. Up to 12 different colored lights are emitted from a device and, after being registered by the eyes, can provoke emotional reactions from a patient. As the lights provoke emotional memories, the patient regressing slowly backwards in time, the psychologist asks them questions about their condition.

QUICK DEFINITION

UltraClear® and **UltraClear Plus®** are metabolic liver detoxification programs in powder form for food-based clearing, made primarily from high protein white rice and safflower oil. **UltraClear Sustain®** provides nutritional support for patients with gastrointestinal dysbiosis and impaired mucosa.

To contact **Constantine A. Kotsanis, M.D.**: MindBody Health Center International, Baylor Medical Plaza, 1600 West College Street, Suite 260, Grapevine, TX 76051; tel: 817-481-3131; fax: 817-488-8903. To contact **Wolfram Kühnau, M.D.**, or to order his book, write: Pases Tijuana, #406, Desp. 104, Primer Piso, Edificio Allen Lloyd, Tijuana, B.C. Mexico, Codigo Postal 22320; tel: 52-66-835151; fax: 52-66-844238. For **UltraClear, UltraClear-Plus,** and **UltraClear Sustain**, contact: Metagenics West, Inc., 12445 East 39th Avenue, Suite 402, Denver, CO 80239; tel: 303-371-6848 or 800-321-6382; fax: 303-371-9303. For more information about **Adrenal Stress Index** saliva test, contact: Diagnos-Tech, Inc., 6620 South 192nd Place, J-104, Kent, WA 98032; tel: 800-878-3787 or 425-251-0596; fax: 206-251-0637. For **phosphatidylserine** (Phosserine), contact: Thorne Research, P.O. Box 3200, Sandpoint, ID 83864; tel: 208-263-1337 or 800-228-1966; fax: 208-265-2488. For more information about **gluten-free** and **casein-free products**, contact: Finegold Association, 127 East Main, Riverhead, NY 11901; tel: 800-321-3287 or 516-367-9340; fax: 516-369-2988.

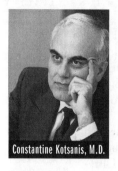

Constantine Kotsanis, M.D.

To Dr. Kotsanis, it is not only important to detoxify the internal organs, such as the liver, pancreas, and intestines, of toxic materials, but also to purge the often repressed emotions of pain, grief, and unresolved trauma, in order to achieve a lasting cure.

For more information about the **Adrenal Stress Index**, see Chapter 2: Testing, p. 63. For more about **hypothyroidism**, see Chapter 6: Reversing Hidden Thyroid Problems, pp. 164-189. For more on **psychological factors underlying CFS**, see Chapter 11: Healing Psychological and Emotional Factors, pp. 292-317.

In Millicent's case, it was revealed that she came from a dysfunctional family, says Dr. Kotsanis. As a child, she was treated like a soldier by her father (a military man) and she felt abandoned by her mother who suffered from a terrible illness. Millicent said also that she had been sexually abused by relatives. As an adult, she married a man much like her authoritative father.

"These difficult emotional memories can contribute to an already debilitating condition and need to be acknowledged by the patient," says Dr. Kotsanis. "The light therapy approach allows your brain to regress to the point where the affliction formed," he adds. "Once you relive the original problem, you completely cleanse yourself of it." Typically, there are 15 color treatments, each lasting one hour, one daily for five days per week. "What psychotherapy takes three years to achieve, this approach can produce in three weeks," Dr. Kotsanis says. The light therapy moved Millicent a couple of steps closer to recovery, he adds.

After these steps—mercury amalgam removal, DMPS, dietary changes, nutritional supplements, detoxification, and light therapy—Millicent was about 60% improved. To complete the recovery, Dr. Kotsanis analyzed Millicent's hormone levels. Using a saliva test called Adrenal Stress Index (ASI), Dr. Kotsanis was able to examine the rhythm and secretory activity of Millicent's adrenal glands. He learned that Millicent's cortisol (SEE QUICK DEFINITION) levels (an adrenal gland secretion indicative of stress) were exceptionally high, which is often the case in CFS. This meant her adrenal glands were virtually exhausted; hence, her chronic fatigue. In addition, Dr. Kotsanis determined that Millicent's thyroid was mildly underactive, a condition called hypothyroidism characterized by many of Millicent's symptoms.

Instead of supplementing the adrenal glands or thyroid, Dr. Kotsanis prescribed a formula that would correct the balance of brain chemicals (neurotransmitters—SEE QUICK DEFINITION) that directly affect the adrenal glands. He had Millicent take a formula (three times daily) containing brain nutrients, such as phosphatidylserine and phosphatidylcholine (both derived from lecithin). Dr. Kotsanis says that had he attempted to correct the brain chemical axis controlling the adrenal glands before removing Millicent's mercury fillings and flushing out residual mercury with DMPS, the treatment would have failed. "The adrenal glands and most of the endocrine system would have been shut down by the mercury."

After ten days on this supplement, the brain chemicals in effect realigned themselves and "her whole life turned around—Millicent's energy level skyrocketed," says Dr. Kotsanis. "She was happy and began telling everyone how wonderful she felt." Millicent's self-esteem soared, her vitality returned to normal, and for the first time in many months, she was glad that she was alive again. Her sexual drive, absent for years, returned. Typically this is the last to return when you are chronically ill, according to Dr. Kotsanis. Millicent's husband was delighted. 'I have my wife back,' he told people. About one month later, Millicent became pregnant and felt herself to be "the happiest woman in town."

This case illustrates Dr. Kotsanis' principle of illness causation and health restoration. "Many factors in Millicent's life led to a gradual breakdown of her immune system. To reverse this, you must clean out the system starting with the basics: clean the colon, liver, and spleen; remove the heavy metals and toxins; resolve the emotional issues; and put the good nutrition back."

It is "extremely essential" to know how the body's detoxification system works. You also must understand that if the immune system is perpetually occupied with inflammation, allergies, and detoxification, it will not have the time or resources to do anything else, such as promote a lasting recovery, Dr. Kotsanis explains. "Everything we do here supports the immune system."

The patient is like a house with three stories, including body, mind, and spirit, says Dr. Kotsanis. "You must keep all three floors clean if you're going to call yourself a holistic physician." Dr. Kotsanis cautions that it's prudent to expect lasting recovery from a

QUICK DEFINITION

Cortisol is a hormone secreted by the adrenal glands which are located atop the kidneys. Cortisol secretion (as well as the adrenal gland's other hormones, DHEA, adrenaline, and aldosterone) occurs in daily cycles, peaking in the morning and having the lowest values at night. Cortisol promotes protein building, regulates insulin and glycogen synthesis, and helps produce prostaglandins. Under conditions of stress, high amounts of cortisol are released; chronic excess secretion is associated with obesity and suppressed thyroid function. Imbalances in cortisol secretion are linked with low energy, muscle dysfunction, impaired bone repair, thyroid dysfunction, immune system depression, sleep disorders, poor skin regeneration, and decreased growth hormone uptake.

A **neurotransmitter** is a brain chemical with the specific function of enabling communications to happen between brain cells. Chief among the 100 identified to date are acetylcholine, gamma-aminobutyric acid (GABA), serotonin, dopamine, and norepinephrine. Acetylcholine is required for short-term memory and all muscle contractions. GABA works to stop excess nerve signals and thus keeps brain firings from getting out of control; serotonin does the same and helps produce sleep, regulate pain, and influence mood, although too much serotonin can produce depression. Norepinephrine is an excitatory neurotransmitter.

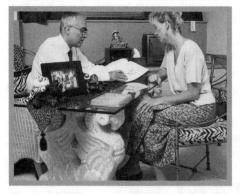

"Many factors in Millicent's life led to a gradual breakdown of her immune system," says Dr. Kotsanis. **"To reverse this, you must cleanse the colon, liver, spleen; remove the heavy metals and toxins; resolve the emotional issues; and put the good nutrition back."**

complex case of chronic fatigue to take at least 9-12 months.

"This case reflects what I call a comeback from Hell," Dr. Kotsanis comments. "Two years ago, Millicent was imprisoned in her own home by longstanding environmental toxins, and her family was on the verge of disintegrating. Remember, the average chronic fatigue patient trusts nobody, but they also tend to jump on the bandwagon anytime someone promises good results. This case taught me how frustrated a patient can be and how a physician must be patient and thorough in his approach."

In retrospect, reflects Dr. Kotsanis, this was one of his most gratifying cases. "After a long journey, Millicent came all the way back to be a vibrant, healthy, and happy person. This is my greatest reward as a physician." ∎

Building Up the Immune System

As Millicent's case illustrates, restoring a depleted immune system is one key to reversing a chronic illness. Dr. Kotsanis employed dietary recommendations, nutritional supplements, and a variety of detoxification methods to accomplish this. Among the array of other immune-building techniques, immunomodulators and traditional Chinese medicine are also highly successful.

An immunomodulator is a substance that can tune, adjust, regulate, or focus—modulate—the activities of the immune system to reverse illnesses. Homeopathic remedies, herbs, hormones, amino acids and other nutritional supplements, and specific dietary changes can all operate as immunomodulators. Here, **Jesse Stoff, M.D.**, describes the immunomodulators he uses to rebuild a depleted immune system:

Immunomodulators for Immune Health

Knowledge of how an individual's immune system is working can be used to precisely direct immune function and restore health. Running standard blood tests (such as the T- and B-cell and NK-cell function tests) to establish the state of the patient's biochemistry and immune function provides the needed information. My focus is on the structure and function of the immune system. It is essential to address both components because a person's immune system can be structurally intact yet not functioning well.

By analogy, this is like having an expensive, perfectly crafted Swiss clock that you forgot to wind; it could keep excellent time, but it isn't even functioning. The test results tell me specifically what areas are malfunctioning or weak and then I can apply the appropriate immunomodulators as treatment. During treatment, I regularly monitor immune status with blood tests so I can track the progress and make changes in treatment as needed.

One example of an immunomodulator is an oral form of transfer factor called NK Daily. Transfer factor is an immunological term indicating a way of passively transferring immunity from one organism to another, thereby stimulating the NK cells. This product uses purified colostrum (first mother's milk after birth) from cows. By stimulating the NK cells, NK Daily gently but thoroughly stimulates immune function.

Another immunomodulator I frequently use is NK Support, a natural immune-building compound which, among other things, contains arabino-galactan, or Larix. Larix is a powdered concentrate of complex carbohydrates derived from the Western larch tree (*Larix occidentalis*). It has been proven to stimulate the activity of NK cells and macrophages (immune cells that "eat" germs). I often prescribe Larix for people with chronic infections, such as chronic fatigue syndrome, pneumonia, or HIV, if their NK function is not at a desirable level of activity. Combining NK Support with vitamin C and iodine activates an immune enzyme needed to dissolve the cell membranes of foreign proteins (such as bacteria or cancer cells) already targeted by NK cells.

In other words, with this simple combination of substances, we can activate a fairly large component of the immune system. Specifically, I typically use ten drops of iodine, three times daily, for four to six weeks; the iodine is in the form of a super-saturated solution of potassium iodide known clinically as SSKI. For vitamin C, I prescribe 1,000 mg, three times daily; for NK Support, one tablespoon in water or juice, three times daily.

It's important to note that if the natural killer cells lack the biochemical support (from nutrients) they need to work appropriately, stimulating them will get you nowhere. You have to provide the key nutrients to stabilize the biochemistry, thereby freeing the immune system to function efficiently. For example, the amino acid (SEE QUICK DEFINITION) L-arginine is helpful to NK cell function; similarly, maintaining the correct ratio of L-arginine and lysine, another amino acid, is also critical. Among dietary sources, L-arginine is available in high amounts in peanuts, almonds, garbanzo beans, soy protein isolate, sunflower seeds, cashews, and other nuts. Lysine-rich foods include cottage cheese, chicken, tuna, turkey, yogurt, steak, and other meat and dairy products.

There are approaches for selectively stimulating B or T immune cells. For B cells, a formula called Immune Boosters is effective as it supports the nutrient needs of these cells throughout the 24-hour (circadian) cycle. A homeopathic remedy called *Stibium* can aid the T cells and help reorganize the troubled, chaotic immune system.

The adrenal hormone precursor DHEA (SEE QUICK DEFINITION) is also effective in activating T4 cells. The DHEA I prescribe is in a long-acting base form, 100 mg daily. The advantage of using a long-acting, slow-releasing form is that otherwise you risk getting a spike of DHEA into the blood, a sudden hormone increase that could depress the brain's pituitary gland. The amino acid L-gluta-

EDITOR'S NOTE

Jesse Stoff, M.D., is medical director of Solstice Clinical Associates. From 1985-1991, Dr. Stoff was editor of the *Journal of Anthroposophic Medicine* and from 1986-1991, he was vice president of the Physicians' Association for Anthroposophic Medicine. Dr. Stoff is coauthor of the best-selling *Chronic Fatigue Syndrome: The Hidden Epidemic* (Harper Collins, 2nd Edition, 1992). To contact Dr. Stoff: Solstice Clinical Associates, Southwest Professional Plaza, 2122 North Craycroft Road, #112, Tuscon, AZ 85712; tel: 520-290-4516; fax: 520-290-6403.

mine (one teaspoonful in juice or water, three times daily) can help maintain white blood cell populations and certain T-cell production at desirable levels. This amino acid provides nitrogen needed for white blood cell function and the health of the small intestines, which is why L-glutamine is considered essential for intestinal health during times of stress and critical illness.

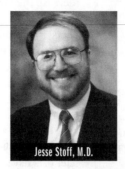

Jesse Stoff, M.D.

It's important to note that if the natural killer cells lack the bio-chemical support (from nutrients) they need to work appropriately, stimulating them will get you nowhere, says Dr. Stoff. You have to provide the key nutrients for the immune system to function efficiently.

Removing the toxic load from the liver is another way to assist the immune system. The liver is the body's main filter of toxins. When the amount of toxins circulating becomes too high and overwhelms the liver, the immune system must then deal with the toxins that ordinarily would have been eliminated from the body. I use an herbal extract called *Carduus marianus* (milk thistle) as an aid for liver detoxification. An individualized formula of Chinese herbs is also useful for liver cleansing.

To focus on the nutrient deficiency side of immune system dysfunction, I employ a daily intravenous nutritional product called Metbal®. Described as a cellular metabolic enhancer or "super vitamin," this natural product pumps nutrients into the cells in very high concentrations in a short time period.

Originally developed in the 1970s to increase the ability of cells to absorb critically needed nutrients, Metbal is made from four natural agents; ribose (150 mg), vitamins B3 (20 mg) and C (75 mg), and the amino acid alanine (15 mg). The product is infused intravenously for five to ten minutes. Metbal appears to trigger the immune system, correct DNA damage by supplying nutrients essential for repairs and rebuilding, and

For more information about *Stibium* and *Carduus marianus*, contact: Weleda Pharmacy, P.O. Box 49, Congers, NY 10920; tel: 800-289-1969 or 914-268-8572; fax: 800-280-4899 or 914-268-8574. For **Immune Boosters, NK Support**, and **NK Daily**, contact: Solstice Vitamin Company, 982 Stuyvesant Avenue, Union, NJ 07083; tel: 800-765-7842 or 908-810-0909; fax: 908-810-9207. For **L-glutamine** (Doctors Brand), contact: Genesist, 1321 South Grant Street, Longmont, CO 80501; tel: 303-651-2522; fax: 303-772-4566. For **Metbal® Vitamin Supplement**, contact: Southwest Nutraceuticals, 1955 West Grant, Suite 125U, Tuscon, AZ 85745; tel: 520-740-1993; fax: 520-624-4028. For **DHEA**, contact: Mountain View Pharmacy, 10565 North Tatum Boulevard, Paradise Valley, AZ; tel: 800-942-7065 or 602-948-7065; fax: 602-948-9489.

For information about **Dr. Stoff's approach to cancer,** see *An Alternative Medicine Definitive Guide to Cancer* (Future Medicine Publishing, 1997; ISBN 1-887299-01-7); to order, call 800-333-HEAL.

increase the ability of cells to assimilate nutrients. An alkaline diet also supports the assimilation of nutrients. A good alkaline diet would include a variety of fruits, vegetables, beans, and nuts; persimmons, seaweed, lentils, and pumpkin seeds are excellent alkaline foods. ■

Beta-1,3-Glucan—Ever since the 1940s, scientists have been honing their knowledge of the remarkable abilities of beta-1,3-glucan as an immunomodulator. It effectively stimulates and activates the immune system and works therapeutically in cases of infection, cancer, ulcers, radiation exposure, and trauma.

Beta-1,3-glucan, a simple sugar derived from the cell wall of a common yeast called *Saccharomyces cerevisiae* (baker's yeast), is now available in a supplement form as MacroForce™. MacroForce's beta-1,3-glucan is a purified isolate and does not contain any yeast proteins that would otherwise provoke allergic reactions in sensitive individuals, according to Leonid Ber, M.D., vice president of research and development for ImmuDyne, Inc., in Houston, Texas, the makers of Macroforce.

The research supporting the claims for beta-1,3-glucan as an immune system activator has been building steadily in recent decades. In 1996 alone, 144 scientific studies were published on the medical uses of beta-1,3-glucan. One fact has consistently emerged from these studies: beta-1,3-glucan produces its multiple broad-scale immune effects because it is a nonspecific immune stimulator. This means it causes a response capable of being directed at many conditions, perhaps all.

Research at Harvard University in the 1980s showed that the macrophage—a key immune system white blood cell that "eats" unwanted, foreign microbes—has a specific receptor for beta-1,3-glucan. In nontechnical terms, we might say the yeast talks directly to the immune cell. When the macrophage is activated by this contact, it starts a "cascade of events turning the cells into 'an arsenal of defense,'" explains Donald J. Carrow, M.D., a physician based in Tampa, Florida, who has used beta-1,3-glucan successfully with many patients.

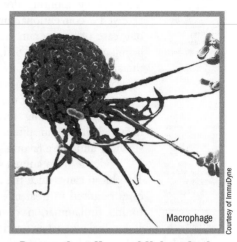

Macrophage

Courtesy of ImmuDyne

Dr. Carrow further notes that the specificity of this macrophage receptor site may explain why beta-1,3-glucan "is one of the most potent stimulators of the immune response." Dr. Carrow says that "there is now evidence to show that beta-1,3-glucan is, from an evolutionary point of view, the most widely and most commonly observed macrophage activator in nature."[1]

Research at Harvard University in the 1980s showed that the macrophage—a key immune system white blood cell that "eats" unwanted, foreign microbes—has a specific receptor for beta-1,3-glucan. In nontechnical terms, we might say the yeast talks directly to the immune cell.

Myra D. Patchen, M.D., of the U.S. Armed Forces Radiobiology Research Institute, suggests that beta-1,3-glucan appears to work as a free-radical scavenger. She believes it may even protect the macrophages from damage by radiation, toxins, heavy metals, invading microbes, and other poisons (collectively called free radicals) in the body. Beta-1,3-glucan's capabilities in resisting infections are well documented.

Scientists at the State University of São Paulo in Brazil tested beta-1,3-glucan's ability to stimulate the immune system against a fungal skin infection. Nine patients with serious fungal infections were given beta-1,3-glucan intravenously once weekly for one month,

Endocrine glands, including the testicles, ovaries, pancreas, adrenals, thyroid, parathyroid, and pituitary, are central to the regulation and normalization of all the body's complex, interconnected systems, from metabolism and heat production to spermogenesis and uterine preparations for pregnancy.

followed by monthly doses for 11 months. They also received a conventional antifungal drug. There was only one case of relapse among these patients, while another group of eight infected patients who were treated only with the antifungal drug had five relapses. The researchers also observed that the nine patients in the first group had far lower residual traces of the fungal infection in their blood chemistry, concluding that "the patients who received beta-1, 3-glucan, in spite of being more seriously ill, had a stronger and more favorable response to therapy."[2]

Evidence from animal studies demonstrates that beta-1,3-glucan can reduce the amount of conventional antibiotics required to treat infectious conditions such as peritonitis (inflammation of the membrane lining of the abdominal and pelvic cavities). In mice infected with a bacteria to produce peritonitis, a combination of beta-1,3-glucan and a standard antibiotic increased their long-term survival by 56%. Bacterial counts were noticeably down within eight hours of the injection and the numbers of key immune cells were markedly higher. "Clinical use of immunomodulators may alter conventional use and dosage of antibiotics," suggested study director William Browder, M.D., of Tulane University in New Orleans.[3]

Resetting the Immune System's Thermostat With Thymus Protein–Located behind the sternum in the chest, the thymus gland is part of the body's endocrine (SEE QUICK DEFINITION) and lymphatic systems. It grows during childhood, reaches its maximum size at puberty, and then begins to gradually shrink for the rest of one's life.

This is unfortunate because one of the thymus gland's principal tasks in the body is to release specialized proteins that stimulate white blood cells, the immune system's prime defense molecules, to resist and resolve infections. With age, then, as the thymus gland becomes smaller, there is often a corresponding gradual reduction in the immune system's potency in protecting the body against infections, illnesses, and disease.

The immune system continues to function, of course, because pre-programmed T cells (a type of white blood cell) are still circulating in the body, but at a reduced level. It's the thymus' job to keep the body supplied with fresh, vigorous T cells. "The thymus is like an immune system thermostat, and it regulates the immune system at an optimal point," says Terry Beardsley, Ph.D., of the University of California at San Diego, who in the 1980s conducted research that led to developing a thymic protein supplement (derived from calf thymus cells) called BioPro Protein A to address the problem of thymic insufficiency.

As early as the 1960s researchers sought to develop an extract of thymus protein capable of stimulating the immune system and the T-lymphocytes (SEE QUICK DEFINITION). But the extracts they came up with contained only small fragments of the targeted thymus protein; Thymosin had 13 amino acids and Thymopoetin had only five amino acids. While these fragment extracts showed some immune-stimulating effects, they were not particularly useful in programming T4 lymphocytes.

"The thymus is like an immune system thermostat, and it regulates the immune system at an optimal point," says Terry Beardsley, Ph.D., who in the 1980s conducted research that led to developing a thymic protein supplement.

Then, in 1983, Dr. Beardsley successfully isolated the *complete* thymic protein (containing 500 amino acids, or protein building blocks) which activates the T4 helper cells (*Proceedings of the National Academy of Sciences*, 1983). Biopro Protein A is derived from calf thymus cells; these live cells are then cloned (copied) in the laboratory, after which the protein is extracted and purified.

Dr. Beardsley's innovation was in preserving an intact, activated protein in the same complete form as would be produced by the human thymus itself. As a result of being a complete protein, Biopro Protein A is effective at programming T4 helper cells to release interleukin 2 (one of the immune system's activators of "killer T cells"). The substance both increases the numbers of these critical white blood cells and enhances their activity. Dr. Beardsley was able to show that thymus cells can be transplanted between species without being rejected and that the extracts remain biologically active, producing a stimulatory effect on the immune system.

As a commercial product, BioPro Protein A comes in single-dose packets (4 mcg) containing 12 trillion biologically active protein molecules in maltodextrin powder. The recommended dose is typically one to three packets per day, depending on your particular needs. If

QUICK DEFINITION

The main types of **T lymphocytes** are: Helper T cells (also known as T4 cells), which locate antigens and secrete immune proteins (particularly, the interleukins and interferon) to stimulate B cells and macrophages, and activate Killer T cells; Killer T cells (T8 cells), which bind to the specific invader and destroy it; and Suppressor T cells, which prevent excessive immune reactions by suppressing antibody activity.

you are not ill, a maintenance dose of one packet every day or two should be sufficient. The extract should be slowly dissolved under the tongue (where it is absorbed directly into the bloodstream), as stomach acids will destroy the fragile structure of the protein.

Another study showed that thymus extract has a beneficial effect on cancer, specifically for four patients with non-Hodgkin's lymphoma, three with Hodgkin's disease, and one with myeloma (*Blut*, 1983). After three months on thymus extract, "the total number and the percentage of T cells increased significantly," stated the researchers. They concluded that treatment with thymus extract was "effective in restoring immunocompetence in patients with T-cell deficiency."

According to certified nutritionist Gayle Black, Ph.D., of New York City, the daily use of thymic protein fortified her immune system as she underwent chemotherapy for breast cancer. Normally, chemotherapy drastically reduces white blood cell counts, thereby dangerously weakening immune competence, but in Dr. Black's experience, during the six months of chemotherapy, her white blood cell count never dropped below 2,500, a relatively healthy level. Even better, her levels of CD4-helper and CD8-killer white blood cells *increased*.

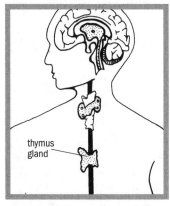

The thymus gland activates bone marrow or stem cells to respond to foreign or abnormal cells (bacteria, toxins, tumor cells, or transplanted tissue). Once activated, these cells develop into T lymphocytes (the "T" stands for thymus-derived), the "workers" of the cell-mediated immune system that will respond to antigens (foreign substances) but not to the body's own tissues.

A similarly favorable report comes from licensed nutritionist and registered radiology technologist Terri Clark, L.N.C., of Miami, Florida. Clark was diagnosed with breast cancer which soon spread to her bones and lungs, requiring twice-monthly drainage of one to two quarts of liquid from her lungs. Clark attributes her successful recovery from this otherwise life-threatening cancer to her use of 8-12 mcg daily of thymic protein over an 11-month period. Clark's cancer markers (blood substances indicating cancer, determined by laboratory tests) fell dramatically: her CEA went from 354 to 5, while her CA15-3 dropped from 900 to 85. "At this time, my lungs are completely free of any signs of disease," states Clark.

Studies with patients using thymus extracts have shown positive results. A small clinical trial involving patients with Epstein-Barr virus (associated with mononucelosis and chronic fatigue syndrome) also shows the strong therapeutic effect of BioPro Protein A. Six participants took 4 mcg of BioPro Protein A, three times daily, for 60 days. After treatment, the Epstein-Barr virus levels for four of the six

For more information on **BioPro Protein A**, contact: Alternative Health Concepts, P.O. Box 18748, Anaheim, CA 92817; tel: 714-283-5898; fax: 714-921-0120.

patients were reduced, in one case by 75%. All patients reported a reduction in symptoms and no adverse side effects. Five said they had increased energy levels and needed less sleep; others said their "energy level increased dramatically–probably 50% or more" and that they had "less tiredness during the day."[4]

Immunocal: Immune Nutrient from Milk Protein–One of the most important substances required by the immune system for optimal functioning is an amino acid complex called glutathione. However, supplementation is made difficult by the complexity of the body's system for delivering glutathione to cells. Canadian researchers figured out a way to deliver gluathione effectively in the form of a natural milk protein supplement called Immunocal™, and early research suggests it has benefits for chronic fatigue syndrome, cancer, AIDS, hepatitis, and age-related conditions such as Alzheimer's, Parkinson's, and arteriosclerosis.

Glutathione is a tripeptide, a small protein consisting of three amino acids (glutamic acid, cysteine, and glycine) bound together. The substance functions as a principle antioxidant, scavenging free radicals and toxins such as lipid peroxides that would otherwise damage, even destroy, cells. It accomplishes this valuable task by working with an enzyme called glutathione peroxidase. Further, glutathione regulates the activities of other antioxidants such as vitamins A, C, and E.

However, when the body is suffering from oxidative stress, supplies of glutathione become depleted. Oxidative stress is a condition in which the body is unable to detoxify itself completely and is overrun by free radicals because antioxidants are depleted. Oxidative stress affects the nervous, immune, and endocrine systems, and it may underlie many of the symptoms associated with chronic fatigue.

Glutathione exerts another protective and scavenging role in concert with the liver, the body's primary organ of detoxification and internal cleansing. In the liver, glutathione combines with toxins, carcinogens, and waste products as a way of more effectively securing their elimination from the body. In addition, glutathione helps red blood cell membranes and other cellular proteins maintain their structure, and aids the production of leukotrienes, immune system cells crucial for working against inflammation.

But glutathione also has an important role in supporting the activity of white blood cells called lymphocytes (the key players in the body's immune response) as well as antibodies (specialized immune defense cells). In fact, for lymphocytes to do their job, glutathione must be present. The tricky fact about glutathione is that you can't simply take in more glutathione as a supplement; it must be made *inside* the cells. In other words, glutathione doesn't enter cells directly; rather, it must be made within them by precursors.

Recognizing this biochemical fact, Canadian researchers developed Immunocal in 1993 to deliver to the cells the necessary *precursors* for glutathione. In the course of researching dietary protein sources capable of boosting the immune system, Gustavo Bounous, M.D., of McGill University in Montreal, Quebec, discovered the substance which later became Immunocal. Today, Dr. Bounous serves as the medical director of Immunotec Research, the manufacturers of Immunocal, located in Vaudreuil-Dorion, Quebec, Canada.

Immunocal is a natural food supplement consisting of concentrated milk protein powder containing unusually high amounts of glutathione precursors, according to Immunotec Research. "Immunocal promotes optimal functioning of the immune system by sustaining normal levels of glutathione and glutathione precursors in the lymphocytes. Glutathione, acting as the cellular antioxidant, allows for a full immune response," says Immunotec literature.

Immunocal contains concentrates of three substances in the whey portion of milk (serum albumin, alph-lactalbumin, and lactoferrin). These contain a large quantity of cystine, an amino acid breakdown product which is a more usable form of cysteine (the amino acid precursor of glutathione). Studies have shown that cysteine levels tend to be the rate-limiting factor (the biochemical bottleneck) in maintaining the ideal level of glutathione.

For more information about **Immunocal**™, contact: Immunotec Research Ltd., 292 Adrien Patenaude, Vaudreuil-Dorion, QC, Canada J7V 5V5; tel: 514-424-9992; fax: 514-424-9993; website: www. immunocal.com.

The problem with cysteine (both a protein building block and an antioxidant) is that it is found in only trace amounts in a limited number of foods, including raw egg whites, milk, and meats. If the body is under immune stress, as happens with a viral infection, dietary sources may not be sufficient to produce enough glutathione.

If you isolate cysteine and take it in large quantities, however, it can be toxic. Rapidly metabolized (burned up, digested by the body), cysteine is unusable as a dietary supplement. Immunocal solves this problem because it contains cystine, which is to say, cysteine in a more practical form. This form is readily released during digestion and transported to target cells, where it can be broken down into cysteine.

Once in the cells, cysteine can then be used as raw material for the synthesis of glutathione, the goal of all this biochemistry. For example, proper amounts of glutathione enable white blood cells (lymphocytes such as T cells, B cells, and natural killer cells) to reproduce in order to make antibodies or to attack foreign substances directly.

Five hundred liters of fresh, raw cow's milk are necessary to produce one kilogram of Immunocal, according to Immunotec. It is produced using a gentle process and low temperatures to preserve the biological activity of the proteins. Recommended dosage is one pouch (10 g) of Immunocal daily. Here you add the powder to 4-6 ounces of milk, water, or juice and shake gently to mix. There are no reported side effects from using Immunocal, says Immunotec.[5]

Traditional Chinese Medicine

William M. Cargile, B.S., D.C., F.I.A.C.A., former chairman of research for the American Association of Oriental Medicine, has treated CFS patients using acupuncture alone, concentrating specifically on building the immune system. Dr. Cargile treats CFS using the acupuncture points which relate to autoimmunity and clearing all the meridians (SEE QUICK DEFINITION) in the body. He also strongly advises patients to undergo allergy testing before acupuncture treatment so they can rid their diets of allergens which may jeopardize treatment.

Dr. Cargile notes that the immune system uses 60% of the body's energy storage compound called ATP (adenosine triphosphate—SEE QUICK DEFINITION), which manufactures proteins to make immune antibodies. "You don't have enough energy because your immune system is using all the ATP for the production of antibodies, until there is none left. That is why you feel so bad," he explains.

One of Dr. Cargile's patients, Emily, a 54-year-old woman with chronic fatigue syndrome, was diagnosed with idiopathic chronic fatigue, meaning her condition did not

To contact **William M. Cargile, B.S., D.C., F.I.A.C.A.:** Center for Preventive Medicine, 2800 Midland Avenue, Suite #106, Glenwood Springs, CO 81601; tel: 970-945-4014; fax: 970-925-4086. For the **American Association of Oriental Medicine,** contact: 433 Front Street, Catasauqua, PA 18032; tel: 610-266-1433; fax: 610-264-2768.

"People with CFS have a compromised immune system which is weak and at the same time hyperactive," says Maoshing Ni, D.O.M., Ph.D., L.Ac. "My objective is to strengthen and simultaneously desensitize, normalize, and regulate the immune system," he explains.

have a known cause such as cancer or thyroid or endocrine abnormalities. "She had a 13-year history, with no relief, and a continuous worsening of the condition," says Dr. Cargile. "She literally did not have the motivation to walk to the kitchen more than once a day." Dr. Cargile used acupuncture to stimulate both Emily's immune system and the production of ATP in her body. Within five treatments, Emily, who previously had spent up to 20 hours a day in bed, was walking three miles daily, with her energy level restored.

Maoshing Ni, D.O.M., Ph.D., L.Ac., of Santa Monica, California, also reports successful treatment of chronic fatigue syndrome with traditional Chinese medicine. "The people who come to see me have been bounced from one internist to another," he says. "They've been through the mill, and been rejected by the Western medical establishment." He concurs with Dr. Cargile that the key to CFS is in improving immune function. "People with CFS have a compromised immune system which is weak and at the same time hyperactive. My objective is to strengthen and simultaneously desensitize, normalize, and regulate the immune system," he explains.

To accomplish this, Dr. Ni uses a combination of acupuncture, Chinese herbs, and lifestyle changes, including diet, exercise, rest, and meditation. He explains, "Herbs are used to support immune functions. They are easily assimilated and adapted by the body. I also implement a low-stress diet. Up to 30% to 40% of the body's energy goes to digestion, so we want to conserve that energy as much as possible." Patients reportedly experience a 65% to 80% relief of symptoms after the treatment period (generally, three months) and are then able

To contact **Maoshing Ni, D.O.M., Ph.D., L.Ac.:** 1131 Wilshire Boulevard, Suite #300, Santa Monica, CA 90401; tel: 310-917-2200; fax: 310-917-2267.

to return to a normal life. After a three-month follow-up treatment, Dr. Ni reports that 90% to 95% of his patients have recovered from CFS. "Acupuncture reprograms the body and the herbs support that reprogramming," states Dr. Ni.

CHAPTER

5 Detoxifying the Body

ALTERNATIVE PHYSICIANS working with chronic fatigue know that removing toxins from the body is an essential phase in restoring their patients to health and vitality. Each year, people are exposed to thousands of toxic chemicals and pollutants in air, water, food, and soil. People living today carry within their bodies a "chemical cocktail" made up of industrial chemicals, pesticides, food additives, heavy metals, general anesthetics, and the residues of conventional pharmaceuticals, as well as of legal (alcohol, tobacco, caffeine) and illegal drugs (heroin, cocaine, marijuana).

Today people are exposed to chemicals in far greater concentrations than were previous generations. For example, over 70 million Americans live in areas that exceed smog standards; most municipal drinking water contains over 700 chemicals, including excessive levels of lead. Some 3,000 chemicals are added to the food supply, and as many as 10,000 chemicals—in the form of solvents, emulsifiers, and preservatives—are used in food processing and storage. These can remain in the body for years.[1]

To make matters worse, food and product labels do not always list every ingredient. When people consume these foods—especially seafood, meat, and poultry—they ingest all the chemicals and pesticides that have remained as accumulated contaminants in the food chain. These pollutants lodge in the body—loading it up with poisons—and manifest in a variety of symptoms, including decreased immune function, nerve cell toxicity, hormonal dysfunction, and psychological disturbances.

The Loading Theory of Toxicity

The "loading theory" of toxicity, according to its formulator, Serafina

Corsello, M.D., director of the Corsello Centers for Nutritional Complementary Medicine in New York City and Huntington, New York, states that no single factor causes a disease, such as exposure to infectious agents or because of psychological traumas that lower immune resistance.

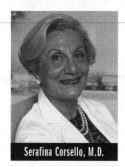

Serafina Corsello, M.D.

Dr. Corsello stresses that if you don't take care of the intestines, eliminate its toxic load and rebalance its bacterial population, "no immune disorder will ever truly get relieved."

Rather, the *cumulative load* of multiple poisons creates an illness.

You don't *suddenly* get sick: it takes a long time for the body to break down. This is compounded of layers of toxicity, malnutrition, and dysfunction, she notes. Nothing alone can cause chronic fatigue. People don't *get* a disease—they develop it, Dr. Corsello explains. "I touch a lot of my chronic fatigue patients. I embrace them. I take care of them. I'm exposed to the virus—but I don't get chronic fatigue from them."

The loading theory outlines a process of many factors acting together in the creation of illnesses. Over time, these multiple factors weigh down the immune system and eventually throw it out of balance. Among the typical multiple stressors there are toxic metals (mercury leaching from fillings, aluminum), petrochemical residues (pesticides and fertilizers), chemical pollutants (in the water and air), electromagnetic pollution (power lines), undiagnosed food allergies, nutritional deficiencies, biochemical imbalances, insufficient exercise, and emotional stress (family, job, and personal).

All these factors impinge on the immune system's natural ability to resist the downhill slide into illness, says Dr. Corsello. "These factors interact and compound each other to break down the immune system. In fact, these stressors may be accumulating for years, over a lifetime, before they send the system into disregulation." The loading theory of illness is the cornerstone of the Corsello Center's approach to patients, from the moment they first call for an appointment.

Increasingly, toxicity is being identified as the predisposing factor in a long list of acute and chronic illnesses, including environmental illness and chronic fatigue, degenerative diseases, and cancer. "The current level of chemicals in the food and water supply and the indoor

A healthy intestine is immunologically *vigilant* against undesirable pathogens and toxins. One that is overburdened and compromised fails to perform its immune defensive role and may start contributing to the emergence of an autoimmune illness or other chronic disease.

and outdoor environment has lowered our threshold of resistance to disease and has altered our body's metabolism, causing enzyme dysfunction, nutritional deficiencies, and hormonal imbalances," says Marshall Mandell, M .D., a pioneer of environmental medicine based in Norwalk, Connecticut.

Where do all the toxins come from? They come from a polluted environment (air, water, and food), lack of water, overconsumption of food, a faulty, nutritionally inadequate diet, lack of exercise, accumulated stress, excess antibiotic use, and chronic constipation and poor elimination. Bioaccumulation (a buildup in the body of foreign substances) seriously compromises physiological and psychological health. Since 1985, hundreds of studies have demonstrated the dangers to health from toxic bioaccumulation.[2] Since 1945, toxins have accumulated in the human system faster than they can be naturally eliminated, which means the body now needs assistance in detoxifying.

Detoxifying the body is another important component in promoting the health of the immune system and addressing other factors which may be contributing to your chronic fatigue. As our environment and food are increasingly saturated with chemicals, the body's mechanisms for elimination of toxins cannot keep up with the chemical deluge. The constant circulation of toxins in the body taxes the immune system which must continually strive to destroy them.

When combined with multiple infections and nutritional deficiencies, this toxic overload may be the proverbial last straw in the development of CFS. Given that many people with CFS have chemical allergies and that environmental illness is a disease reaction to 20th century chemicals, it is advisable to take measures to remove the toxins stored in the body.

The Immune Vigilance of the Intestines

In addition, intestinal toxicity is intimately related to immune dysfunction. The large and small intestines are actually part of the immune system. In fact, "the intestinal mucosa and some of its submucosal structures constitute the largest immunological system of the body," states Dr. Corsello. The intestines' mucus layers trap debris and pathogens and represent the active front of immune function. The large and small intestines—at 25 feet long, they are the body's largest internal organ—together represent a key part of the body's immune system, says Dr. Corsello, accounting for perhaps 80% of our body's lymphatic-immune resources. "The digestive system is one of the first screening systems against the daily load of contact with bacteria, viruses, and parasites, that, if left unchecked, would constitute a grave threat to our entire immune system."

A healthy intestine is immunologically vigilant against undesirable pathogens and toxins. One that is overburdened and compromised fails to perform its immune defensive role and may start contributing to the emergence of an autoimmune illness or other chronic disease. "A large onslaught of infective agents can overcome the immune vigilance of most people, even in the presence of so-called 'normal' immune systems," Dr. Corsello notes.

The intestines consist of a complex and delicately balanced population of mixed microflora in which the friendly, beneficial bacteria should outnumber the harmful ones. But this ecology is easily upset, says Dr. Corsello, leading to a condition of imbalance called dysbiosis. "At the Center, we have observed an almost immediate relationship between stressful events and the exponential growth of dysbiotic organisms such as *Candida albicans* and other pathogens."

Another factor that upsets intestinal ecology is parasites, as discussed in Chapter 3. These enter the body (or the numbers of resident ones increase) from contaminated water and food supplies (both domestic and from foreign travel) and/or repeated courses of antibiotics that diminish the proportion of friendly intestinal bacteria. Despite this, "there is an overwhelming lack of awareness of this by Western physicians, especially American-trained physicians, who refuse to acknowledge that parasitosis [parasite infestation] is a major factor in systemic illness."

Dr. Corsello notes that physicians at her center have observed a strong correlation in their patients between having intestinal parasites and a range of chronic conditions such as arthritis, respiratory problems, heightened allergies, menstrual disorders, and prolonged bowel disorders. Such people with chronic, untreated parasitic states are highly prone to develop autoimmune disorders. "I've yet to see a menopausal woman with severe symptoms who doesn't have parasites."

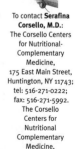

To contact **Serafina Corsello, M.D.:** The Corsello Centers for Nutritional-Complementary Medicine, 175 East Main Street, Huntington, NY 11743; tel: 516-271-0222; fax: 516-271-5992. The Corsello Centers for Nutritional Complementary Medicine, 200 West 57th Street, New York, NY 10019; tel: 212-399-0222; fax: 212-399-3817.

An imbalance among the intestinal microflora can lead to food allergies, both acute and delayed, Dr. Corsello says. You might eat a food today and experience an allergic reaction to it 24 to 36 hours later, yet fail to make the connection—but your body always does. "Dysbiosis and delayed food allergies are almost universally present in people with autoimmune disorders."

Otherwise healthy foods become branded as foreign and undesirable by the intestine's immune guards; these foods do not get properly digested and, enwrapped by immune system proteins, they may pass inappropriately into the blood circulation as an immune complex (SEE QUICK DEFINITION). This is the increasingly common condition called leaky gut syndrome. Undigested foods then become part of the overall suppressive load on the immune system.

If the intestines are unbalanced (dysbiotic) and "leaky," bacteria and parasites "can overcome the defensive intestinal barrier and, through the circulatory system, both the lymph and blood, invade organs. The circulating immune complexes can then trigger a variety of diseases affecting the connective tissue (collagen) layer of the body, such as arthritis and lupus," Dr. Corsello says. Dr. Corsello stresses that if you don't take care of the intestines, eliminate its toxic load and rebalance its bacterial population, "no immune disorder will ever truly disappear."

Surviving the Toxic Immune Syndrome

With these general observations about toxicity established, we move deeper into the subject with the clinical recommendations of **William R. Kellas, Ph.D.**, and **Andrea S. Dworkin, N.D.**, of the Center for Advanced Medicine in Encinitas, California. They are the authors of the reference works *Surviving the Toxic Crisis* (1996) and *Thriving in a Toxic World* (1996). Here are the recommendations of Drs. Kellas and Dworkin for surviving what they call "the toxic immune syndrome":

At the Center for Advanced Medicine, our focus is to help our patients get their lives back on track by getting to the root causes of their illness. The idea for this approach evolved out of the medical problems I (William Kellas) faced in the early 1970s when I developed a crippling autoimmune disease called ankylosing spondylitis in my twenties.

At the time, my doctors told me I would probably remain in a wheelchair for the rest of my life. I refused to accept this verdict and immediately started to search for answers. I had all my mercury amalgam fillings removed; I flushed all the parasites out of my intestines; I did chelation therapy to remove the mercury from my system; I had my dental bite balanced; I had whiplash and nose injury problems corrected. It took me about ten years to regain my health, but that's because I had to piece it all together on my own. Now that we know what's required, we can produce the same results in our patients in less than a year.

It was my study of healing methods for myself that led me to the philosophy of our clinic: always look for the root, underlying cause of any illness. Along the way, I met other practitioners with health problems who were similarly searching for alternative methods of healing. "We fit in where our patients want to be, because all of our doctors or their families were also once patients," says Gary Shima, M.D., our former medical director.

Our clinic serves patients who prefer a more natural alternative to health and healing, supported by sound medical principles. We offer the best of technology and natural healing methods, including immunotherapy, ten different kinds of intravenous therapy, colonics, acupuncture, allergy therapy, clinical nutrition, massage, craniopathy, naturopathy, chiropractic, and Feldenkrais bodywork.

Our principle is this: *What you don't see may be sinking your ship.* This ship, of course, is your body and health. Disease occurs after your immune system breaks down; this happens as the result of an onslaught of toxic suppressors and the accumulation of biochemical deficiencies, all of which allow unwanted microorganisms to invade and flourish in the body. The result is chronic illness, which we define as a health problem you've had for 120 days or more.

Have you already been to doctors and heard them say, "You're not really sick," yet you know you're not well? Most chronic patients we see have consulted at least ten physicians and still haven't received lasting help. Getting to the root causes rather than just aiming for relief of symptoms is the main characteristic of comprehensive health care and the only way to get real help.

There are many steps in a patient's road to bad health. We call these cumulative steps "primary toxic suppressors" and they include such factors as mercury dental amalgams (SEE QUICK DEFINITION), chemical toxins, surgeries, electromagnetic radiation, poor nutrition, structural problems, and others. These in turn adversely affect the

137

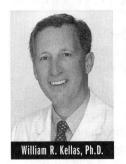

There are many steps in a patient's road to bad health, says Dr. Kellas. We call these cumulative steps "primary toxic suppressors" and they include such factors as mercury dental amalgams, chemical toxins, surgeries, electromagnetic radiation, poor nutrition, structural problems, and others.

William R. Kellas, Ph.D.

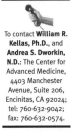

To contact **William R. Kellas, Ph.D.**, and **Andrea S. Dworkin, N.D.**: The Center for Advanced Medicine, 4403 Manchester Avenue, Suite 206, Encinitas, CA 92024; tel: 760-632-9042; fax: 760-632-0574.

immune system, the key to your body's optimal functioning, and produce what we call the toxic immune syndrome. This is a multifaceted condition of weakness and susceptibility that sets up a domino effect of poor health.

Here's how it works. Let's say you have a structural problem with your back, spine, neck, or overall posture. This restricts the nerve supply to your organs and digestive system; the result of this is poor digestion, which can lead to putrefaction of food materials in your intestines. From this, you might develop food sensitivities as the healthy food becomes toxic. Add to this the negative influence of antibiotics from dental work, surgery, or medications, and you begin knocking out the beneficial bacteria in your system that should be screening out harmful influences.

You may experience symptoms such as pain, stiffness, fatigue, infection, weight gain, allergies, or headaches. These symptoms may vary according to your weakest genetic link or vulnerability.

Now you are open to microbial invasion and long-term internal infections. This can then throw your hormonal system out of balance, blocking the smooth action of your digestive and lymph systems. As a result, toxins overload your body's natural filters and you are unable to detoxify. In effect, your body becomes poisoned from within and begins to develop illnesses in the various organs, such as jaundice in the liver, urinary infection in the bladder, and constipation in the intestines.

Your body is now more vulnerable to petrochemicals in your foods and environment, leading to, for example, chronic fatigue, reduced sperm count, or infertility. Following this, your tissues become inflamed and more deeply-set illnesses develop, such as cancer, fibromyalgia, and edema. All of this then feeds back to your brain, producing contractions in the membranes covering your brain and spinal cord, which then misalign the vertebrae and skull.

Dental problems, produced by mercury amalgam fillings, electrical charges from dental work, and misalignments in the jaw, are major players in a surprising number of health conditions. Other dental-related problems that contribute to this negative domino effect include whiplash, which can imbalance the bite; cranial sutures out of alignment; patient sensitivity to dental materials; bite imbalance; and infected, toxic root canals. Here the medical and dental branches should work together on diagnosis (medical) and treatment (dental) of these problems.

The good news about this circle of ill effects is that it also shows us how to regain health by way of reversing the stages in the toxic loop, although you'll need to take several steps at once to see improvement. When you clear up one problem, this enables the other parts of the interrelated system to function better, which in turn helps to clear up further problems all the way around the circle. To be effective, a clinic must help stop the influx of toxins, remove the toxins from all the body systems, and support the body nutritionally and biochemically in healing disease.

The U.S. Centers for Disease Control divide the causes of illness into these categories: heredity, 18%; environment, 19%; medical intervention, 10%; and lifestyle, 53%. This means that 82% of the causes of disease are within your control: improving your environment, avoiding medical interventions, and changing how you live. That 82% is the focus of our treatments at the clinic.

Our philosophy is that chronic degenerative disease, which takes years to develop and show its effects, is best prevented and treated by *comprehensive* health care, along the lines I've outlined above. Our patient care is coordinated with all our different practitioners, who share a similar philosophy of healing and who have equal access to the patient charts and test results. Our staff meets regularly to discuss the best way to work together for the patient's health.

Comprehensive health care removes the obstacles to the body's

QUICK
DEFINITION

Mercury fillings, or amalgams, have been used in dentistry since the 1820s, but not until 1988 did the routine use of mercury raise serious enough questions for the Environmental Protection Agency (EPA) to declare scrap dental amalgam a *hazardous waste*. Evidence now shows that mercury amalgams are the *major* source of mercury exposure for the general public, at rates six times higher than that found in fish and seafood. Studies by the World Health Organization show that a single amalgam can release 3-17 mcg of mercury per day, making dental amalgam a major source of mercury exposure. A Danish study of a random sample of 100 men and 100 women showed that increased blood mercury levels were related to the presence of more than four amalgam fillings in the teeth. Mercury toxicity has been shown to have destructive contributory effects on kidney function, in cardiovascular disease, neuropsychological dysfunction, reproductive disorders, and birth defects, to name a few. Symptoms of mercury toxicity make a very long list: anorexia, depression, fatigue, insomnia, arthritis, multiple sclerosis, moodiness, irritability, memory loss, nausea, diarrhea, gum disease, swollen glands, headaches, and many more.

The good news about this circle of ill effects is that it also shows us how to regain health by way of reversing the stages in the toxic loop, although you'll need to take several steps at once to see improvement.

natural healing processes, but it's important to remember that healing usually occurs as a series of "baby steps." As it took a long time to reach your present state of ill health, it will probably take some months, possibly years, to restore it as completely as possible. Even so, we are getting dramatic improvements in people with fibromyalgia, chronic fatigue, and multiple sclerosis in less than a year. ■

Detoxification Therapy

"A body with a healthy immune system, efficient organs of elimination and detoxification, and sound circulatory and nervous systems can handle a great deal of toxicity," states Leon Chaitow, N.D., D.O., of London, England.

"But if a person's immune system has been damaged from chronic exposure to environmental pollutants, restoring these functions, organs, and systems can be accomplished only through detoxification therapies, including fasting, chelation, and nutritional, herbal, and homeopathic methods, which accelerate the body's own natural cleansing processes." Intestinal detoxification is also an important method of removing toxins from the body and, as discussed earlier, the intestines are in themselves an essential part of the immune system.

Most alternative medicine physicians agree that detoxification is essential and that it brings many benefits to the person undertaking it. One of the most important and longest lasting effects of detoxification therapy is the reduction of stress on the immune system, says Elson Haas, M.D., director of the Preventive Medical Center of Marin in San Rafael, California. Other benefits can include increased vitality, reduced blood pressure and blood fats (cholesterol and triglycerides), improved assimilation of vitamins and minerals, and mental clarity.

Everyone has a natural, specific level of tolerance for toxins that cannot be exceeded if good health is to be maintained. When the body gets overwhelmed with toxins, the immune system mechanisms malfunction, and

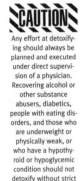

CAUTION

Any effort at detoxifying should always be planned and executed under direct supervision of a physician. Recovering alcohol or other substance abusers, diabetics, people with eating disorders, and those who are underweight or physically weak, or who have a hypothyroid or hypoglycemic condition should not detoxify without strict medical supervision.

Dr. Kellas' Six Steps to Detoxification and Healing

1. Eliminate intake of toxins and cleanse all toxic suppressors from the body.
First, you must stop bombing your body with more toxins. Toxic suppressors can include heavy metals (mercury, aluminum, cadmium, copper, lead, arsenic, nickel), chemicals (carcinogens, fluoride, chlorine, food additives), and radiation (electromagnetic, microwave, nuclear, solar, X rays, computer screens). They can also include ingested hormones, steroids, drugs, alcohol, toxic water, caffeine, processed foods, inhaled or absorbed pesticides, perfume, smog, nicotine from cigarettes, noise, and stress.

The toxic suppressors must be eliminated before medications and other natural approaches will have permanent effect.

2. Detoxify the body and unblock detoxification pathways.
Even though you have reduced the entry of new toxins into your body, old toxins are still in your bloodstream, lymph nodes, and organs. Our treatments involve chelation therapy to remove metals from the blood, intravenous vitamin C (to detoxify the blood), sauna (to remove chemicals), and detoxification diets (to remove allergens and yeast-supporting conditions). We also prescribe fasting, organ flushes, enzymes, amino acids, physical therapy, lymph drainage, constitutional water therapy (to cleanse the lymph system), exercise, and colonics, and provide counseling for the patient's emotional and spiritual issues.

3. Provide the body with biochemical and nutritional support.
Now that the cleansing is completed, it's time to support your body's natural restoration and defense. To support the body's biochemistry, we prescribe minerals, enzymes, vitamins, pure water, oxygen therapy, amino acids, herbs, and essential fatty acids.

4. Align and rebalance all body structures.
We use chiropractic, osteopathy, and dental work to rebalance the nervous system; trigger points to realign the electrical system; gamma globulin, cyclic AMP, transfer factor, allergy antigens, and low dosage immunotherapy to support the immune system; and Feldenkrais, soft tissue and lymph manipulation, and craniosacral work to rebalance the muscles and their movements. When you rebalance the bite and remove the toxins from the mouth you have already won 60% of the detoxification battle.

5. Eliminate harmful microorganisms and disease-producing parasites from the body.
Once the primary suppressors and toxins are removed from your environment and your body, it's time to go after the secondary suppressors, or opportunistic microorganisms. Harmful microbial organisms within your system, such as bacteria, worms, protozoans, mycoplasmas, fungus, parasites, and viruses, must be flushed out. We've found that certain conventional drugs (Flagdyl and Fasigyn) work best, in conjunction with tetracycline, *acidophilus*, and sometimes an herbal formula and/or bismuth gel, over a 21-day intensive program. In addition, you must kill the parasites outside the body, in the skin, under the nails, and in the hair; for this we use iodine baths every five days.

6. Rebuild, restore, and regenerate the health of the body's interrelated systems.
The key to achieving this step is to strengthen the immune system. Here we use "probiotics" (beneficial micro-organisms) such as *L. acidophilus* and *L. bifidus*. We also provide emotional counseling to help fortify the patient's psychological attitude during the process to accept the healing and to rework a new way of looking at themselves and life.

fatigue, confusion, aggression, or mental disorder may occur. Other symptoms indicating that you may need detoxification are headaches, joint pain, recurrent respiratory problems, back pain, inhalant allergy symptoms (nasal or sinus), insomnia, mood changes, food allergies, and digestive ailments.

Scrubbing and Repopulating the Intestines

Taking care of a patient's intestinal system is the first order of business in the Corsello Center's treatment plan, explains Dr. Corsello. Their intestinal cleansing plan consists of a blend of 80% insoluble and 20% soluble fiber from flaxseed and fruit pectin mixed with vitamin C powder and fruit juices. This formula begins to disinfect and scrub the intestines, removing layers of yeast, bacteria, and parasites.

The next step is to repopulate the intestines with more friendly bacteria (SEE QUICK DEFINITION), or probiotics, such as *Lactobacillus acidophilus* and *Bifidobacterium*. Repopulating causes a 'gentle war' in your intestines, says Dr. Corsello. The unwanted yeasts and bacteria are killed off and the probiotics establish themselves as the predominant species. Research has proven that giving probiotics to rebalance the intestinal immune defenses reduces inflammation of the intestinal lining and is helpful in both treating and preventing food allergies, notes Dr. Corsello. "Since gut immune suppression is often responsible for systemic immune suppression, this approach may have life-or-death repercussions."

To aid this process, Dr. Corsello prescribes a salad dressing made from flaxseed oil and extra virgin cold-press olive oils mixed with vitamin E and garlic. This supplies the intestines with needed essential fatty acids (both omega-3s and omega-6s) and it helps to heal the damaged mucosal layers.

For more about **Serafina Corsello, M.D.**, see "Reversing Lupus and Diabetes," *Digest* #22, pp. 44-53.

The third step in restoring intestinal efficiency is to give the patient injections or slow-drip intravenous infusions of B vitamins, selenium, zinc, manganese, and liver-protecting substances (taurine, glutathione). If your intestines are in dysbiosis and you take B vitamins orally, they become food for all the infective agents resident in the intestines; but if you inject them, the B vitamins bypass intestinal barriers and enter the bloodstream directly, says Dr. Corsello. "Most people who are ill suffer from malab-

Testing for Your Detoxification Capabilities

Determining how efficiently the body can detoxify itself is especially useful for CFS sufferers. Here are two laboratory tests that can help.

Detoxification Profile—If your liver is unable to adequately detoxify your body's store of toxins and waste products, this situation may contribute significantly to the emergence and continuation of your chronic fatigue. Excess free radicals and by-products of incomplete metabolism resulting from poor detoxificiation (called "toxic intermediate metabolism") can create problems in the cells. Specifically, these toxins can interfere with the movement of substances across the cell membrane and induce damage to the mitochondria, the

For information about the **Detoxification Profile** and **Oxidative Stress Profile**, contact: Great Smokies Diagnostic Laboratory, 63 Zillicoa Street, Asheville, NC 28801; tel: 828-253-0621 or 800-522-4762; fax: 828-252-9303.

For more on **glutathione and detoxification**, see Chapter 4: Restoring Immune Vitality, pp. 127-129.

cells' "energy factories." The Detoxification Profile helps to identify places where your system is impaired in its ability to detoxify.

Oxidative Stress Profile—When your ability to detoxify is impaired and/or you are deficient in antioxidants, free radicals run unchallenged throughout the body, damaging cells. They tend to affect the immune, endocrine, and nervous systems, damaging mitochondria, interrupting communication among cells, and depleting key nutrients and antioxidants. This is called oxidative stress. The Oxidative Stress Profile assesses the degree of free radical damage in the body and measures the body's level of glutathione, an amino acid complex central to detoxification.

sorption," she adds. Nutrient infusions maximize absorption and produce quicker results; the infective agents eventually starve to death.

The fourth step involves major dietary changes. "If patients are eating junk foods, then no matter what I do, their dietary choices will harm the process of restoring their intestines." The dietary plan is based on three factors: first, eliminate all foods known to produce allergic reactions in the patient; second, match the diet to the patient's blood type; and third, match the diet with the biochemistry of the specific disease process. "Our nutritional interventions have a precise biochemical knowledge behind them and are very specifically tailored."

How to Soak Out Your Toxins with Detoxifying Baths

In this section, **Joseph Dispenza**, director of the Parcells Center in Santa Fe, New Mexico, explains the benefits and techniques of using therapeutic bathing as a way of cleansing and healing:

The skin is the largest organ of the body and 65% of body cleansing is accomplished through it. Cleansing the skin with detoxifying baths is a science, according to the late naturopathic pioneer Hazel Parcells, N.D., D.C., Ph.D. Her therapy of detoxifying baths was developed over a period of 50 years of clinical observation and application. With a program of good nutrition, they stand as proven methods to help the body regain and remain in good health.

"Cleanse the body, give it the right building materials, and nature will heal and build," said Dr. Parcells. She also said: "If you want to be healthy, you have to trade your wishbone for a backbone and get to work." The principle of Dr. Parcells' therapeutic baths is based on the chemical axiom that "the weak will draw from the strong." In this case, cool water will draw toxins out of a heated body. The hot water solution draws toxins out of the body to the surface of the skin. Then, as the water cools, the toxins are pulled from the surface of the skin by the change in temperature, and go into the water. Specifically, here are Dr. Parcells' bath formulas:

Formula #1: Environmental Radiation or X Rays–Do this bath if you have been exposed to environmental radiation or X rays. Air travel, for instance, will increase levels of radiation in your body; dental X rays will leave deposits in the body that interfere with healthy functioning. This bath is indicated if you have been feeling general muscular aches, mild nausea, fatigue, headaches, slight dizziness, or a disturbance in equilibrium.

Dissolve one pound of sea salt or rock salt and one pound of baking soda in a tub of water as hot as can be tolerated. Mix salt and soda thoroughly with the water, then stay in the bath until the water has cooled.

For more about **Hazel Parcells, N.D.**, see "You Too Can Live to Be 100," *Digest* #8, pp. 18-22.

EDITOR'S NOTE

Joseph Dispenza, director of the Parcells Center and the author of ten previous books, is the author of *Live Better Longer: The Parcells Center Seven-Step Plan for Health and Longevity* (1997), Harper San Francisco. Hazel Parcells practiced naturopathic medicine for nearly 60 years until her death at the age of 106 in January 1996.

Formula #2: Heavy Metal Exposure–If you have been exposed to heavy metals (such as aluminum), carbon monoxide or unburned carbons, or pesticide sprays, this bath can help detoxify your body of these substances. Cooking with aluminum will bring on symptoms; frequent airplane commuters absorb carbon monoxide through the skin, which then gets inside the body; eating foods that have not been cleaned of pesticide contamination can lead to an accumulation of pesticides in the cells.

This bath is indicated if you are experiencing decreased energy, shortness of breath, lightheadedness, impaired equilibrium, or a general feeling of being "out of sorts."

Add one cup of regular brand Clorox™ bleach (with the blue-and-white label) to a full tub of water as hot as can be tolerated. Mix thoroughly with the water. Stay in the bath until water has cooled; do not shower for at least four hours following the bath. The bath can, and will, remove toxins with utmost

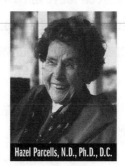

Hazel Parcells, N.D., Ph.D., D.C.

"Cleanse the body, give it the right building materials, and nature will heal and build," said Dr. Parcells. She also said: "If you want to be healthy, you have to trade your wishbone for a backbone and get to work."

effectiveness. You'll feel the difference. If you are sensitive to chlorine, don't do this bath.

Formula #3: Low-Grade Radioactive Materials—If you have been exposed to low-grade radioactive materials in the atmosphere or have consumed food irradiated by cobalt 60, this bath will be useful. It is prudent to assume that residues of cobalt 60 are found in a wide range of foods, from fresh fruits and vegetables to grains and packaged meats; don't expect to find them labeled as such. Conditions that would benefit from this bath include soreness of the gums or mouth, swollen glands, sore throat, and indigestion (an inability to treat food comfortably in the stomach).

Dissolve two pounds of baking soda in a tub of water as hot as can be tolerated; mix thoroughly. Stay in the bath until water has cooled; do not shower for at least four hours following the bath.

Formula #4: General Toxicity—Try this general detoxifying bath if you are suffering from general muscle aches and pains, or fatigue brought about by physical exertion or mental or emotional stress. It is particularly useful to raise the acid level in the body to help build immunity and to ward off a feeling that you are about to be ill.

Add two cups of apple cider vinegar (pure, not the "flavored" variety) to a tub of water as hot as can be tolerated; mix thoroughly. Stay in the bath until water has cooled. Do not shower for at least four hours following the bath.

General Tips on Detoxifying Baths—Therapeutic bathing is most effective

Therapeutic bathing is most effective when done before bedtime, because the body detoxifies during sleep. The baths can be continued without harm until a relief from symptoms is noticed.

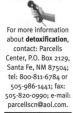

For more information about **detoxification**, contact: Parcells Center, P.O. Box 2129, Santa Fe, NM 87504; tel: 800-811-6784 or 505-986-1441; fax: 505-820-0990; e-mail: parcellscn@aol.com.

when done before bedtime, because the body detoxifies during sleep. Use only one bathing formula per evening. Do not mix ingredients from different formulas; each bath is recommended *only* for specific indications, as described. The baths can be continued without harm until a relief from symptoms is noticed. If redness, dryness, or roughness of the skin develops, it is an indication that the body is working to remove toxins. These aspects of cleansing are not uncommon.

To minimize discomfort, rub a little olive oil or almond oil or non-petroleum-based baby lotion on your skin after bathing. If you feel you have need for all the baths, alternate them on different evenings. If these baths are in any way too rigorous or unpleasant, cut back on your use of them, or discontinue. ■

More Detoxification Baths with Salts and Herbs

Jacqueline Krohn, M.D., M.P.H., who practices medicine in Los Alamos, New Mexico, offers the following techniques for using hot herbal baths as an effective way to detoxify the body. The hot water stimulates blood flow near the skin surface, opens pores, and increases perspiration, thereby supporting the faster release of toxins, Dr. Krohn explains in her book, *The Whole Way to Natural Detoxification*. She suggests starting with a trial series of plain-water hot soaks as a preparation because, depending on one's toxic load, detoxification baths "can make you feel very ill" as the toxins move out of your body.

Dr. Krohn advises an initial five-minute immersion in water as hot as you can tolerate, then build in five-minute increments to a 30-minute soak. Before taking the bath, shower and scrub your body thoroughly using soap and a loofah sponge, and take another cleansing shower after the soak; follow the same procedure for the detoxification baths, described below. Always use extreme care when stepping out of a hot bath, as standing up abruptly may cause temporary dizziness.

Dr. Krohn cautions that if you experience dizziness, headache, exhaustion, fatigue, nausea, or weakness, stop the bath and wait a few days before resuming the program. If you experience none of these symptoms, then proceed with three detoxification baths per week. Dr. Krohn recommends taking some vitamin C before and after each bath (to help remove toxins) and drinking an eight-ounce glass of pure water during each bath (to encourage sweating). Dr. Krohn suggests using only one of the following protocols per bath; each substance has a different detoxifying benefit.

■ Epsom Salts—Start with ¼ cup of Epsom salts added to the bath water, and build gradually to four cups per bath.

■ Apple Cider Vinegar—Start with ¼ cup added to the water, then increase gradually to one cup.

■ Hydrogen Peroxide—Add up to eight ounces of food-grade 35% hydrogen peroxide to a tub half full of warm water.

■ Baking Soda—Eight ounces of baking soda (sodium bicarbonate) may be used; alternatively, mix equal amounts of baking soda and sea salt, gradually increasing to one pound of each.

■ Ginger Root—Peel and slice a small piece of fresh ginger root into numerous pieces, boil in water, then steep for 30 minutes and strain. Add the resulting herbal broth to your bath water.

■ Clay—Although clay is traditionally used for a facial cleansing pack, it can also detoxify when ½ cup is added to a tub of hot water.

■ Burdock Root—Slice a handful of burdock root into small pieces. Boil it in two quarts of water for 30 minutes, strain the liquid, then add it to the bath.

■ Oatstraw—Add a heaping handful of this herb to two quarts of water and boil for 25 minutes, says Dr. Krohn; strain and pour it into the bath.

■ Herbal Teas—Herbs such as catnip, yarrow, peppermint, boneset, blessed thistle, pleurisy root, chamomile, blue vervain, and horsetail may also work as detoxifiers when added to your bath, Dr. Krohn says. She advises mixing one cup of a single brewed herb tea (boiled, simmered, and filtered) to the bath; use only one herb at a time, she adds.

> ## Lead Poisoning and Chronic Fatigue
>
> Undiagnosed lead exposure may be a contributing cause to chronic fatigue syndrome. A woman, 47, was admitted to the hospital with confusion and headaches and a ten-year history of constipation, fatigue, and weight loss. Her blood lead level was ten times above what is considered "safe." Further investigation revealed that, for 28 years, she had used water from a hot water heater contaminated with deteriorated lead solder, according to *The Lancet* (April 27, 1996).

How To Do a Natural Liver Flush

The healthy and efficient functioning of the liver is central to well-

Jacqueline Krohn, M.D., M.P.H., Frances Taylor, M.A., Jinger Prosser, L.M.T., *The Whole Way to Natural Detoxification: Clearing Your Body of Toxins* (1996). Available from: Hartley & Marks Publishers, Inc., Box 147, Point Roberts, WA 98281; tel: 800-277-5887 or 360-945-2017; fax: 800-707-5887 or 604-738-1913; e-mail: hartmark@direct.com.

being and disease prevention, which explains why it's advisable to periodically flush the organ clean using natural substances, says master herbalist and acupuncturist Christopher Hobbs, L.Ac. The liver is the body's chief detoxification organ so it must be kept in optimal condition. "Liver flushes are used to stimulate elimination of wastes from the body, to open and cool the liver, to increase bile flow, and to improve overall liver functioning," says Dr. Hobbs. "I have taken liver flushes for many years now and can heartily recommend them."

Here are Dr. Hobbs' instructions for preparing and administering a liver flush:

■ Citrus Juice—Squeeze enough fresh lemons or limes to produce one cup of juice, says Dr. Hobbs. A small amount of distilled or spring water may be added to dilute the juice, but the more sour it tastes, the better it will perform as a liver cleanser. Orange and grapefruit juices may also be used, provided they are blended with some lemon or lime juice.

■ Garlic and Ginger—To the citrus juice mixture add the juice of 1-2 cloves of garlic, freshly-squeezed in a garlic press, and a small amount of freshly grated raw ginger juice, Dr. Hobbs advises. Grate the raw ginger on a cheese or vegetable grater, then put the shreds into a garlic press, and squeeze out the juice.

■ Olive Oil—Add one tablespoon of high-quality olive oil (such as extra virgin) to the citrus, garlic, and ginger juice. Either blend or shake the ingredients to guarantee complete mixing.

■ Taking the Flush—The liver flush is best taken in the morning, preferably after some muscle stretches and breathing exercises, says Dr. Hobbs. Do not eat any foods for one hour following the flush, he adds.

■ Cleansing Herbal Tea—After an hour has elapsed, Dr. Hobbs recommends taking two cups of an herbal blend he calls "Polari Tea." It consists of dry portions of fennel (one part), flax (one part), burdock (¼ part), fenugreek (one part), licorice (¼ part), and peppermint (one part). Simmer the herbs (excepting the peppermint) for 20 minutes, then add the peppermint and allow to steep for ten minutes. For convenience, you may prepare several quarts of the tea in advance, says Dr. Hobbs.

■ Continuing the Flush—Dr. Hobbs suggests doing the liver flush twice yearly, in the spring and fall, for two full cycles each. A cycle consists of ten consecutive days of taking the flush ingredients, followed by three days off, then another ten days on. "I have never seen anyone experience negative side effects from this procedure."

■Detoxification Phases—In cleansing the liver there are two phases, known as Phase I and Phase II. These refer to the natural two-step process the liver conducts to rid the body of toxins. During Phase I, the liver converts toxic compounds

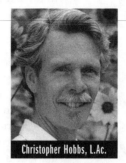

Christopher Hobbs, L.Ac.

"I have taken liver flushes for many years now and can heartily recommend them," says Christopher Hobbs, L.Ac. "I have never seen anyone experience negative side effects from this procedure."

into intermediate toxins. In Phase II, the liver converts these intermediate toxins into substances that can be eliminated from the body, delivering them to the colon (via the gallbladder) or bladder for excretion.

Christopher Hobbs, L.Ac., and Foundations of Health, *Healing With Herbs & Foods* (1994), Botanica Press. Available from: Interweave Press, Inc., 201 East Fourth Street, Loveland, CO 80537; tel: 970-669-7672; fax: 970-667-8317.

Seven Steps to Promote Detoxification

William Lee Cowden, M.D., of the Conservative Medicine Institute in Richardson, Texas, and coauthor of *An Alternative Medicine Definitive Guide to Cancer*, suggests the following seven steps that anyone can adopt to assist their body in eliminating toxins and to promote immune and digestive health:

1. Make Dietary Changes. Start eating a diet that is high in fiber and fresh raw vegetables and fruits, and very low in mucus-producing foods. It would be preferable to completely stop eating all milk products from cows and all refined white flour products, such as pastas, breads, and baked goods. At least for the duration of this program, it is also advisable to reduce your intake of sugar, eggs, meats, fowl, most fish, nuts, seeds, and unsprouted beans and grains.

2. Reduce Your Stress Load. Practice stress-reduction techniques before each meal. These might include muscle relaxation, deep breathing, or the visualization of a favorite natural setting. Listening to a stress-reduction audiotape before the meal can be helpful. It is also advisable to eat in a calm, pleasant environment, either by yourself or with a companion whose presence does not produce stress or discomfort in you.

3. Practice Lymphatic Drainage. It is important to take steps to clean out your lymphatic system, especially the lymph vessels that attach

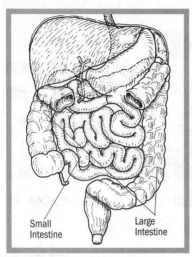

The small and large intestines

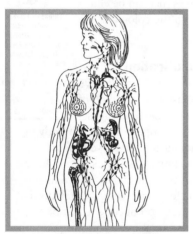

Lymph nodes are clusters of immune tissue that work as filters or "inspection stations" for detecting foreign and potentially harmful substances in the lymph fluid. Acting like spongy filter bags, lymph nodes are part of the lymphatic system, which is the body's master drain. While the body has many dozens of lymph nodes, they are mostly clustered in the neck, armpits, chest, groin, and abdomen. Lymph fluid (1-2 quarts) accounts for 1% to 3% of body weight. Exercise can increase lymph flow by 15 times.

to the intestines. You can do this by gently bouncing on a mini-trampoline or rebounder for five to 15 minutes once daily. This will stimulate the numerous lymph nodes in your neck, chest, and groin to start draining toxins into the bloodstream for removal from the body.

4. Brush Your Skin. In the early morning, soon after you get up, take a wooden brush with stiff natural bristles and lightly brush your skin. Move the brush across the skin toward the center end of each collarbone, as important lymph drainage sites are located here. Spend eight to ten minutes dry brushing your entire body. This procedure will mechanically aid your lymph system in its detoxification efforts. Do the dry brushing before taking a bath, but be aware that skin brushing just before bedtime can make it difficult to fall asleep.

5. Do Ozonated Bathing. Many of the toxins that build up in the body are fat soluble and gather in the fatty tissues. If you immerse yourself in a tub of warm ozonated water for 30 minutes once daily for two to three weeks this will aid in removal of the toxins from your body. Ozone (SEE QUICK DEFINITION) purifies the bath water by killing living viruses, bacteria, fungi, and parasites. It will also oxidize the water-insoluble toxins on the skin, turning them into water-soluble toxins. Once water soluble, they may be flushed from the system.

Here's how to do it. Purify the

tapwater by running it through a KDF solid charcoal showerhead filter as you fill the tub. A KDF solid charcoal showerhead filter can remove up to 99% of the toxic substances found in tap water. Next, bubble ozone (O_3, a form of oxygen) into the water using an ultraviolet ozone generator and an ozone-diffusing bath bubbler.

Do not use an electric spark ozonating system because this produces more nitrates and other harmful chemical substances. This converts the ozone that is accumulating in the air above the bubbling water back into oxygen so that it is not irritating to the lungs. During the 30-minute soak, scrub your entire skin surface three times with a loofa sponge or natural fiber brush. Bubble the ozone for 15 minutes before you get into the tub and also during your 30-minute soak.

Adding to your bath water ½ cup of Body Soak Gold, increasing this amount to one cup over two to three weeks; this will usually produce a faster removal of toxins from the body than ozonated water alone. After you have used one full bottle of Body Soak Gold, you may gain additional detoxification benefit by switching to ¼ cup of Liquid Needles Foot Soak added to the bath water; over a period of several days, increase this amount to one cup for each 30-minute bath. Best results are obtained if both Soaks are added to KDF charcoal-filtered water. As a variation on skin brushing, use a loofa sponge to brush your skin.

QUICK DEFINITION

Ozone (o_3) is a less stable, more reactive form of oxygen, containing three oxygen atoms. This extra atom enables ozone to more readily oxidize other chemicals. In oxidation, the extra oxygen atom breaks off, leaving ordinary oxygen (o_2), thereby favorably increasing the oxygen content of body tissues or blood. Ozone is a commonly occurring natural substance. Medical-grade ozone is used as part of oxygen therapy to increase local oxygen supply to lesions, to speed wound healing, to reduce infections, and stimulate metabolic processes. Ozone may be administered intravenously, by injection, or applied topically as a gas or dissolved in water or olive oil; it may also be taken orally or rectally as ozonated water.

6. Fortify Yourself With Nutrients. It is important to take at least 400 IU of vitamin E, 25,000 IU of beta carotene and/or mixed carotenoids, 2,000 mg of vitamin C, and 100 mg of grape seed extract (pycnogenol) either 30-40 minutes before your ozonated bath or 10-15 minutes after it.

7. Use Special Supplements. Take one lozenge of superoxide dismutase (SOD) and 100 mg of L-glutathione powder. Dissolve both substances under your tongue before each bath; this enables them to be absorbed faster and more completely. These nutrients will facilitate toxin removal from your system. SOD is an antioxidant enzyme that protects the system against free-radical damage from chemicals or radiation. L-glutathione is a sulfur-containing peptide (made of amino acids, which are protein building blocks) and antioxidant essential to the body's toxic waste disposal system.

A Five-Month Intestinal Detoxification Program

Dr. Cowden often recommends a five-month gentle detoxification program. Here, you are required to maintain a diet low in foods known to produce mucus while taking herbs and fiber that help to break up the intestine's mucoid lining. This program, which takes three to five months to clean out the intestine's false lining (mucoid plaque), is effective for people with allergies, irritable bowel syndrome, yeast and fungal overgrowth, parasitic infection, severe liver or kidney disease, or for anyone seeking an improved state of health.

Preliminaries—Begin a low-mucus-forming diet and practice dry skin brushing once daily for the first three months, then decrease to twice weekly.

Herbal Fiber—Take an herbal fiber product as a bowel-bulking agent two times daily at first, building up to 3-4 times daily after one week. Dr. Cowden developed the NatureSpring Friendly Flora and Fiber formula specifically for this purpose. This product may be taken daily for maintenance after the three- to five-month cleanse.

Along with this formula, start taking an herbal product called NatureSpring Intestinal Cleanse at the rate of one capsule twice daily, building up gradually to 1-2 tablets taken 3-4 times daily. The goal is to have 2-3 bowel motions daily. The herbs—slippery elm, cascara sagrada, papain, cayenne, and ginger—will help to break down the mucoid lining of the intestines and stimulate the intestines to push toxic feces out. Some may find this product unnecessary, and most should taper off after 4-5 weeks.

⚠CAUTION⚠

All protocols are for adult dosage only and are generalized; that is, dosages and conditions will vary with the individual. Listen to your body; build up the dosage slowly and carefully and only go at a rate you can tolerate. Before beginning any treatment, consult a qualified health-care professional. This is especially important if you are pregnant or nursing children.

Mucoid Remover—On the third day, add NatureSpring Bowel, Blood and Body Cleansing Formula starting with ½-1 tablet, two times daily; build gradually to three tablets taken 3-4 times daily. This formula has 30 ingredients that break down the mucoid lining, cleanse the blood, drain the lymphatics, and stabilize the function of various organ systems. Based on transient symptoms that you notice once you begin this program—toxin release, frequency and size of bowel movements—you, the user, are able to decide the rate of advancement in terms of dosage. Be sure to drink copious amounts of pure water (nonchlorinated, nondistilled) while on this program.

Additional Internal Cleansing Programs

In addition to the commercial products mentioned above, there are several others available over the counter, enabling anyone to start a self-care detoxification program to cleanse not only the intestines, but other organs as well. However, people with CFS are cautioned to do so only under the guidance of a physician.

A.M./P.M. Ultimate Cleanse™–"When was the last time you cleaned your liver, your heart, your lungs, or your body's sewage system?" asks nutritionist Lindsey Duncan, C.N., chief nutritionist for Home Nutrition Clinic in Santa Monica, California. Duncan offers a practical way to accomplish this, using a series of inner detoxification products, including Super Cleanse™, Ultimate Fiber™, and A.M./P.M. Ultimate Cleanse™.

The A.M./P.M. Ultimate Cleanse program is set up as a two-part vegetarian detoxification formula. It involves 29 cleansing herbs, amino acids, antioxidants, digestive enzymes, vitamins, and minerals, and five kinds of fiber. Both Multi-Herb™ and Multi-Fiber™ formulas (components in the program) are taken in the morning and evening, in gradually increasing dosages, for several weeks. Positive signs that the detoxification program is working include flu-like sensations, runny nose, transient pimples, headaches, "brainfog," or fatigue, all of which will pass in one or two days.

"The goal is to stimulate, feed, and detoxify the complete internal body, not just the bowel," states Duncan. "My objective was to address all five channels of elimination, as well as all of the vital organs and tissues in the body." By the end of the program, a person should be having two to three bowel movements every day.

Once the internal system is cleaned out, nutrient absorption can proceed much more efficiently. The key to the effectiveness of the Ultimate Multi™ formula, Duncan explains, is the timing: the morning formula stimulates, the evening formula relaxes. Following your body's natural digestive and cleansing cycles is the key to proper detoxification and supplementation, says Duncan.

For information on **Dr. Cowden's cancer protocol**, see *An Alternative Medicine Definitive Guide to Cancer* (Future Medicine Publishing, 1997; ISBN 1-887299-01-7); to order, call 800-333-HEAL.

For information and sources of **NatureSpring** products and other products mentioned by Dr. Cowden, contact: Health Restoration Systems, Inc., P.O. Box 832267, Richardson, TX 75083-2267; tel: 972-480-8909; fax: 972-480-8807. HRS offers a six-day residential educational/ detoxification intensive program with professional medical supervision in Dallas, Texas. This program is helpful for people with chemical toxin overload or cancer that is rapidly spreading and for women with silicone implant toxicity. **Body Soak Gold** (containing water, sea minerals, and glycerin) and **Liquid Needles Foot Soak** (containing electrolytes from mineral particles in a clear solution) are also available from HRS. For a source of **SOD** as Opti-Guard™ (Antioxidant/S.O.D. Enzyme Enhancer), contact: Optimal Nutrients, 1163 Chess Drive, Suite F, Foster City, CA 94404; tel: 415-525-0112 or 800-966-8874; fax: 415-349-1686.

For more information about **A.M./P.M. Ultimate Cleanse™**, contact: Nature's Secret, 4 Health, Inc., 5485 Conestoga Court, Boulder, CO 80301; tel: 303-546-6306; fax: 303-546-6416. For more information about **Nature's Pure Body Program™**, contact: Pure Body Institute of Beverly Hills, 423 East Ojai Avenue, #107, Ojai, CA 93023; tel: 800-952-7873 or 805-653-5448; fax: 805-653-0373.

Nature's Pure Body Program™—Another inner cleansing herbal formula is called Nature's Pure Body Program™ made by Pure Body Institute of Beverly Hills, California. The program is a blend of 27 herbs specifically chosen for their ability to flush toxins out of the organs and old fecal matter from the intestines. For example, buckthorn bark stimulates bile secretion; chickweed and black cohosh root combat blood toxicity; *Cascara sagrada* bark promotes intestinal peristalsis (the intestine's natural contraction rhythms); yarrow flower regulates liver function; peach leaves are a natural laxative; and licorice root stimulates the adrenal glands.

The program consists of two sets of pills: colon and whole-body blends. Users start with one colon and three whole-body pills taken twice daily with water, 30 minutes before breakfast and 30 minutes before dinner. The colon pills can be increased to three pills twice daily, or more, until the bowels move twice daily; the whole-body pills are increased to 4-7, taken two times daily. Users need to double their intake of pure water (to at least 64 ounces daily), take one day off from the pills every week, and take a daily multivitamin.

The key here is to go slowly and be patient. The program is designed to last about 30 days, although first-time users may find that three courses are required for complete inner cleansing and detoxification. Even if you consider yourself healthy, given the degree of toxins in our outer and inner environments, an inner cleansing can be beneficial for everyone. "When poor diet, stress, or lack of exercise tax the body beyond its natural abilities to digest, absorb, and eliminate wastes, it is time for a general, internal 'house-cleaning,'" says company president, Ken Wright.

Cleanse Thyself™: The Arise & Shine Program—One of the cardinal principles of alternative medicine is that a healthy colon is the key to lasting wellness and vitality. It's not hard to see why when you consider the fact that the small and large intestine together comprise about 25 feet of internal storage space in the body.

While food is meant to pass through the colon in about 14 hours (called "transit time"), poor diet, lack of fiber intake, stress, excessive antibiotics, and other factors can slow matter to almost a standstill, allowing only a small portion of waste matter to be actually eliminated from the body. It may be shocking to know that autopsies have found 20-30 pounds of old fecal matter still lodged in the myriad intricate folds of the small and large intestine.

Fecal matter that remains for long term storage in the colon becomes the seedbed for many illnesses, and this is why periodic colon cleansing is widely recommended by alternative health practitioners, including naturopath Richard Anderson, N.D., N.M.D. In 1986, he introduced the Cleanse Thyself self-care colon cleansing program. The program enables you to "clean your entire alimentary canal from your tongue to your stomach, to your organs, all the way down to your colon," says Dr. Anderson, whose Arise & Shine company, makers of Cleanse Thyself, is based in Mt. Shasta, California.

How the Colon Gets Clogged and Toxic. One of the prime places to see the effects of inappropriate choices in diet over the years is in the state of the colon. Many people continually eat high levels of acid-forming foods such as sugars, processed grains, eggs, and meat, says Dr. Anderson.

These foods deplete the body of electrolytes (SEE QUICK DEFINITION) which in turn make the bile, the intestinal fluid that helps digestion, more acidic. Bile that is acidic cannot digest food normally, and this causes the buildup of mucoid plaque, an abnormal fecal substance, on the inner wall of the intestines. This plaque (also known as false mucoid lining) can diminish digestive performance and cause a buildup of toxins in the intestines and liver. The process then feeds on itself, as the formation of plaque further inhibits normal digestion, and this causes toxins and disease-causing organisms to be absorbed by the body through the intestines rather than eliminated.

As digestion becomes less efficient, the body is not able to produce sufficient amounts of helpful substances needed for functioning, and this leads to still higher levels of toxins in the bowel, explains Dr. Anderson. Liver function becomes compromised, no longer efficiently filtering out toxins, and the body's immune defenses are taxed by this toxic overload and become less competent at resisting illness.

There is a psychological dimension to colon toxicity, too, says Dr. Anderson. Negativity and heavy emotions get "stuck" in the body, as if anchored by the old mass in the intestines. The result can be the propagation of outmoded feelings, attitudes, and thoughts—"negative thought patterns," says Dr. Anderson—all of which can negatively influence one's health. "If we do not cleanse our bowels and

Electrolytes are substances in the blood, tissue fluids, intracellular fluids, or urine which conduct an electrical charge, either plus or minus. Examples include acids, bases, and salts, such as potassium, magnesium, phosphate, sulfate, bicarbonate, sodium, chloride, and calcium. Electrolytes provide inorganic chemicals for cellular reactions and control mechanisms such as the conduction of electrochemical impulses to nerves and muscles. Electrolytes are also needed for key enzymatic reactions involved in metabolism, or the release of energy from food.

Negativity and heavy emotions get "stuck" in the body, as if anchored by the old mass in the intestines. The result can be the propagation of outmoded feelings, attitudes, and thoughts—"negative thought patterns," says Dr. Anderson—all of which can negatively influence one's health.

replenish the electrolyte reserves, our body's ability to heal itself is greatly diminished."

Cleaning Out Your System. The Cleanse Thyself program will impress many as a well-considered approach, embodying the principles of naturopathic detoxification. Dr. Anderson recommends that the prospective user first test both saliva and urine for pH balance using pH tester papers included in the kit. pH is the degree of acidity and alkalinity of a solution, measured on a scale of one (acidic) to 14 (alkaline).

The results of the pH test, which indicate your body's electrolyte levels, determine what level of the Cleanse Thyself program should be used, from the Mildest Phase to the Master Phase. More specifically, the Mildest Phase of the Cleanse Thyself Program is designed for those whose bodies are weaker, chronically or severely ill, or elderly enough that they need a very gentle approach to cleansing, Dr. Anderson explains.

"Persons who use the mildest phase generally show a severely over-acidic condition prior to preparing for cleansing. For such a person, the first step before beginning to cleanse must be to begin to alkalinize so that the body has enough resources to handle cleansing in a positive manner." The Master Phase of the cleanse involves fasting from solid foods while taking the supplements along with fresh juices. "The Master Phase should only be attempted by persons whose bodies have already attained an adequate reservoir of electrolytes and strength to handle this powerful level of cleansing," says Dr. Anderson.

For example, those starting on the Mildest Phase should have a breakfast that consists of fresh fruit, while their lunch and dinner should emphasize alkaline-forming foods, such as salad greens, raw vegetables, potatoes, and more fresh fruits. The user on this phase also consumes two Cleanse Thyself Shakes, consisting of liquid bentonite (a purifying clay), psyllium husk powder (a fibrous bulking agent), and pure water. The Mildest Phase is well-suited both for people who can't take the time off from work for a more demanding clean-out and for those who are too toxic and weak to handle a stronger regimen, says Dr. Anderson.

To soften and break up toxic waste material while detoxifying cells, the program provides two customized elements, called Chomper and Herbal Nutrition. Chomper is an herbal laxative (in tablet form) containing plantain, *Cascara sagrada*, barberry, peppermint, sheep sorrel, fennel seed, ginger root, myrrh gum, red raspberry, rhubarb root, goldenseal, and lobelia.

Herbal Nutrition is a vitamin supplement (containing alfalfa, dandelion, shavegrass, chickweed, marshmallow root, yellow dock, rosehips, hawthorne, licorice root, Irish moss, kelp, amylase, and cellulase) that helps strengthen and nourish the body during the detoxification process. Both Chomper and Herbal Nutrition are taken daily, says Dr. Anderson.

Each successive stage in the Cleanse Thyself program involves stricter dietary controls, a higher intake of program supplements, and a correspondingly deeper cleansing. Typically, the overall cleansing program takes four weeks, in which three are devoted to the Pre-Cleanse, and one week to the Power or Master Phase. The Pre-Cleanse is essential, Dr. Anderson says, because it allows the herbs enough time to prepare the mucoid plaque for removal and to start neutralizing stored intestinal toxins such as pesticides, drugs, and heavy metals.

> **QUICK DEFINITION**
>
> The term **pH**, which means "potential hydrogen," represents a scale for the relative acidity or alkalinity of a solution. Acidity is measured as a pH of 0.1 to 6.9, alkalinity is 7.1 to 14, and neutral pH is 7.0. The numbers refer to how many hydrogen atoms are present compared to an ideal or standard solution. Normally, blood is slightly alkaline, at 7.35 to 7.45; urine pH can range from 4.8 to 7.5, although normal is closer to 7.0.

Fecal matter that remains for long term storage in the colon becomes the seedbed for many illnesses, and this is why periodic colon cleansing is widely recommended by alternative health practitioners.

Mucoid plaque tends to be anywhere from $1/64$ to one inch thick, with a texture from stiff and hard to soft, flexible, or gooey. It is often blackish green in color and somewhat resembles rubber or leather, says Dr. Anderson. It is the strange product of many years of inappropriate diet, malabsorption, and colonic stagnation. "It is not uncommon for pieces to come out more than 2-4 feet long, but the average is 6-18 inches," Dr. Anderson says. Based on figures obtained from customer testimonials, out of a total user base of about 70,000 people, Dr. Anderson estimates that about 95% of the program's users have eliminated mucoid plaque.

For more information about the **Cleanse Thyself™ program**, contact: Richard Anderson, N.D., N.M.D., Arise & Shine, 401 Berry Street, P.O. Box 1439, Mt. Shasta, CA 96067; tel: 916-926-0891 or 800-688-2444; fax: 916-926-8866.

It is common to have physical reactions to the detoxification process, such as headaches, vomiting, diarrhea, fatigue, or dizziness, says Dr. Anderson. For all the discomfort, this is actually a sign that the process is working and that you are eliminating toxins from your body. If these symptoms occur, don't move on to either of the higher phases before your body has a chance to recover, cautions Dr. Anderson. He recommends that users wait to progress to the next phase until they have been without these symptoms for at least three days.

Intensifying the Detoxification. The Gentle Phase, also called Pre-Cleanse, is the step most commonly used, says Dr. Anderson. Even if you are continuing with the other two phases (Power and Master), Dr. Anderson recommends staying on this phase for at least one week and up to three weeks to prepare your system for the more demanding cleansing ahead.

"What took months, years, or a lifetime to create cannot be cleaned up in a week's time," he says. This phase prepares the mucoid plaque in the intestine for removal and reduces the stress on your liver by giving it time to process more waste.

The second step, called Power Phase, is appropriate only for those who have completed the Pre-Cleanse, cautions Dr. Anderson. Here "you are likely to remove many feet of toxic mucoid plaque and pounds of toxic waste." In this stage, a new component called Flora Grow is added to replenish beneficial intestinal bacteria depleted by antibiotics and years of poor eating habits, says Dr. Anderson.

The third step, called Master Phase, produces the most powerful detoxification. No meals are allowed in this phase, but it includes five Cleanse Thyself Shakes, five doses of Chomper and Herbal Nutrition, one dose of Flora Grow, and an enema twice daily. If you have cleansing reactions when starting this phase, you are not ready to begin the Master Phase and should go back to the Gentle Phase, Dr. Anderson cautions.

"As you begin to cleanse your digestive system, other parts of your body will respond as well," says Dr. Anderson. "You'll not only rid yourself of toxic, pathogenic waste, you'll also release toxic feelings and emotions." A common refrain from users new to colon cleansing is "I eliminated more than I ever thought I had in me." According to a testimonial from a user in Australia, "The main improvements I have noticed are energy levels, vision, hair, skin, mental attitude, ability to cope with stress situations—generally I'm a much happier and healthier person." Other benefits cited by users include cessation of menstrual pain, migraines, and joint pain, fewer colds, resolution of lifelong sinus congestion, itching, ulcers, and a breast cyst, weight loss, and better concentration, among many others.

Probiotics for the Intestines—The human body contains an estimated several trillion beneficial bacteria comprising over 400 species, all necessary for health. Many of these "friendly" bacteria, also called probiotics, reside in the intestines where they are essential for proper nutrient assimilation. Among the more well-known of these are *Lactobacillus acidophilus* and *Bifidobacterium bifidium.*

Prior to 1945 and the introduction of mass market foods and chemicalized agriculture, Westerners normally obtained adequate amounts of probiotics from fresh vegetables. Friendly bacteria are actually soil-based organisms which are incorporated into plants and then eaten by humans. However, overly acidic bodily conditions, chronic constipation or diarrhea, dietary imbalances, consumption of overly processed foods, and the excessive use of antibiotics and hormonal drugs can interfere with probiotic function and even reduce the number of these. When the body's probiotic population drops, conditions are set for illness, unless steps are taken to replenish them.

Life Science Products of St. George, Utah, took steps in this direction when they developed Nature's Biotics™, a blend of 61 nutrients, including at least six selectively bred strains of soil-based probiotic organisms. In addition, the supplement contains amino acids, phytoplanktons, plant pigments and enzymes, minerals, trace elements, essential fatty acids, and starches.

Once the mixture makes contact with water, the friendly bacteria become active in the stomach. The intent is to "steer your digestive system toward proper absorption, thereby increasing your body's ability to stay healthy from the inside," says David Doudart, company president. According to Doudart, the product helps to remove waste, debris, and toxins from the intestines; it improves digestion and assimilation; it works against harmful molds, yeasts, fungi, and viruses; and it stimulates the immune system which in turn releases more B lymphocytes.

During the first week of using Nature's Biotics, it's advisable to take one capsule 30 minutes before the evening meal with 10 ounces of pure water. Then during the second week, Doudart recommends taking one capsule 30 minutes before lunch and dinner; during the third week, this pattern is continued and a capsule is taken before breakfast. In general, probiotic supplements are useful both for maintaining good health and for gaining improvement from chronic health conditions such as acne, skin problems, allergies, arthritis, high cholesterol, yeast infections and intestinal disturbances.

In fact, researchers at the University of Washington School of Medicine recently reported that microorganisms

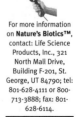

For more information on **Nature's Biotics™**, contact: Life Science Products, Inc., 321 North Mall Drive, Building F-201, St. George, UT 84790; tel: 801-628-4111 or 800-713-3888; fax: 801-628-6114.

Overly acidic bodily conditions, chronic constipation or diarrhea, dietary imbalances, consumption of overly processed foods, and the excessive use of antibiotics and hormonal drugs can interfere with probiotic function and even reduce the number of these.

with therapeutic properties (probiotics) can be used successfully to treat and prevent selected vaginal, urinary tract, and intestinal infections, such as diarrhea associated with antibiotics, infantile diarrhea, and candidiasis. Probiotics, formerly a "neglected" modality, now "may offer an alternative to conventional antimicrobials to which many pathogenic microorganisms eventually develop resistance," stated Gary W. Elmer, Ph.D., author of the research report.[3]

FOS: Health Food for Friendly Bacteria—Alternative medicine physicians have long recognized the benefit of supplementing with "friendly" bacteria, or probiotics, to restore the balance of flora in the intestines and thus promote intestinal health. Probiotics are especially important after an intestinal detoxification program. A new approach to restoring the balance of intestinal flora was developed in Japan in the mid-1980s.

Called prebiotics, it involves introducing nutrients that directly feed the beneficial bacteria already in place in a person's large intestine, most typically, *Bifidobacteria* and *Lactobacilli*. Japanese researchers determined that a naturally occurring form of carbohydrate, called fructo-oligosaccharides (FOS), found in certain foods in minute amounts, could be a perfect food for *Bifidobacteria*.

FOS acts like an intestinal "fertilizer," selectively feeding the friendly microflora in the large intestine so that their numbers can usefully increase. *Bifidobacteria* work to lower the pH (SEE QUICK DEFINITION) in the large intestine to a slightly more acidic condition; this discourages the growth of unfriendly bacteria. Feeding the friendly bacteria is a crucial step in maintaining the correct balance of intestinal microflora; when they are out of balance, a condition called dysbiosis (SEE QUICK DEFINITION), intestinal function is compromised.

Studies have demonstrated that taking ¼ teaspoon (1 g) of NutraFlora® FOS powder daily for four weeks led to a five-fold increase in the total count of beneficial bacteria. A Japanese study found that when 23 hospital patients, 50-90 years old, took 8 g of FOS daily for two weeks, their *Bifidobacteria* levels increased by ten times. Benefits from increasing *Bifidobacteria* levels include relief of constipation or diarrhea, promotion of regularity, serum cholesterol reduction, control of blood sugar levels, immune function enhancement, improved calcium absorption and B vitamin synthesis, better digestability of milk proteins, and a reduction of the detoxification load on the liver, among others.

NutraFlora contains 95% pure FOS, in dry powder form or as a syrup, to be used as a dietary supplement. While FOS is found in garlic, honey, Jerusalem artichokes, soybeans, burdock, chicory root, asparagus, banana, rye, barley, tomato, onion, and triticale, according to nutrition expert Robert Crayhon, M.S., C.N., "There is not enough FOS in foods in the average diet to get an optimal or therapeutically significant dose."

Technically, you would have to eat 429 garlic cloves to get the same amount of FOS in one teaspoon of NutraFlora powder. That's why FOS is synthesized using a natural process that optimizes the yield. Recognizing this, in Japan today over 500 commercially prepared foods contain FOS (known there as "neosugar"), with the endorsement of Japan's Minister of Health. FOS, which is made by fermenting sucrose with a fungus called *Aspergillus niger* (*Aspergillus oryzae* is used to make miso and soy sauce), is about 30% as sweet as sucrose.[4]

Toxicity and the Health of the Cells

Francine, 10, was diagnosed with a mysterious, severe neurological disorder. She was tired all the time, had chronic muscle pains, couldn't walk or stand easily, and wasn't able to concentrate at school. For convenience, her doctors called it fibromyalgia. They gave Francine antibiotics to treat bacteria that they discovered in her system, but this was not the cause, says Thomas Rau, M.D., director of the Paracelsus Clinic in Lustmühle, Switzerland. "It was only a secondary infection which the antibiotics made worse." Soon she developed colitis and was eventually brought to Paracelsus by ambulance.

QUICK DEFINITION

Intestinal dysbiosis refers to an imbalance of intestinal flora. Specifically, these flora are friendly, beneficial bacteria, called probiotics, such as *Lactobacillus acidophilus* and *Bifidobacterium bifidum*, and unfriendly bacteria in the intestines such as *Escherichia coli* and *Clostridium perfringens*. In dysbiosis, the unfriendly bacteria predominate; they begin fermentation producing toxic by-products such as ammonia, amines, nitrosamines, phenols, cresols, indole, and skatole, which interfere with the normal elimination cycle. Dysbiosis is considered a primary cause or major cofactor in the development of many health problems, such as acne, yeast overgrowth, chronic fatigue, depression, digestive disorders, bloating, food allergies, PMS, rheumatoid arthritis, and cancer.

For more about **detoxification methods**, see Chapter 9: Addressing the Allergy Connection, pp. 232-258.

For more information about **FOS** and **NutraFlora®**, contact: GTC Nutrition Company, 1400 West 122nd Avenue, Suite 110, Westminster, CO 80234; tel: 303-254-8012; fax: 303-254-8201.

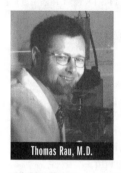

Thomas Rau, M.D.

"This is biological thinking," says Dr. Thomas Rau. "Bacteria, viruses, or fungi can only change form and flourish if they have the suitable cellular conditions. They develop from *within* the organism; they do not invade it from without."

To contact **Thomas Rau, M.D.**: Paracelsus Clinic, CH-9062, Lustmuhle bei St. Gallen, Switzerland; tel: 41-713-357171; fax: 41-713-357100.

Oxidation-reduction refers to a basic chemical mechanism in the cell by which energy is produced from foods. Electrons (negatively charged particles in an atom) are removed from one atom, resulting in "oxidation" of this first atom, and then are added or transferred to another atom, resulting in "reduction" of this second atom. The molecules that give up their electrons are referred to as oxidized; the molecules that accept electrons are referred to as oxidants. This continual process of energy metabolism is actually a flow of electrons, or a minute electrical current within the cell.

There, she was helped by an approach called biological medicine, which involves looking at the condition of the body's cells. This information will lead you to understand why the body is sick. When cells become imbalanced, conditions are set for infection, illness, or chronic disease to begin; when cells are rebalanced, conditions are set for healing and a return to health. "As we see it, sickness is not caused by bacteria, but the bacteria come with the sickness," Dr. Rau says. "This is biological thinking. Bacteria, viruses, or fungi can only change form and flourish if they have the suitable cellular conditions. They develop from *within* the organism; they do not invade it from without."

Correcting the cellular imbalance is at the core of biological medicine, a concept founded by the Clinic's namesake, Paracelsus, a 16th-century alchemist, physician, and medical troublemaker. The idea is that knowing the biochemistry of the cells—the pH balance of acidity and alkalinity, the oxidation-reduction (SEE QUICK DEFINITION) potential—is of paramount importance to the physician's treatment plan. Biochemical changes can be the result of outside influences, such as faulty diet, inadequate nutrition, chemical or heavy metal exposure, chronic organ toxicity, stress, or trauma.

As the first stage in Francine's treatment, Dr. Rau put her on a detoxification program to flush the toxins, including mercury, out of her body. He used a combination of DMPS (SEE QUICK DEFINITION) and sodium bicarbonate infusions (an alkalinizing preparation) to remove mercury from Francine's body and to reduce the extreme acidity of her cells. Although her blood pH was 7.38 and thus alkaline, Francine's urine had a pH fluctuating between 4.0 and 5.0, which is very acidic. The pH norm for urine is about 6.8, says Dr. Rau.

In addition, Dr. Rau's team gave Francine daily intravenous infusions of vitamins B, C, and E, plus magnesium and other trace elements. They prescribed a specific diet and administered both homeopathic and Enderlein (SANUM—SEE QUICK DEFINITION) remedies, all in an effort to improve the acid-base conditions of her cells. After about three weeks on this program, Francine was able to walk and speak normally again. After four weeks, she was able to ride a bicycle; and six months after beginning treatment, she was in school again as a normal, healthy child, after having been seriously ill for 18 months prior to seeing Dr. Rau.

Reversing neurological problems specific to children is a specialty at Paracelsus Clinic. Tourette's syndrome, attention deficit disorder, and hyperactivity often have a strong toxicity factor involved, says Dr. Rau. Frequently, aluminum toxicity is the cause. Poor nutrition, a diet based on highly processed foods, and sodas containing phosphoric acid lead to a deficiency in trace elements. This, in turn, upsets the cellular terrain, making it too acidic and enables aluminum to enter the tissues and wreak havoc. "Aluminum only gets into your body if the terrain is acid," says Dr. Rau. Once again, whether you're concerned with diagnosis or healing, the terrain is everything.

QUICK DEFINITION

DMPS (2,3-dimercapto-propane-1-sulfonate) is the chelating (binding-up) agent of choice for the removal of elemental mercury from the human body. It can be given orally, intravenously, or intramuscularly and is useful for people who have been exposed to mercury amalgam through their dental fillings or those who show evidence or suspicion of heavy metal toxicity from other sources.

SANUM remedies, developed by Guenther Enderlein, M.D., Ph.D. (1872-1968), are produced by SANUM-Kehlbeck GmbH & Co. KG, D-2812 Hoya, Germany. In the United States, contact: Pleomorphic Product Sales, Inc., 5160 W. Phelps Rd., #B, Glendale, AZ 85306; tel: 602-439-7977; fax: 602-439-7996. The line includes about 100 preparations of benign microorganisms or protein particles identified by pleomorphic practice. For example, "Mucokehl" is Mucor racemosus, a fungus that regulates microorganisms affecting the thickness of blood. These remedies injected around the tumor site, adjust the pH and cellular terrain and help the pathogenic microorganisms revert back to harmless forms. In effect, the SANUM remedies help the body restore the optimal cellular terrain for health.

CHAPTER

6

Reversing Hidden Thyroid Problems

A MAJOR AND OFTEN overlooked cause of chronic fatigue syndrome is an underactive thyroid gland (located in the neck), a condition known as hypothyroidism. Although, according to conventional medicine, hypothyroidism is a separate illness from CFS and a diagnosis of one precludes a diagnosis of the other, many people with CFS have not been properly tested for thyroid problems.

Putting each illness into its own category does not serve the interests of the patient. Since thyroid hormones are integral to maintaining optimal body energy levels and are required for proper immune system function and nearly all aspects of body function, hypothyroidism can be central among the multiple factors involved in creating CFS. If that is the case, successfully reversing the syndrome

> **Broda O. Barnes, M.D., Ph.D., stated that untreated thyroid problems are responsible for 64 common medical ailments suffered by about 40% of the population.**

will require discovering the hidden thyroid imbalance along with all the other contributing factors.

Knowledge of the importance of the thyroid to human health has been known by Western doctors since the 1950s, but most have chosen to ignore it. It was Broda O. Barnes, M.D., Ph.D., a pioneer in thyroid research and the author of 100 medical articles on this gland, who made the remarkable claim that was ignored by the medical establishment then and is still not sufficiently heeded today. Dr. Barnes stated that untreated thyroid problems are responsible for 64

The Thyroid Gland

The **thyroid gland**, the largest of the body's seven endocrine glands, is located just below the larynx in the throat and has interconnecting lobes on either side of the trachea. The thyroid is the body's metabolic thermostat, controlling body temperature, energy use, and, for children, the body's growth rate. The thyroid controls the rate at which organs function and the speed with which the body uses food; it affects the operation of all body processes and organs. Of the hormones synthesized in and released by the thyroid, T3 (tri-iodothyronine), represents 7%, and T4 (thyroxine), accounts for almost 93% of the thyroid's hormones active in all of the body's processes. Iodine is essential to forming normal amounts of thyroxine. The secretion of both these hormones is regulated by thyroid-stimulating hormone, or TSH, secreted by the pituitary gland in the brain. The thyroid also secretes calcitonin, a hormone required for calcium metabolism.

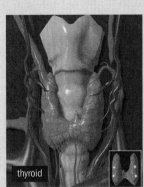

thyroid

Hypothyroidism is a condition of low or underactive thyroid gland function that can produce numerous symptoms. Among the 47 clinically recognized symptoms are: fatigue, depression, lethargy, weakness, weight gain, low body temperature, chills, cold extremities, general oversensitivity to cold, infertility, rheumatic pain, menstrual disorders (excessive flow, cramps), repeated infections, colds, upper respiratory infections, skin problems (itching, eczema, psoriasis, acne, dry, coarse, scaly skin, skin pallor), memory disturbances, concentration difficulties, paranoia, migraines, oversleep, "laziness," muscle aches and weakness, hearing disturbances, burning/prickling sensations, anemia, slow reaction time and mental sluggishness, swelling of the eyelids, constipation, labored difficult breathing, hoarseness, brittle nails, and poor vision.

common medical ailments suffered by about 40% of the population. Many alternative physicians agree with Dr. Barnes and believe that, given the increasing prevalence of chronic and degenerative illness, we need to pay more attention to Dr. Barnes' conclusions.

Thyroid problems may be on the rise due to the increasingly toxic environment in which we live. Radiation is probably the greatest environmental cause of hypothyroidism and other thyroid problems, including tumors and thyroid cancer, states Lita Lee, Ph.D., an enzyme therapist based in Lowell, Oregon, who frequently treats thyroid-generated problems. The incidence of childhood thyroid cancer has increased 100 times in those areas of Ukraine, Belarus, and Russia most acutely exposed to the Chernobyl nuclear accident in

April 1986, stated experts from the United Nations in November 1995. Childhood thyroid cancer is the fastest way in which the impact of radiation exposure shows up in the body.

Mercury toxicity can also produce hypothyroidism, according to Dr. Lee. This heavy metal, comprising up to 50% of mercury amalgam dental fillings (SEE QUICK DEFINITION), poisons an enzyme critical in converting the inactive form of the thyroid hormone, thyroxine (T4), into the active form, tri-iodothyronine (T3). Other thyroid inhibitors include fluoride (common in water, foods, and toothpaste); synthetic and genetically engineered hormones (such as estrogen) in meat, dairy products, poultry, and eggs; excess polyunsaturated fats such as soybean, safflower, canola, corn, and flaxseed oils; and excess iodine.

In this chapter, you will learn how hypothyroidism and other thyroid disorders can contribute to CFS and how they can be reversed with alternative medicine. In the following section, **Stephen E. Langer, M.D.**, of Berkeley, California, discusses the effects of thyroid dysfunction and relates two medical case histories, one of CFS and the other of Hashimoto's autoimmune thyroiditis (HAIT), which shares many of the symptoms of CFS:

The Thyroid and Chronic Fatigue

There is a hidden reason why chronic fatigue, muscle pain, depression, weight problems, and other conditions are so hard to diagnose. It's called the thyroid gland. The thyroid is the largest of the body's seven endocrine glands, and its role in all aspects of healthy body functioning is paramount, yet it is also probably the most overlooked factor in a great many health problems, from chronic fatigue to obesity, depression to skin problems.

Since I began medical practice in 1967, the single most important element in my approach has been attention to the thyroid gland and two hormones it secretes. The thyroid controls how fast energy is burned in every cell, a process called metabolic activity. The healthy functioning of the thyroid is central to everything else in the body and, as Dr. Barnes said, problems here can contribute to numerous medical conditions.

Yet the "cure" is surprisingly simple: nothing has so low a toxicity level and is as easy and inexpensive to use as thyroid hormone, correctly administered by a physician. There is much more room for therapeutic intervention with thyroid-based health conditions than with other glandular problems because, while the thyroid is central to so many body functions, hormonal adjustments can be made with minimal disturbance of the overall system.

To contact **Stephen Langer, M.D.:** 3011 Telegraph Avenue, Suite 230, Berkeley, CA 94705; tel: 510-548-7384. Dr. Langer is coauthor (with James F. Scheer) of *Solved: The Riddle of Illness* (New Canaan, CT: Keats Publishing, 1995).

The Whole Body Becomes Underactive

The list of thyroid-related health problems is long and disturbing [see sidebar: "The Thyroid Gland," p. 165]. When the thyroid is underactive, everything in the body gradually becomes hypoactive as well, from circulation to libido. But here's the problem: It's my estimation that a large number of clinically severe thyroid conditions go undetected for long periods of time and some, regrettably, are never picked up.

In addition, people are often erroneously treated for chronic health conditions that are really based on the thyroid and that would respond well and quickly to a small dose of thyroid hormone. For example, take skin problems. One of the first things the body does when the thyroid is underactive is reduce the blood supply to the skin to conserve energy. As a result, a person with this problem will perspire less, bacteria can flourish on the skin, and acne lesions can develop. If you aggressively treat the acne and ignore the thyroid, you won't see much permanent change.

As another example, consider depression. I treated a patient who had been depressed for 60 years; yet when he took thyroid hormone, his depression was gone within a month. Whatever his previous physicians prescribed focused on his depression but missed the underlying thyroid cause, so he was miserable for most of his lifetime. Incidentally, although medical research and statistics suggest that an underactive thyroid is more common in women, I contend there is as much underactive thyroid and thyroiditis (inflamed thyroid) in men as in women.

Success Story:
Reversing Ten Years of Hypothyroidism

When Frank, 47, first came to my office, he had near total body failure—in other words, he was almost permanently bedridden. He had chronic fatigue, intermittent headaches, light sensitivity, multiple chemical sensitivities, heart palpitations, mood swings, and anxiety

"There is a hidden reason why chronic fatigue, muscle pain, depression, weight problems, and other conditions are so hard to diagnose. It's called the thyroid gland," says Stephen Langer, M.D.

fluctuating with depression. Frank was cold all the time, his appetite was poor, his mental abilities were sluggish, and he'd been sick for most of the previous ten years. He was also on prescription antidepressants.

I ordered standard laboratory tests for Frank's thyroid function, to evaluate the status of his T3, T4, TSH, and FTI (free thyroxine index, to see how much thyroxine was actually active). Some physicians only look at T4 levels. Taken alone, this is pointless. TSH is the most sensitive indicator of thyroid function, but the whole thyroid panel should be run. Of the four, Frank's TSH levels were elevated; the normal range is 0.35 to 5.5, but his was 10.6. Any elevation of TSH means the thyroid gland is failing functionally, because it has had to compensate in order to sustain the body's multiple functions.

Frank started taking a quarter of a grain daily of natural thyroid hormone derived from animals. Over the next three months, I gradually increased the dosage to almost two grains per day. My preference was to run a series of allergy sensitivity tests, but Frank's budget didn't allow for this. As a way of working around this, he began a low-fat diet that was high in complex carbohydrates and low in "glycemic" foods, which means foods whose carbohydrate (or simple sugar) composition is absorbed too rapidly into the bloodstream.

Frank tracked his diet to see which foods provoked problems, and identified wheat, corn, and dairy as allergenic foods to be eliminated. In addition, he took a high-potency multivitamin/mineral supplement and about 1,000 mg total of the essential fatty acids omega-3 and omega-6 (SEE QUICK DEFINITION). These were in the form of gamma linolenic acid (GLA) from borage oil (240 mg, twice daily) and eicosapentaenoic acid (EPA; 240 mg, twice daily). Frank also took daily doses of Ester C (a form of vitamin C; 500 mg), calcium (125 mg), and magnesium (65 mg). I increased his dietary protein intake so that more amino acids (the building blocks of proteins) would be available to his brain where

The Thyroid and Its Hormones

The thyroid has four principal hormones: T1, T2, T3, and T4. Thyroid hormones are stored in the thyroid and released to the body as needed. T1 (mono-iodothyronine) and T2 (di-iodothyronine) are not considered especially active. T4 (thyroxine) contains iodine, is produced exclusively in the thyroid gland, and accounts for almost 93% of the thyroid's hormones active in all of the body's processes; its chief function is to increase the speed of cell metabolism, or energy conversion.

Iodine and the amino acid tyrosine are essential to forming normal amounts of T4. When the body requires more T3 (tri-iodothyronine), T4 can give up its iodine to form T3 which, while representing only about 7% of the thyroid hormone complement, has a greater biological activity by a factor of three to four times. About 80% of the body's T3 comes from converting T4, typically in the liver and kidneys. When T4 conversion runs smoothly— that is, the enzyme cascade (sequencing of enzymes in chemical reactions) is correct—normal body temperature and metabolic rates are maintained.

If the thyroid is functioning poorly, however, T4 breaks down to form reverse tri-iodothyronine, or rT3 (a different chemical version of T3). Stress, fasting, illness, or elevated cortisol (from the adrenal glands) can contribute to the occurrence of this faulty conversion. As rT3 levels increase, metabolism and body temperature decrease, and various enzymes fail to function properly. In addition, as rT3 levels build, levels of T3 decrease, leading to low T3 syndrome, thyroid dysfunction, and a skewed ratio of T3 to rT3.

continued on next page

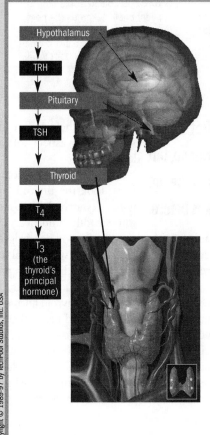

Hypothalamus

TRH

Pituitary

TSH

Thyroid

T$_4$

T$_3$
(the thyroid's principal hormone)

The Thyroid and Its Hormones (cont.)

This condition of elevated rT3 is known as Wilson's Syndrome.

Total blood levels of T3 and T4 consist of only 1% biologically active components (called the free levels), while 99% is the metabolically inactive portion bound to proteins. In a healthy person, total T4 levels as indicated in a blood test (or thyroid panel) are 4.5-12.5, but for someone with hypothyroidism (underactive thyroid), those values will be less than 4.5. For Free-T4, the normal range is 0.9-2; hypothyroid, less than 0.9. For Free-T3, normal is 80-220; hypothyroid, less than 80. TSH is normally 0.3-6; for hypothyroid, greater than 6.

The formation and secretion of T3 and T4 are regulated by a complex sequence of hormonal causes and effects, set off by the brain's hypothalamus gland. The hypothalamus secretes a substance called thyrotropin-releasing hormone (TRH), which in turn directs the pituitary gland to produce thyroid-stimulating hormone, or TSH (thyrotropin). Because TSH has a direct effect on the production of T4 and T3, TSH blood levels are conventionally taken as the best index for thyroid dysfunction, both hypo and hyper (overactive). When thyroid function is low, TSH levels normally go up.

Frank was a classic "basket case" before taking the thyroid hormone, but now he is a functional human being, doing a world better than he was before.

they could help offset the biochemical aspect of his depression.

Over the three months Frank took the thyroid hormone, I watched his condition steadily improve. His stamina, energy, digestion, muscular function, and mood got progressively better. All of his systems had been operating at suboptimal levels; restoring the correct level of thyroid hormone was like stoking the flames in all his cells.

Frank was a classic "basket case" before taking the thyroid hormone, but now he is a functional human being, doing a world better than he was before. He's able to fend for himself, prepare his own meals, and exercise regularly without being drugged to the eyeballs on conventional medications which gave him practically every side effect possible. In fact, Frank's mental processes improved so much with the thyroid hormone that he was able to stop taking all his prescription drugs.

Success Story:
Ending Three Years of Painful Thyroiditis

A second major health problem relating to an underactive thyroid is called Hashimoto's autoimmune thyroiditis, known as HAIT (SEE QUICK DEFINITION) or simply as thyroiditis. Here the thyroid gland is enlarged, though usually without pain. However, the autoimmune factor is involved because the body releases antibodies against its own thyroid as if it were a foreign object in the body.

HAIT seems to run in families, with most patients being between the ages of 13 and 40. Typical symptoms include fatigue, memory loss, depression, and a sense of nervousness that can range from mild anxiety to serious panic attack. You can also have allergies, irregular heartbeat or palpitations, muscle and joint pain, sleep disturbances in which you wake up with your mind racing and heart beating fast, reduced sexual interest, menstrual irregularities, headaches, digestive disorders, and intestinal problems from diarrhea to constipation. Also, you are likely to have the sensation of a lump in your throat; this is actually your inflamed, slightly swollen thyroid gland.

When I am confronted with this symptom picture, I routinely have the patient's thyroid antibodies (SEE QUICK DEFINITION) checked. For example, a person's thyroid hormone levels (such as T4) may be normal but their thyroid antibodies are elevated. Many physicians miss this; in my opinion, thyroid antibody tests should be run routinely on anyone with a chronic health problem. If a patient has a low elevation of thyroid antibodies, I will start this person on a low dose of thyroid hormone even if their thyroid hormone levels are supposedly normal. Let me explain this by presenting a case.

Theodora, 43, came to me with multiple symptoms. She had chronic fatigue, joint and muscle pain, headaches, insomnia, numerous infections, frequent sore throats, nasal congestion, and was always on the verge of having a cold. She also had intermittent heart palpitations, irregular periods, intestinal gas, indigestion, constipation, and diarrhea. Her muscle pain was so widespread she felt that every muscle in her body hurt.

Testing revealed that while her thyroid hormone levels were normal, her level of thyroid antibodies was sky-high. I started her on a low dose of thyroid hormone, at a ¼ of a grain (15 mg) per day, then gradually increased this to three grains over the next year. My HAIT patients often ask me if they must remain on thyroid hormone indef-

QUICK DEFINITION

Hashimoto's autoimmune thyroiditis (HAIT) is a disease in which the body releases antibodies that attack the thyroid gland as if it were a foreign enemy. Characterized by an enlarged thyroid, other symptoms of HAIT include deep fatigue, memory loss, depression, anxiety, digestive disorders, sleep disturbances, muscle and joint pain, and allergies, among others. HAIT strikes predominantly women between the ages of 13 and 40. Most sufferers gradually develop hypothyroidism.

An **antibody** is a protein molecule containing about 20,000 atoms, made from amino acids by B lymphocyte cells in the lymph tissue and set in motion by the immune system against a specific foreign protein, or antigen. An antibody is also referred to as an immunoglobulin and may be found in the blood, lymph, colostrum, saliva, and the gastrointestinal and urinary tracts, usually within three days after the first encounter with an antigen. The antibody binds tightly with the antigen as a preliminary for removing it from the system or destroying it.

For more on **nutritional supplements** for CFS, see Chapter 10: Ending Nutritional Deficiencies With Supplements, pp. 260-291.

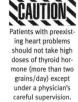

CAUTION

Patients with preexisting heart problems should not take high doses of thyroid hormone (more than two grains/day) except under a physician's careful supervision.

initely. I have been able to wean many of my HAIT patients from a thyroid supplement in a relatively short time—within three to six months—by bolstering their immune system nutritionally.

A lab test indicated Theodora was deficient in three amino acids, plus vitamin B5, inositol, and zinc. Rather than prescribing amino acid supplements, I had her increase her dietary protein intake. To address the other deficiencies, I started Theodora on a high-potency multivitamin/mineral. Another test indicated that Theodora had elevated *Candida albicans* yeast in her intestines.

To address this, Theodora started a high complex carbohydrate diet and avoided refined sugars, sweets, and fruits. She began rotating her foods so that her system was not constantly having to process the same foods. Through food allergy testing, I determined that Theodora was sensitive to a long list of foods, including kidney beans, rye grain, cheddar cheese, egg yolk, wheat, almonds, figs, kale, and others. I also gave her grapefruit seed extract (500 mg, three times daily) to help detoxify her intestines; *L. acidophilus* capsules (two capsules, three times daily) to recolonize her intestines with the appropriate "friendly" bacteria (SEE QUICK DEFINITION); and high-potency garlic (one tablet, twice daily). All of this helped to remedy her intestinal problems. In general, people with thyroid problems tend to have sluggish intestines.

After about six months on this program, many of Theodora's symptoms were much reduced, and after a total of 12 months, she was about 75% improved. Her muscle pains were greatly diminished, her energy level was much better, all signs of flu and cold were gone, she was able to exercise comfortably, and all her digestive processes were practically normal. ■

Thyroid Problems and Nutritional Deficiencies in CFS

As Dr. Langer has demonstrated, diagnosing an underactive thyroid is crucial in successfully reversing a chronic illness such as CFS. Addressing nutritional deficiencies is equally vital. We have seen in cases throughout this book that deficiencies of this type are usually a feature in CFS. Here, founder and medical director of the Center for Progressive Medicine in New York City, **Raphael Kellman, M.D.**, describes how he addresses these factors. He also explains his four-point program for reversing CFS and discusses the impact of the psychological component he calls "the meaning dimension":

From my clinical experience, it seems clear that two key factors in chronic fatigue syndrome are often overlooked as contributing causes. These are an underactive thyroid gland and undiagnosed nutrient deficiencies. About 40% of the patients I see in my practice who have chronic fatigue are actually suffering from hypothyroidism. Nutrient tests reveal that many chronic fatigue syndrome patients have numerous vitamin deficiencies, notably vitamin C and the B-complex vitamins. Knowing about these two hidden factors enables me to use thyroid hormones and precise nutrient prescribing to help reverse the symptoms of chronic fatigue syndrome.

Success Story:
Fatigued From an Underactive Thyroid

The case of Kristi, 34, excellently illustrates how an underactive thyroid gland can contribute to many of the symptoms associated with chronic fatigue syndrome and, for Kristi, to an unusual and highly premature stroke for which she had to be admitted to the hospital. When she consulted me, Kristi was able to work, but needed about eleven hours of sleep every night and was still deeply tired all the time. She reported that she had been overweight much of her life and that in recent months she had developed various gastrointestinal problems, including constipation and abdominal pain.

Kristi's conventional doctors were unable to account for her stroke nor could they explain (or treat) her fatigue. Kristi also suffered from allergies, rashes, and occasional hair loss, had difficulty concentrating, and often felt unaccountably cold. Most of these symptoms are straightforward markers for a thyroid deficiency, which means the thyroid gland is not producing enough hormones to sustain its multiple functions. However, to determine whether the thyroid is underworking, you need to use the right thyroid test.

For more information about **thyroid testing**, see Chapter 2: Testing, pp. 34-72. For more about **magnesium and CFS**, see Chapter 10: Ending Nutritional Deficiencies With Supplements, pp. 281-284.

Although my clinical experience shows that a significant number of chronic fatigue patients have underlying hypothyroidism, this fact is often not picked up in the standard thyroid hormone tests. I often correlate TSH results with the patient's body temperature (less than 97.8° F sug-

Is Your Thyroid Underactive?
Two Simple Tests That Will Tell You

Broda Barnes, M.D., in his classic work *Hypothyroidism: The Unsuspected Illness* (New York: Harper & Row, 1976), introduced the axillary (under the arm pit) temperature test as an easy way to determine adequate thyroid function. Dr. Barnes said that a resting body temperature below 97.8° F indicates hypothyroidism; menstruating women should take the underarm temperature only on the second and third days of menstruation. However, according to Lita Lee, Ph.D., a different approach might be better.

"From clinical experience, I believe the oral temperature is much more accurate than the axillary temperature. The oral temperature should be 98° F in the morning before you become active and should increase to 98.6° F to 99° F for at least ten hours daily. The best time to do this test is about 20 minutes after lunch, because that's when the temperature and pulse are at their optimum levels. Women should do this during their menstrual periods to insure missing the rise of temperature during ovulation."

Another way to tell if you are hypothyroid is to measure your resting pulse, advises Dr. Lee. The healthy resting pulse should be about 85 beats per minute (the national average is around 72); but if your pulse is less than 80, you may have an underactive thyroid. Babies have a pulse greater than 100 until around the age of eight years when the pulse slows down to around 85.

"The idea of a slow pulse being healthy is folklore," Dr. Lee explains. "Studies of healthy people who have no heart disease were found to have an average pulse of 85 beats per minute. Studies of the smartest high school students showed a pulse of 85 versus a pulse of 70 in below average students. On the other hand, some low thyroid people have a high pulse of over 100 beats per minute. These are people who literally run on adrenaline."

gests a thyroid problem) and the results of a thyroid sonogram, which indicates if the thyroid is enlarged. Clinically, the bottom line is that when we treat many chronically fatigued people, basing treatment on the assumption of an underactive thyroid, they get much better, thereby confirming the diagnosis.

The TRH stimulation test is inexpensive (about $100) and is performed by most laboratories.

In Kristi's case, her TSH level according to a TRH (thyrotropin releasing hormone) stimulation test was at 25, way above normal. Armed with this information, I put Kristi on a synthetic thyroid supplement called Synthroid, starting at a dosage of 0.125 mcg daily. To complement this, I gave her an animal-derived glandular called

Thyrosine Complex (containing pancreas, spleen, and liver extracts). Kristi took this three times daily. Tyrosine (which she also took as an additional supplement at 1,000 mg daily) is a precursor to the T4 thyroid hormone. It is likely that Kristi's underactive thyroid was the predisposing factor in her stroke, a link that Dr. Barnes first proposed in the 1950s.

A vitamin and nutrient status blood test indicated that Kristi was deficient in vitamins C and B complex. For patients with hypothyroidism and poor gastrointestinal function and nutrient absorption, I supply nutrients by intravenous infusion rather than through oral supplements. Once weekly, for about six weeks, Kristi received an IV infusion of B complex and magnesium (4 cc each), and 6-10 g of vitamin C. At the same time I gave her grape seed extract (200-300 mg daily), and a bioflavonoid (SEE QUICK DEFINITION) that enhances the concentration of vitamin C between cells. It also helps the cells pick up, absorb, and retain the vitamin C, thereby saturating the tissues, rather than having it excreted into the urine.

In addition to the IV intake, Kristi took oral vitamin C at 500 mg, six times daily, along with a complete vitamin B complex (125 mg) and magnesium (1,000 mg daily in two divided doses). Often, patients with chronic

Is Thyroid Disease Due to an Excess of Conventional Drugs?

One of the major contributing causes to thyroid disease may be an excess of conventional drugs and environmental substances, says medical researcher Lynne McTaggart.

For example, lithium, taken for manic-depressive disorder, can produce hypothyroidism in up to 33% of long-term users, while the heart drug Cordarone can produce either an overactive or underactive thyroid condition which cannot be detected for 18 months, at which point it is well-established. The long-term use of interferon-alpha for hepatitis can also generate either form of thyroid imbalance; certain drugs for lowering cholesterol have rendered a thyroid underactive. Research shows that other drugs such as cough mixtures, antiseptics, and radiographic contrast agents can render the thyroid either hypo or hyper.

Some evidence exists linking smoking with depressed thyroid function, while most illnesses and surgical procedures can upset the thyroid's function. The thyroid is particularly sensitive to events carrying a strong emotional charge such as a death or divorce. One of the "greatest culprits," says McTaggart, is the widespread use of iodized salt. Here some populations may consume too much iodine, as some regions have sufficient natural iodine in the soil and diet. An excess of only a few milligrams daily can unbalance the thyroid.[1]

fatigue have low levels of magnesium in their red blood cells. As a further boost to her energy levels and to support her immune system, Kristi started taking the Chinese herb astragalus (500 mg, twice daily). Astragalus is a tonic for strengthening the immune system, enabling it to better resist disease and infection.

Kristi noticed some improvement immediately on this program, and within four weeks she felt a significant difference. After four months, she was 100% better. She had lost 45 pounds, her hair had grown back, and she felt "vital" for the first time in her life. Today, eight months later, Kristi feels like a "new" person. This case shows how the TRH test made all the difference in outcome. Had Kristi undergone this test some years earlier, it is possible the stroke and obesity could have been prevented.

Success Story:
Fatigued from Nutrient Deficiencies

In perhaps 40% to 50% of my CFS patients, an underlying thyroid problem is the root cause, while a nutritional deficiency or central nervous system imbalance may be the source of the rest of the symptoms. The latter was the case with Tonya. Tonya, 31, had suffered from mild but chronic depression for almost four years and required at least ten hours of sleep a night.

During the day, she usually felt tired, which led to her missing many days of work. There were week-long stretches when her fatigue worsened. In her case, the TRH stimulation test came out negative, which meant she did not have an underactive thyroid. But a vitamin and essential nutrient test indicated deficiencies. I started Tonya on the same IV and oral nutrient program I used with Kristi, but without thyroid hormones or glandular extracts (SEE QUICK DEFINITION). At the same time, I implemented a four-part regimen which I often use for CFS patients.

1. Gastrointestinal—Addressing gastrointestinal function is a basic step in reversing nutrient deficiencies. If you're not absorbing nutrients, no matter what supplements you take, they will not have the intended effect. Though some of the recommendations here may be obvious, they are crucial to eliminating deficiencies. Eat about 50% less food and do not eat "garbage" foods—processed foods devoid of nutrients—which overwhelm and toxify the intestines. Eat whole grains, organically raised fresh fruits and vegetables, beans, and small amounts of fish, chicken, or turkey. These high-fiber dietary changes alone will do much to start cleansing the bowel of toxins and impacted matter.

Specific supplements can improve intestinal function and nutrient absorption. I often prescribe betaine hydrochloric acid (the stomach's primary digestive "juice") and digestive enzymes to enhance digestion. B-complex vitamins (125 mg daily) and *Lactobacillus acidophilus* and other "friendly" bacteria aid the gastrointestinal tract in absorbing nutrients, as does consuming at least ten glasses of pure water daily. Once you've established better intestinal function, then it's far more likely that nutrients taken as supplements will be more completely absorbed.

2. Circulation—You have to ensure that blood circulation is working efficiently because blood flow is what heals, delivering essential nutrients and removing toxins. Often CFS patients are overweight, which means there is stagnation and poor circulation. I often use the herb hawthorn (250 mg, three times daily) to improve blood circulation to the extremities (legs, feet, arms, hands). The herb *Ginkgo biloba* (120 mg, twice daily) enhances blood circulation to the brain and thereby improves memory. Regular exercise should be encouraged, too, as it stimulates circulation and, despite a patient's tiredness, the exertion will ultimately help them feel better.

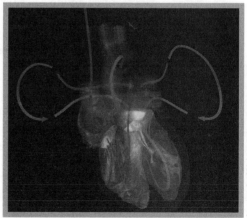

You have to ensure that blood circulation is working efficiently because blood flow is what heals, delivering essential nutrients and removing toxins.

3. Immune System—You need to support the immune system, but it's tunnel vision to assume that it is only the immune system that has anything to do with healing. The immune system is not separate from the body's other systems and the body

"Clinically, the bottom line is that when we treat many chronically fatigued people, basing treatment on the assumption of an underactive thyroid, they get much better, thereby confirming the diagnosis," says Raphael Kellman, M.D.

itself does not know of an "immune" system distinct from all its other operations. They are interconnected.

As discussed above, astragalus (500 mg, twice daily) and vitamin C (500 mg, four times daily) with grape seed extract (200 mg daily) are indicated as excellent immune supporters. In addition, Siberian ginseng (500 mg daily) combined with a liver extract has been shown to enhance the activity of T lymphocytes (white blood cells). To gain this advantage, Kristi took Aqueous Liver Extract, which contains vitamin B12, Siberian ginseng extract, and 11,000 mg of raw liver (but free of fat or cholesterol) in each capsule. Also helpful and regular features of my program are echinacea (250 mg, four times daily), coenzyme Q10, and, on occasion, garlic.

4. Central Nervous System—This approach to supporting the central nervous system is sometimes called neurotransmitter precursor therapy. Neurotransmitters (SEE QUICK DEFINITION) are key brain chemicals that convey important functional "messages," while precursors are substances, often amino acids (protein building blocks), that are necessary for synthesizing the brain chemicals. There are clinical grounds for suggesting that in some chronic fatigue patients a neurotransmitter deficiency is a contributing factor.

Specifically, I find chronic fatigue patients deficient in norepinephrine, serotonin, and dopamine. This helps explain the problems in mental functioning and processing often encountered in these patients. It's common for such patients to have trouble concentrating and remembering. They sometimes feel mentally bombarded by external noises and cannot filter out extraneous sounds from essential ones (such as a human voice). This, in turn, increases their stress and anxiety levels.

When you increase the levels of precursors required to make the key brain chemicals, this increases the patient's brain energy levels and general cognitive abilities. The amino acids tyrosine (which I give at 500-2,000 mg daily) and phenylalanine (500-1,000 mg daily) are precursors to dopamine and norepinephrine. When giving these amino acids, you must also provide vitamin B6 and vitamin C which are needed for the body to convert the precursors to neurotransmitters.

When patients respond to this form of treatment, it confirms our diagnosis and also shows that, for them at least, the source of chronic fatigue is in the brain. Patients with reduced libido respond especially well to enhancing dopamine levels, while memory and cognitive problems seem associated with deficiencies of either norepinephrine or acetylcholine. To boost mental performance, acetylcholine, choline, lecithin, DMAE (300-500 mg daily), and N-acetyl cysteine (100-400 mg daily) are helpful.

Some chronic fatigue patients also have a problem with their liver, called fatty infiltration, which means too much fat is deposited in the liver. Often a patient with this problem is overweight because they can't metabolize fat. Nutrients helpful in reversing this are milk thistle (70-140 mg, three times daily), lecithin (12 mg, three times daily),

Some Key Supplements in Tonya's Nutritional Program

N-acetyl cysteine (NAC) is an antioxidant made from the amino acid cysteine that works against cellular damage caused by toxins and free radicals; specifically, NAC can protect the liver from toxicity derived from drugs and chemical exposures.

DMAE (dimethyl amino ethanol) is a mind-enhancing, nervous system–restoring nutrient normally present in small amounts in the human brain and abundant in sardines and anchovies. It is believed to help elevate mood, improve memory, concentration, and learning, aid sleeping at night, and increase daytime energy.

Milk thistle (silymarin) is often suggested for cases of chronic hepatitis, and drug-induced liver disease. As a potent antioxidant, it protects the liver, which is the second largest organ in the body and is responsible for processing all nutrients, toxins, and drugs.

Lecithin (found in grains, beans, and egg yolks) is a high source of choline, which is needed to make the brain chemical acetylcholine and to help metabolize fats; if there is insufficient choline in the body, fats get trapped in the liver and block metabolism.

Inositol (a fiber component) is considered a B vitamin and works closely with choline, especially in cases of liver disorders, diabetes, and depression; it helps remove fats from the liver, preventing stagnation of liver fats and bile.

Phosphatidylcholine (a combination of two fatty acids, choline and phosphate) is needed to maintain cell membranes and to help reduce multiple liver symptoms from hepatitis and cirrhosis, and fatty liver from alcohol or diabetes.

"Some CFS patients have a decreased sense of meaning in their lives and, for these people, the lack of meaning can be a prime cause of the physical problem," states Dr. Kellman.

For more information about **Thyrosine Complex** and **Aqueous Liver Extract**, contact: PhytoPharmica, P.O. Box 1745, Green Bay, WI 54305; tel: 414-469-9099 or 800-553-2370; fax: 414-469-4418. For **Betaine HCL Caps** (with Pepsin), contact: Twin Labs, 2120 Smithtown Avenue, Ronkonkuma, NY 11779; tel: 516-467-3140 or 800-645-5626; fax: 516-467-3080. For **clinical information**, contact: Thyroid Foundation of Canada, 1040 Gardiners Road, Suite C, Kingston, Ontario K7P 1R7 Canada; tel: 613-634-3426; fax: 613-634-3483; e-mail: thyroid@ican.net; website: http://home.ican.net/~thyroid/Canada.html.

inositol (600 mg daily), and phosphatidylcholine (1,200 mg, four times daily).

So this was Tonya's complete program, which I introduced in stages. She responded excellently at the point we added the central nervous system component. That made a big difference. After six weeks, she was about 80% improved. After about four months on the program, Tonya was completely recovered. Her successful outcome, joined with that of many other patients, convinces me that a broader theory of health is emerging to embrace the idea that a *web* of causes leads people to illness and that we need a web of treatments to achieve wellness.

The Meaning Dimension

In some cases, a patient's response to treatment is not as good as it could be. There seems to be something preventing their body from responding better. Often, I discover that the source is what I call "the meaning dimension." When people have a decreased sense of meaning in their lives, that lack of meaning can be a prime cause of the physical problem and interfere with treatment. This is a clear demonstration of the interrelatedness of the body, mind, and spirit. It is difficult to reverse a chronic illness without restoring health on all three levels, as Katerina's case shows.

Katerina, 54, complained of chronic fatigue. I put her on our nutritional and detoxification program, yet she did not respond well to the treatment, even after several months. Although Katerina did not complain of depression, I sensed that she felt her life was virtually meaningless. To provoke a strong emotional response as a basis for finding meaning in her life, I suggested she watch Steven Spielberg's movie *Schindler's List*, which is about Holocaust victims in 1940s Europe. At first, Katerina thought this would depress her, but the morning after watching the film, she woke feeling energized. She had rediscovered the meaning dimension.

Nobody complains of fatigue when they have just won the lottery. Similarly, you don't feel fatigued in moments of compassion, joy, laughter, or grief—moments in which life feels meaningful. Katerina saw that she did not have enough of these moments in her life, but that she could if she chose to.

Katerina eventually changed her job but, in the short term, she began experiencing life differently, with a new attitude, and it was this attitude shift and the emergence of personal meaning in her life that made all the difference in Katerina's recovery. Within three months, she was free from fatigue. Mere recognition of the lack of meaning, bringing the problem to the forefront, is often sufficient to release the hold on the body and allow it to respond to treatment. ∎

The Importance of Pinpointing Thyroid Dysfunction

The following two cases show how pinpointing thyroid dysfunction can lead to a successful reversal of all the patient's symptoms. The first case comes from Raphael Kellman, M.D., and shows the importance of using the *correct test* to prove thyroid dysfunction.

Year-Long Extreme Fatigue

Mona, 42, had suffered with extreme fatigue for a year, waking in the morning, after 8-10 hours of sleep, feeling more tired than when she went to bed. During the day she often needed a nap. While she ate relatively little, Mona was steadily gaining weight, and she also experienced bloating, constipation, and occasional abdominal pains; her skin was dry; her hair was thinning; her menstruation was irregular and was preceded by PMS. Mona also reported that she had difficulty concentrating, was forgetful, and felt depressed, even though she had no strong psychological or emotional reasons for it.

Iodine, the Thyroid, and the Goiter Belt

In the early 1970s, U.S. health authorities referred to the "goiter belt," meaning those regions in the U.S., mostly in the Midwest, in which the incidence of goiter (enlarged thyroid gland) was unusually high. This problem was later traced to iodine deficiency.

Iodine is essential to forming normal amounts of thyroxine (T4); as long as one consumes about 50 mg per year of iodine, the thyroid gland should be able to make all the T4 it needs. Since that time, most people in the U.S. have used iodized table salt from which they obtain the miniscule amount of iodine needed to keep their thyroid gland theoretically healthy and functional.

"Theoretically" is an important distinction because there is still a high incidence of thyroid problems, or "hidden hypothyroidism," in the 1990s, despite dietary fortification with iodized salt. For a variety of reasons, the thyroid gland of an increasing number of people is becoming dangerously underactive, upsetting systems throughout the body and mind.

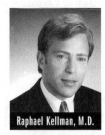

Raphael Kellman, M.D.

Nobody complains of fatigue when they have just won the lottery. Similarly, you don't feel fatigued in moments of compassion, joy, laughter, or grief—moments in which life feels meaningful.

EDITOR'S NOTE

Raphael Kellman, M.D. is an internist who blends conventional and holistic/alternative medicine, a fusion he calls "post-modern medicine." He also holds a degree in philosophy. He can be contacted at the Center for Progressive Medicine, 140 West 69th Street, New York, NY 10023; tel: 212-721-6633; fax: 212-721-6714.

When Mona's conventional physician performed a routine thyroid hormone test (for T3 and T4 levels), the results came back "normal." Although, on the basis of these results, she was advised to "rest and not worry," Mona thought otherwise, and sought a different thyroid test to measure TSH levels. But this test yielded "normal" results, too. Mona's doctor, noticing her anxiety and depression, wrote her a prescription for Prozac.

"Her life seemed to be spiraling downwards," comments Dr. Kellman. "Her depression subsided a little on the Prozac, but her fatigue, weight, and other problems got worse." Dr. Kellman immediately ran the TRH thyroid test on Mona; her TSH level was 22 after stimulation, objectively indicating an underactive thyroid. He started Mona on Synthroid (a synthetic form of T4) and Thyrostim (a natural supplement containing amino acids, vitamins, and thyroid extract) to convert T4 to T3.

In addition, Mona began a nutritional program to help her body regain normal thyroid function. Dr. Kellman observes, "It's not enough to replace the low T4 with synthetics. The underlying causes of the underactive thyroid must be addressed as well." Many of these causes—including nutrient deficiencies, overload of toxins and free radicals, hormonal imbalances (such as high cortisol), and mental and physical stress—benefit from improvements in diet and nutrition. By adding the nutritional program, Dr. Kellman was able to gradually lower Mona's doses of Synthroid, and eventually stop the medication altogether.

"Within two weeks Mona began to feel more energy and more alive," notes Dr, Kellman. "A few weeks later, her brain fog began to lift and her attention span was significantly better. In no time, she was back to her old self and began noticing weight loss and thicker, fuller hair, and her skin was normal again. Soon her periods were more regular and her PMS became tolerable, and in six weeks, Mona's mood was much better and her energy level was, in her words, 'The best I can ever remember.'"

Burgeoning Fatigue Following Pregnancy

The second case involving an underactive thyroid comes from Martin Feldman, M.D., who practices in New York City.

Mara, 32, gave birth after an untroubled pregnancy, but three weeks after delivery, she began to notice a drop in her energy. By mid-afternoon every day, Mara needed a nap, and she had to rest again in the early evening; in addition, she developed an intolerance to cold. The energy drain progressed steadily for the next three months, at which point she consulted Dr. Feldman. Mara told him that prior to her pregnancy, she had not experienced any of these symptoms.

Routine blood tests for Mara's thyroid function (T3, T4, and TSH) came back "normal." This is a common problem, observes Dr. Feldman. "The blood levels are fine, but the thyroid is not right." To refine his diagnostic picture of Mara's thyroid function, Dr. Feldman ran an antimicrosomal antibody test and an antithyroglobulin antibody test, but these also yielded supposedly normal results. Both of these tests measure the body's possible autoimmune response to its own thyroglobulin (a protein present in the thyroid gland), thereby indicating a thyroid imbalance.

Finally, Dr. Feldman had Mara do the basal body temperature test for thyroid function by placing a thermometer under her arm as soon as she woke up in the morning and before getting out of bed. Her temperature was lower than the norm for this test (97.7° F), thereby confirming some degree of thyroid sluggishness. As a corollary, Dr. Feldman ran Mara through the Ragland Postural Blood Pressure test.

For this, you rest horizontally for five minutes and your blood pressure is recorded, explains Dr. Feldman. Then you stand up and your blood pressure is recorded again. In a healthy person, the values increase slightly, or remain constant. In Mara's case, her blood systolic pressure (measured when the heart contracts, as opposed to diastolic, when the heart rests and fills with more blood) dropped slightly, indicating that her adrenal gland function was suboptimal.

Knowing that both thyroid and adrenals were underfunctioning. Dr. Feldman recommended certain key "repair ingredients to allow the thyroid to put itself back into optimal function." His preference, which he achieves in two thirds of his cases, is to avoid giving the external pharmaceutical form of thyroid hormone because the drug does the natural work of the thyroid and the thyroid will shut down. The body then becomes dependent on the pharmaceutical thyroid hormone.

To start his thyroid revival program, Dr. Feldman prescribed a liq-

If Mara had been on conventional drugs, she might have felt some improvement, but no permanent improvement, because it wouldn't have addressed "the root cause—an underactive thyroid," says Dr. Feldman.

To contact **Martin Feldman, M.D.**: 132 East 76th Street, New York, NY 10021; tel: 212-744-4413; fax: 212-472-5139. For **#8THY**, contact: Nutri-West, P.O. Box 950, Douglas, WY 82633; tel: 800-443-333 or 307-358-5066; fax: 307-358-9208. For **Thyroid Plus** (also called N14), contact: Health Industries (distributors), tel: 800-626-3386. For **Thyrophin PMG**, contact: Standard Process, 1200 West Royal Lee Drive, Palmyra, WI 53156; tel: 800-848-5061 or 414-495-2122; fax: 414-495-2512. For **Azeotrophic Adrenal tablets,** contact: ICN Pharmaceuticals, Inc., 3300 Hyland Avenue, Costa Mesa, CA 92626; tel: 800-327-8355 or 714-545-0100; fax: 714-641-7205.

uid herbal blend called #8THY, containing skullcap, parsley, uva ursi, and dulse. As a starting dose, Dr. Feldman advised Mara to put five drops of the tincture in very warm but not boiling water then let it sit for perhaps ten minutes for the alcohol in the tincture to evaporate. Mara took this blend at the rate of five drops, three times daily, then progressed to ten and eventually 15 drops, three times daily.

Next, Dr. Feldman gave Mara the mineral selenium (200 mcg to start, building to 400 mcg, daily) to enhance the conversion of T4 to T3. Glutathione is an amino acid that also helps in this conversion of thyroid hormone, although the dosage must be determined individually, says Dr. Feldman.

He also gave Mara zinc picolinate (22 mg, then increasing) because zinc is part of the thyroid formation system; riboflavin, or vitamin B2 (75 mg daily), as it also helps convert T4 to T3; the amino acid L-tyrosine (500 mg, building to 1,000 mg, daily), because it's needed to produce thyroid hormone; the mineral rubidium (80 mcg daily in four divided doses) to help the L-tyrosine; and glutamic acid (variable dosage) to help the glutathione.

The third element of Dr. Feldman's thyroid revival program was a homeopathic sarcode called Thyroid Plus. A sarcode is a homeopathic preparation made from animal tissue or secretions, in this case, from an animal's thyroid. Thyroid Plus, which contains eleven different homeopathically prepared substances, comes in drop form and must be taken directly in the mouth, not mixed with water, says Dr. Feldman. Mara took this at the rate of 5 drops, three times daily, building to 10 drops, then to 15 drops.

Dr. Feldman's fourth element involved glandular supplements. He gave Thytrophin PMG, which is thyroid hormone from cows processed to remove its thyroxine, making it a food, not a hormone, he says. Mara took four tablets daily, then increased to six (each containing 45 mg). Dr. Feldman emphasizes that the dosage and even the selection of a thyroid glandular is highly specific to the individual patient. Finally, to reset the adrenal glands, Dr. Feldman started Mara on an adrenal supplement.

Progress came quickly for Mara. After ten weeks on this multifaceted program, her energy had returned to normal and her basal body temperature was within the normal range. If Mara had been on conventional drugs, she might have felt some improvement, but no permanent improvement because it wouldn't have addressed "the root cause—an underactive thyroid," says Dr. Feldman.

Reversing a Case of CFS Linked with Hypothyroidism

Clark, 53, enjoyed an active lifestyle—jogging, playing golf, and lifting weights—until chronic fatigue syndrome brought his fitness regimen to a halt. Over the course of a few months, Clark developed severe fatigue, headaches, night sweats, sensitivity to light and cold, low body temperature, short-term memory loss, and disorganized thought processes. He received a diagnosis of CFS. Clark sought the help of Jesse Stoff, M.D., of Tucson, Arizona, coauthor of *Chronic Fatigue Syndrome: The Hidden Epidemic*. Dr. Stoff's protocols were the subject of Chapter 1.

"After I read his book," Clark says, "I felt that he was the doctor to help me fight and eventually beat this disease." In fact, Clark was so impressed with Dr Stoff's writings on the subject that he moved from Washington state to Tucson to undergo his treatment.

To determine the cause of Clark's CFS, Dr. Stoff ran extensive blood tests. The tests showed that Clark had numerous vitamin and mineral deficiencies, in addition to hypothyroidism and candidiasis. Based on this information, Dr. Stoff prescribed a treatment plan which combined thyroid hormone, herbal remedies, vitamin supplements, diet, and stress reduction. After two years with Dr. Stoff, Clark's fatigue had reduced considerably, but he still experienced constant symptoms. Not satisfied with only partial recovery, Dr. Stoff referred Clark to John Dommisse, M.D., another Tucson physician who has had success in treating CFS.

Dr. Dommisse determined that, while Clark's T3 level had improved under Dr. Stoff's care, his T4 was still low. Adding T4 supplements to Clark's treatment was "one of the main contributions I was able to make to Clark's recovery," Dr. Dommisse observes. He also identified and corrected a few remaining vitamin and mineral deficiencies. Following these final adjustments in treatment, Clark was able to go back to jogging, playing golf, and lifting weights sever-

Dr. Feldman's preference, which he achieves in two thirds of his cases, is to avoid giving the external pharmaceutical form of thyroid hormone because then the drug does the natural work of the thyroid and the thyroid will shut down.

al times a week. "I give total credit for my full recovery to Drs. Stoff and Dommisse," Clark says. "I feel positive that this disease has been beaten and that my future will be CFS free."[2]

She Tested Normal But Was Still Exhausted

Bette, 47, felt drained of energy all the time. Her body temperature registered subnormal (95° F to 96° F) in the morning and even though she ate a low-fat diet and exercised six times weekly, she was unable to lose weight (both are typical signs of hypothyroidism). At 188 pounds, which was far too much weight for her height, Bette's feet were always sore. In addition, she suffered from a chronic infection, skin problems, and depression.

Bette's physician ran a TSH (thyroid stimulating hormone) test to check her thyroid, but the results came back "normal." In his mind, this resolved the question of hypothyroidism. Instead of testing further, he suggested she try Weight Watchers and put her on a conventional weight loss drug. The drug lowered her blood pressure to dangerous levels (78/57; an average healthy reading is 120/80).

Consultation with John Dommisse, M.D., set Bette on a different course. "I would never use the TSH blood level as the sole test for screening for hypothyroidism or monitoring its treatment," says Dr. Dommisse. He reports that he usually treats for hypothyroidism if the TSH results are even in the middle of the normal range (greater than 2 mIU) and that, provided the thyroid treatment is not excessive, he "always sees a definite clinical advantage to this approach."

Dr. Dommisse ran three thyroid tests (Free-T3, Free-T4, and 3rd-Generation TSH) on Bette to more accurately assess the state of her thyroid. While the results for Free-T4 and 3rd-Generation TSH were in the normal range, Bette's Free-T3 was below normal. Tests on vitamin and mineral status revealed that Bette was deficient in zinc, manganese, vitamin B12, and chromium, but had an excess of copper.

Dr. Dommisse started Bette on supplements to redress her nutrient deficiencies. He advised her not to drink her tap water or use it in cooking because the copper plumbing in her house was the likely source of the excessive copper in her body. For thyroid imbalances,

Dr. Dommisse typically relies on combinations of T4 (Levoxyl, Synthroid), T3 (Cytomel), and Armour Thyroid (natural desiccated hog thyroid). He finds these effective, especially when the Free-T3 level is lower than the Free-T4, as in Bette's case.

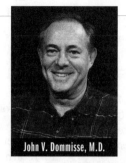

John V. Dommisse, M.D.

Dr. Dommisse reports that he usually treats for hypothyroidism if the TSH results are even in the middle of the normal range and that, provided the thyroid treatment is not excessive, he "always sees a definite clinical advantage to this approach."

Within a few months of starting Dr. Dommisse's program, Bette's fatigue disappeared, her infection and skin problems cleared up, her depression lifted, her feet no longer hurt, and she lost 50 pounds.[3]

Human Growth Hormone in the Treatment of CFS

The proper balance of hormones is vital to health. An underactive thyroid can lead to a hormonal imbalance or deficiency that can, in turn, lead to CFS. But CFS patients who suffer from an underactive thyroid may find relief in a new technique that is starting to catch on with physicians nationwide: human growth hormone (HGH) therapy.

According to Leonard Haimes, M.D., medical director of the Haimes Centre Clinic in Boca Raton, Florida, who devoted six months to a thorough review of the research on HGH, recent research shows an expanding range of conditions for which HGH appears effective, including thyroid problems and chronic fatigue.

Adults who have an underactive thyroid gland appear to be deficient in growth hormone, says Dr. Haimes. When such patients are given adequate HGH, they show gains in energy, muscle strength and mass, mental abilities, and psychological attitude. For those CFS sufferers who have been diagnosed with an underactive thyroid, HGH therapy can replace the growth hormone they've lost as a result, thereby restoring energy and stamina to their bodies.

To contact **John V. Dommisse, M.D.**: 1840 East River Road, Suite 210, Cambric Corporate Center, Tucson, AZ 85718; tel: 520-577-1940; fax: 520-577-1743. To contact **Leonard Haimes, M.D.**: Haimes Centre Clinic, 7300 North Federal Highway, Suite #100, Boca Raton, FL 35487; tel: 561-995-8484; fax: 561-995-7773. For doctors knowledgeable in **HGH therapy**, contact: Natural Health Centers of America, 3450 Park Central Boulevard North, Pompano Beach, FL 33064; tel: 954-955-9458; fax: 954-977-0180. Also **E. Y. Chein, M.D.**: Palm Springs Life Extension Institute, 2825 Tahquitz Canyon Boulevard, Building Plan A, Palm Springs, CA 92262; tel: 619-327-8939.

What is Human Growth Hormone?

Human growth hormone (HGH), naturally secreted by the pituitary gland in the brain, is a small protein-like hormone similar to insulin. HGH is secreted in very brief pulses during the early hours of sleep and remains in circulation for only a few minutes. During adolescence, when growth is most rapid, production of HGH is high. After age 20, HGH production declines progressively at an average rate of about 14% per decade; by age 60, it is not uncommon to measure a growth hormone loss of 75% or more.

Originally, growth hormone, which consists of 191 amino acids (protein building blocks), was used in the early 1980s to correct disturbances in normal growth; later it was synthesized for adult use. Benefits from HGH include increased muscle mass, improved physical strength, reduced fatigue, decreased fat (especially abdominal fat), increased bone strength, revitalization of liver, kidney, spleen, and brain functions, increased exercise capacity, improved kidney blood flow and efficiency, improved cardiac function, and reduced risk from cardiovascular problems, and a general enhancement in the sense of well-being.

The short-term therapeutic effects of HGH (foremost among which is its ability to stabilize the immune system) are impressive, says Dr. Haimes. One of his patients, a 33-year-old man, had suffered from chronic fatigue syndrome for three years, yet after only 20 days of HGH therapy (about ten injections), he was able to return to work, his symptoms alleviated.

HGH is not an altered product, such as a bioengineered tomato in which the genetic structure has been changed, Dr. Haimes explains. Rather, it is grown or duplicated from the "genetic blueprint" of the naturally-occurring hormone found in the human pituitary gland; thus, it is identical to it. HGH therapy is expensive (it can cost $250 a week), but there are many who regard this investment in health as worth the money.

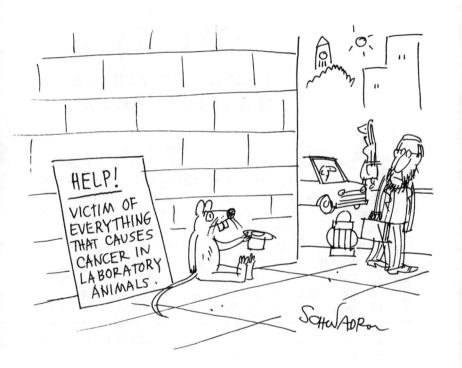

Eliminating Heavy Metal Toxicity

YOUR MERCURY FILLINGS MAY BE FATIGUING YOU

CASES DISCUSSED in previous chapters showed how mercury toxicity contributes to chronic fatigue, immune breakdown, and hypothyroidism. These are just a few of the health disorders associated with dental mercury and yet mercury amalgam is still widely used in the United States to fill cavities in teeth.

Euphemistically called "silver" fillings, mercury amalgam fillings are actually only 35% silver. Mercury, a heavy metal, makes up 50% of the mix, with tin (9%), copper (6%), and a trace of zinc comprising the rest. Mercury amalgams have been used in dentistry since the 1820s; every year, more than 100 million mercury amalgam fillings are put into the mouths of U.S. dental patients, despite the fact that, in 1988, the Environmental Protection Agency (EPA) declared scrap dental amalgam a *hazardous waste*.

Even the American Dental Association (ADA), which has so far refused to ban amalgams, now instructs dentists to "know the potential hazards and symptoms of mercury exposure such as the development of sensitivity and neuropathy," to use a no-touch technique for handling the amalgam, and to store it under liquid, preferably glycerin or radiographic fixer solution, in unbreakable, tightly sealed containers.[1]

Evidence now shows that mercury amalgams are the *major* source of mercury exposure for the general public, at rates six times higher than mercury from fish and seafood. Studies by the World Health

Organization show that a single amalgam can release 3-17 mcg of mercury per day. A Danish study of a random sample of 100 men and 100 women showed that increased blood mercury levels were related to the presence of more than four amalgam fillings in the teeth.

Mercury toxicity has been shown to have destructive contributory effects on kidney function, in cardiovascular disease, neuropsychological dysfunction, reproductive disorders, and birth defects, to name a few. Symptoms of mercury toxicity make a very long list: anorexia, depression, fatigue, insomnia, arthritis, multiple sclerosis, moodiness, irritability, memory loss, nausea, diarrhea, gum disease, swollen glands, headaches, and many more. Following are a few highly revealing case presentations in which mercury toxicity played a major role in the development of chronic fatigue.

Success Stories: CFS Reversed by Mercury Amalgam Removal

The following are clinical accounts of people whose chronic fatigue syndrome was dramatically reversed *after* they had their mercury amalgam dental fillings removed.

All His Symptoms Gone

After he underwent a root canal at the age of 15, Earl suffered severe fatigue and anxiety. At 28, he had a nervous breakdown. At the age of 32, suffering from fatigue, anger, anxiety, back problems, low blood sugar, nervousness, ringing in his ears, concentration loss, and prematurely graying hair, he consulted acupuncturist David J. Nickel, O.M.D., L.Ac., of Santa Monica, California.

Dr. Nickel performed a mercury vapor analysis on Earl's teeth and found that the level of toxic fumes from Earl's six mercury amalgam fillings was 42 times higher than the Environmental Protection Agency's maximum allowable limit. A hair analysis indicated that Earl also had aluminum, copper, and mercury at toxic levels in his tissues and that he had an exceptionally slow metabolic rate.

Dr. Nickel put Earl on a nutritional supplement program after which there was significant improvement in his metabolic rate and blood sugar levels, but limited improvement in his other symptoms. After Earl had all six mercury amalgams and his root canal tooth removed, he began to

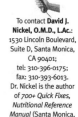

To contact **David J. Nickel, O.M.D., L.Ac.:** 1530 Lincoln Boulevard, Suite D, Santa Monica, CA 90401; tel: 310-396-0175; fax: 310-393-6013. Dr. Nickel is the author of *700+ Quick Fixes, Nutritional Reference Manual* (Santa Monica, CA: Health Acu Press, 1994).

"Almost all my patients who have had their mercury-based fillings removed show moderate to dramatic improvement in their health in usually less than one month," states David J. Nickel, O.M.D., L.Ac.

experience major changes, states Dr. Nickel. In a month, his energy level returned to near what he had enjoyed over 15 years earlier and he was able to exercise, work, and play strenuously with no exhaustion. His other symptoms improved as well. "I don't remember when I have ever felt so good," Earl said.

According to Dr. Nickel, removing the mercury fillings and root canal were responsible for Earl's return to health. "Of the 90% of my patients with amalgam dental fillings, most have a mercury-induced copper toxicity, high calcium levels, and reduced thyroid and adrenal function," states Dr. Nickel. "Mercury is associated with 258 different symptoms and copper with over 100. Almost all my patients who have had their mercury-based fillings removed show moderate to dramatic improvement in their health in usually less than one month."[2]

Acupuncture meridians are specific pathways in the human body for the flow of life force or subtle energy, known as *qi* (pronounced *CHEE*). In most cases, these energy pathways run up and down both sides of the body, and correspond to individual organs or organ systems, designated as Lung, Small Intestine, Heart, and others. There are 12 principal meridians and eight secondary channels. Numerous points of heightened energy, or *qi*, exist on the body's surface along the meridians and are called acupoints. There are more than 1,000 acupoints, each of which is potentially a place for acupuncture treatment.

Undoing Seven Years of Fatigue

By the time he came to acupuncturist M. M. van Benschoten, O.M.D., of Reseda, California, Albert, 37, had been beset by chronic fatigue syndrome for seven years. He reported headaches, chest pain, fatigue, lymph node swelling, muscle aches, irritability, and light-headedness. Although Albert had elevated blood levels of Epstein-Barr virus, normally associated with chronic fatigue syndrome, Dr. van Benschoten's analysis of Albert's acupuncture meridians (SEE QUICK DEFINITION) showed several bacterial and viral infections capable of producing his symptoms.

In addition, he found mercury toxicity from dental amalgams to be the fundamental underlying cause of the suppression of Albert's immune system. To arrive at this conclusion, Dr. van Benschoten used a diagnostic technique in an analytical approach called "acupoint biophoton diagnostics." Toxic metals, such as mercury, interfere with the normal energy patterns in various acupuncture channels; harmful energies set up interference patterns in the meridians, explains Dr. van Benschoten.

Dr. van Benschoten prescribed a series of Chinese herbs to clear the bacterial, viral, and heavy metals, including chrysanthemum, angelica dahurica, isatis, bupleurum, cnidium, astragalus, salvia, platycodon, siler, taraxacum, ligustrum lucidum, and fructus lycium. After taking these herbs for six weeks, Albert was headache free and had relief from fatigue and chest pain. The degree to which mercury toxicity was interfering with his energy pathways also was reduced. Three months later, Albert had 14 mercury amalgams removed.

However, on Albert's next visit, Dr. van Benschoten found that the mercury interference had increased. "Overzealous removal of all amalgam fillings can significantly increase the patient's mercury levels if done without adequate precautions during amalgam removal and proper mercury detoxification therapy," notes Dr. van Benschoten. He instructs his patients to wear an oxygen mask during amalgam removal, in addition to having their dentists use a rubber

To contact **M. M. van Benschoten, O.M.D.:** 19231 Victory Boulevard, Suite 151, Reseda, CA 91335; tel: 818-344-9973.

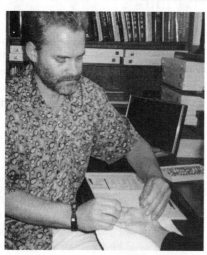
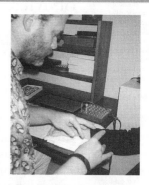
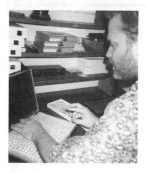

Toxic metals, such as mercury, interfere with the normal energy patterns in various acupuncture channels; harmful energies set up interference patterns ("biophoton" emissions) in the meridians, says Dr. van Benschoten, shown here testing patients' energy patterns.

"I don't feel comfortable using a substance designated by the Environmental Protection Agency to be a waste disposal hazard. I can't throw it in the trash, bury it in the ground, or put it in a landfill, but they say it's okay to put it in people's mouths. That doesn't make sense," says Richard D. Fischer, D.D.S.

dam and high speed suction with water.

After mercury amalgam removal, Chinese herbal medicines can successfully detoxify the patient and restore immune function, says Dr. van Benschoten. For Albert, he prescribed a second series of herbs, including moutan, taraxacum, prunella, glycyrrhiza, grifola, ligustrum lucidum, and verbena to clear the mercury from his system. After taking them for several months, Albert reported he was free from chronic fatigue and that he had a stronger resistance to infection.[3]

CAUTION

For those contemplating removal of their mercury dental fillings, extreme care must be taken to protect the body from mercury poisoning during the amalgam removal process. Further, mercury residues throughout the body must be carefully removed through the use of some form of chelating agent, such as garlic, seaweeds, vitamin C, etc. that will bind with the mercury and help to remove it safely from the body.

The Toxic Dangers of Mercury Fillings

Some dentists, such as Richard D. Fischer, D.D.S., of Annandale, Virginia, refuse to work with mercury amalgams. Dr. Fischer even had his own silver fillings removed to make the point. "I don't feel comfortable using a substance designated by the EPA to be a waste disposal hazard," he says. "I can't throw it in the trash, bury it in the ground, or put it in a landfill, but they say it's okay to put it in people's mouths. That doesn't make sense."

The use of mercury in fillings is banned or severely curtailed in numerous European countries. According to the German Ministry of Health, "Amalgam is considered a health risk from a medical viewpoint due to the release of mercury vapor."[4] But for a long time, the ADA asserted that the mercury amalgam was a tightly-bound chemical complex that would not permit any leakage or release of mercury.

This was conclusively proven wrong in 1985 when studies showed that the air inside a mouth with mercury fillings continually contained elemental mercury vapor and that chewing substantially increased this vapor level. Amalgams can also erode and corrode with time (ideally they should be replaced after seven to ten years), adding to their toxic output. Studies by the World Health Organization (WHO) show that

Selected Health Symptom Analysis of 1,569 Patients Who Eliminated Mercury-Containing Dental Fillings

The following represents a summary of 1,569 patients in six different studies evaluating the health effects of replacing mercury-containing dental fillings with non-mercury fillings. The data was derived from the following sources: 762 Patient Adverse Reaction Reports submitted to the FDA by patients; and 807 patients reports from Sweden, Denmark, Canada, and the United States.[6]

% of Total Reporting	Symptom	Number Reporting	Number Improved or Cured	% of Cure or Improvement
14	Allergy	221	196	89
5	Anxiety	86	80	93
5	Bad temper	81	68	84
6	Bloating	88	70	80
6	Blood pressure problems	99	53	54
5	Chest pains	79	69	87
22	Depression	347	315	91
22	Dizziness	343	301	88
45	Fatigue	705	603	86
15	Intestinal problems	231	192	83
8	Gum problems	129	121	94
34	Headaches	531	460	87
12	Insomnia	187	146	78
10	Irregular heartbeat	159	139	87
8	Irritability	132	119	90
17	Lack of concentration	270	216	80
6	Lack of energy	91	88	97
17	Memory loss	265	193	73
17	Metallic taste	260	247	95
7	Multiple sclerosis	113	86	76
8	Muscle tremor	126	104	82

a single amalgam can release 3-17 micrograms of mercury per day.[7]

Since mercury vapors are continuously released from amalgam fillings, as long as you have mercury dental fillings, you inhale mercury vapor 24 hours a day, 365 days a year. The resulting level of mercury in the body has serious health consequences. Research has demonstrated that the body's tissues—especially in the brain, kidneys, jaw, lungs, gastrointestinal tract, and liver—absorb and store mercury. Mercury toxicity has been shown to have destructive effects on kidney function and contribute to cardiovascular disease, neuropsychological

Exposing the Mercury Hazard in Your Mouth

A Danish dentist has added another valuable piece to the mounting evidence that mercury in dental fillings can be injurious to health.

H. Lichtenberg, D.D.S., of Hilleroed, Denmark, tested 103 of his dental patients, with an average age of 47, for oral mercury vapor emission from their mercury amalgams. Dr. Lichtenberg used a Jerome 413X mercury vapor analyzer (Texas Instruments). On average, each of the patients had at least 14 symptoms associated with mercury poisoning; each patient also had an average of 22 amalgam surfaces.

Dr. Lichtenberg found that the concentration of mercury vapor varied from 3 mcg/cubic meter of air to 329 mcg/m³, with an average of 54.6. Individuals with mercury vapor readings exceeding 50 had an average of 26.8 mercury amalgam surfaces and 1.2 gold and/or porcelain fillings or crowns, while those whose readings were less than 50 had an average of 19.8 amalgam surfaces. In other words, the amount of amalgam surface per mouth is directly related to the amount of mercury vapor likely to be released.

In Denmark, levels up to but not exceeding 50 mcg/m³ of mercury vapor are permitted in a workplace for people working 40 hours a week. Thus, with Dr. Lichtenberg's patients, the mercury exposure not only exceeded Denmark's "safe" amount, but it represented an exposure sustained for 168 hours a week (24 hours a day), indefinitely. Safety levels are relative, however, because Switzerland and Russia allow only 10 mcg/m³ while the U.S. allows 100 mcg/m³. A recent Canadian conference proposed a Tolerable Daily Intake (TDI) for mercury of 1.0 mcg for a person weighing about 150 pounds. Dr. Lichtenberg's patients, on average, were exposed to a TDI that was over 50 times this norm.

Dr. Lichtenberg also reported that more than half of his patients complained of one or more symptoms commonly associated with mercury toxicity, including general fatigue, headaches, irritability, poor memory and concentration, bloating, joint pain, cold hands and feet, and muscle fatigue. As the mercury vapor concentration values increased, so did symptoms of intestinal cramps, irritability, dizziness, and leg cramps, said Dr. Lichtenberg. "It would seem that the number of individual symptoms varies depending on the number of amalgam surfaces present," he stated.

Dr. Lichtenberg further reported that, since about 1976, dentists have tended to use an amalgam with 10% more copper content. However, this type of amalgam can release up to 50 times more mercury and copper vapor than older amalgam types, he says. Dr. Lichtenberg's research also demonstrated that patients with gold fillings or crowns and metal or porcelain crowns experienced a mixing of metals in the mouth that leads to additional corrosion of the mercury fillings, thereby releasing yet more mercury vapor. Summarizing his findings. Dr. Lichtenberg states that "mercury poisoning from the amalgam fillings is widespread throughout the population."[5]

dysfunction, reproductive disorders, and birth defects, to name a few. Like other heavy metals, mercury has been shown to cause damage to the lining of arteries.

This means that if amalgam fillings are present, your circulatory system is constantly being exposed to the damaging effects of this heavy metal. It's interesting to note that cardiovascular disease has become widespread only since the 1920s, about the time of increased use of heavy metals in dental therapy, but long after humans began consuming eggs, meat, milk, butter, and cheese, which are commonly thought to contribute to heart disease.

According to Edward Arana, D.D.S., current president of the American Academy of Biological Dentistry, in Carmel Valley, California, among the other problems caused specifically by mercury amalgam fillings are:

- chronic fatigue syndrome and lack of energy
- tendency toward chronic inflammatory changes, including fibromyalgia, rheumatoid arthritis, and phlebitis
- chronic neurological illnesses, especially when numbness is one of the leading symptoms
- lowering of the pain threshold
- disturbances of the immune system

Mercury poisoning can also lead to symptoms such as anxiety, depression, confusion, irritability, and the

> **Patients with chronic fatigue syndrome or with allergies, thyroid dysfunction, or a lack of resistance to infections all improve after their fillings are properly removed, says Charles Gableman, M.D.**

inability to concentrate, all of which are symptoms of CFS. Such poisoning often goes undetected for years because the symptoms presented do not necessarily suggest mercury as the initiating cause.

Charles Gableman, M.D., a former practitioner of environmental medicine, now living in Lake Forest, California, always advised the removal of his patients' amalgam fillings. Patients with chronic fatigue syndrome or with allergies, thyroid dysfunction, or a lack of resistance to infections all improve after their fillings are properly removed, says Dr. Gableman. He believes it is possible that these patients have suffered from basic allergies their entire lives, and that the mercury toxicity from the fillings simply adds to the body's toxic load and "pushes them over the edge," resulting in chronic medical problems.

Extensive clinical evidence based on patient case histories from many alternative doctors attests to the effects of mercury amalgam toxicity. For example, a patient of biological dentist (SEE QUICK DEFINITION) Hal Huggins, D.D.S., of Colorado Springs, Colorado, had for years endured fatigue, mononucleosis (for which she was hospital-

Biological dentistry stresses the use of nontoxic restoration materials for dental work and focuses on the unrecognized impact that dental toxins and hidden dental infections can have on overall health. Typically, a biological dentist will emphasize the following: the safe removal of mercury amalgams; in many cases, either the avoidance or removal of root canals; the investigation of possible jawbone infections (cavitations) as a "dental focus" or source of body-wide illness centered in the teeth; and the health-injuring role of misalignment of teeth and jaw structures.

ized at age 16), bladder infections, and, eventually, Epstein-Barr virus, candidiasis, food allergies, and muscle spasms. Finally, her own investigation led her to consider the possibility of mercury poisoning and she consulted with Dr. Huggins. He found a tooth with a root canal that had been filled with a dental amalgam. Once the amalgam was removed, her symptoms abated.

The Domino Effect of Mercury Toxicity

"When I see a patient with mercury fillings, I always think, 'It's the teeth, stupid!'" says Bruce Shelton, M.D., M.D.(H), Di.Hom., director of the Allergy Center in Phoenix, Arizona. "Mercury amalgams are as close as you can get to the center of the illness universe; their use in dentistry has set us up for most of the health problems we see today."

In his practice, Dr. Shelton frequently observes a domino effect of illness that begins with mercury toxicity. He reports that 90% of his patients who come in with allergies have an overgrowth of the yeastlike fungus *Candida albicans*. This overgrowth can be due to heavy metals in the body, principally from mercury in the teeth, continually draining in minute amounts into body tissues, Dr. Shelton says.

"Although dental work tends to be very expensive, if you can get a patient to have their teeth corrected, they will get well," reports Dr. Shelton.

"The body is smart and wants to protect itself at all costs. One of the natural absorbers of heavy metal is *Candida*. The body attracts this yeast (and parasites) into the intestines to act as a natural sponge for the mercury. The body, in trying to protect itself against mercury, creates another problem—a yeast infestation."

The next stage of the domino effect is that patients in this predicament typically develop leaky gut syndrome. "If we do not totally digest and absorb our foods before they are broken to basic chemicals, then we have a 'leaky gut.' For example, a little piece of fish that is still chemically fish instead of amino acids will trigger an immune reaction." In this way, leaky gut syndrome leads, in turn, to food allergies, Dr. Shelton says. Soon the person becomes a universal reactor, allergic to multiple chemicals, to seemingly everything. Environmental illness is then the end-product of a string of health problems that stem from mercury and build, one upon the other.

"Although dental work tends to be very expensive, if you can get a patient to have their teeth corrected, they will get well," reports Dr. Shelton. Unfortunately, in his experience, only the more serious patients, the ones who have been scared by their illnesses, are generally willing to have the necessary

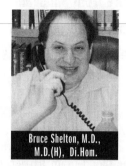

Bruce Shelton, M.D., M.D.(H), Di.Hom.

"Mercury amalgams are as close as you can get to the center of the illness universe; their use in dentistry has set us up for most of the health problems we see today," says Bruce Shelton, M.D., M.D.(H), Di.Hom.

dental work. Those who do not and retain their mercury fillings do improve, but often need six-month therapeutic "tuneups," he says.

According to Dr. Shelton, mercury toxicity can also result in an underactive thyroid, another contributing factor to chronic fatigue. Specifically, in thyroid cases, the fifth tooth from the midline of the mouth (between the two front teeth), upper and lower, in both directions, frequently has a mercury filling or a root canal, or is in a state of degeneration. In other words, potentially four different teeth can have a thyroid connection.

How Mercury Disrupts the Body

Heavy metals such as mercury act as free radicals (SEE QUICK DEFINITION), which are highly reactive, charged particles that can cause damage to body tissues. Since mercury is a cumulative poison, building up in the body with repeated exposure,[8] its effects can be devastating. It can prevent nutrients from entering the cells and wastes from leaving, and block enzymes necessary for the body's detoxification processes.

Mercury can bind to the DNA (deoxyribonucleic acid) of cells, as well as to the cell membranes, distorting them and interfering with normal cell functions.[9] When this happens, the immune system no longer recognizes the cell as part of the body and will attack it. This is the basis of an autoimmune disease, of which CFS is one.

A **free radical** is an unstable molecule with an unpaired electron that steals an electron from another molecule and produces harmful effects. Free radicals are formed when molecules within cells react with oxygen (oxidize) as part of normal metabolic processes. Free radicals then begin to break down cells, especially if there are not enough free-radical quenching nutrients, such as vitamins C and E, in the cell. While free radicals are normal products of metabolism, uncontrolled free-radical production plays a major role in the development of degenerative disease, including cancer and heart disease. Free radicals harmfully alter important molecules, such as proteins, enzymes, fats, even DNA. Other sources of free radicals include pesticides, industrial pollutants, smoking, alcohol, viruses, most infections, allergies, stress, even certain foods and excessive exercise.

After elemental mercury from amalgam fillings is inhaled or ingested, it is converted to methylmercury, the organic form of mercury. As toxic as elemental mercury is, methylmercury is 100 times more toxic.

After elemental mercury from amalgam fillings is inhaled or ingested, it is converted to methylmercury, the organic form of mercury. Methylmercury, because it easily crosses the blood-brain barrier, has been associated with neurodegenerative diseases such as Alzheimer's, multiple sclerosis, and amyotrophic lateral sclerosis. It is important to mention that as toxic as elemental mercury is, methylmercury is 100 times more toxic.

Once it has leached from the dental fillings and infiltrated the body, mercury becomes a neurotoxin, according to Dietrich Klinghardt, M.D., Ph.D., a specialist in neural therapy (SEE QUICK DEFINITION) based in Seattle, Washington. Strangely, a neurotoxin is a substance the nerve cells voluntarily absorb, even though it is poisonous. They do this out of curiosity, Dr. Klinghardt explains.

Nerve endings in the peripheral nervous system constantly scan their environment, engulfing foreign particles and bringing them across the cell membrane for inspection. "These substances may then travel all the way up from the foot to the spinal cord and get presented to the nerve cells there," he says. If the substance is judged to be harmful, the body tries to produce an antitoxin to neutralize it and eliminate it from the body.

But there are two problems here when it comes to mercury, Dr. Klinghardt cautions. "First, as it travels up the nerve, mercury destroys the body's mechanism, a substance called tubulin, for transporting along nerves. Burning the bridges behind it, as it were, it effectively destroys the nerve. Second, the body has not yet learned how to make an antineurotoxin against mercury."

Laboratory research has shown that within 24 hours of injecting a minute dose of mercury into a muscle anywhere in the body (monkeys were used in the study), it is present in the spinal cord and brain. The mercury is also present in the kidneys, lungs, bloodstream, connective tissue, and adrenal and other endocrine glands. In the brain, it tends to congregate in the hypothalamus, which regulates the sympathetic nervous system, and in the limbic system (associated with the brain-

Neural Therapy Can Relieve Fibromyalgia

K atie, 42, had suffered from whole-body pain for five years before receiving treatment for fibromyalgia from Ross A. Hauser, M.D., of Oak Park, Illinois. A series of previous diagnoses, physical therapy rounds, and anti-inflammatory medications and antidepressants (such as Elavil) had brought her no relief. Her neck pain was so intense she had to wear a neck brace; she also had pain in her jaw, arms, legs, and back, and the ligaments in these regions were especially tender.

Dr. Hauser treated Katie with neural therapy (also known as prolotherapy), which involves the injection of local anesthetics (in her case, dextrose or lidocaine) into the junctions of either the bone and ligament or bone and tendon to encourage repair of damaged tissue, and to stimulate the growth of new cells and collagen. Dr. Hauser made his injections at the tender spots over the ligaments and tendons of Katie's arms, legs, jaw, back, and neck. Six weeks later, she no longer needed the neck brace and was able to go swimming and walking. Six months later (after a second neural therapy treatment), Katie experienced pain only with strenuous exercise but was otherwise "doing great," notes Dr. Hauser. After a third prolotherapy treatment, all her symptoms abated. "Katie has been doing fine since—sleeping like a baby—and she has a smile on her face again," Dr. Hauser says.

From the patient records of Ross A. Hauser, M.D. To contact **Dr. Hauser**: Caring Medical & Rehabilitation Services, S.C., 715 Lake Street, Suite 600, Oak Park, IL 60301; tel: 708-848-7789; fax: 708-848-7763.

stem), believed to be the organic seat of emotions.

While mercury levels slowly dissipate in a predictable amount of time from other body tissues and even from the teeth (in six weeks, its levels might be halved), mercury does not have a "half-life" in the nervous system or brain. Instead, it binds firmly to a specific chemical compound which happens to exist there in the body's highest concentrations.

"The main devastating effect of mercury in the nervous system is that it interferes with the energy production inside each cell," says Dr. Klinghardt. "The nerve cell is impaired in its ability to detoxify itself [and excrete the mercury] and in its ability to nurture itself. The cell becomes toxic and dies, or lives in a state of chronic malnutrition. A multitude of illnesses, usually associated with neurological symptoms, result." Among these are chronic viral and fungal illnesses, recurrent episodes of bacterial infections, and chronic fatigue.

By a curious self-preservation reflex of the body, the emergence of these conditions can be viewed as a way of accommodating the heavy

Laboratory research has shown that within 24 hours of injecting a minute dose of mercury into a muscle anywhere in the body (monkeys were used in the study), it is present in the spinal cord and brain.

metal presence, speculates Dr. Klinghardt. "Most, if not all, chronic infectious diseases are not caused by a failure of the immune system, but by a conscious adaptation of the immune system to an otherwise lethal heavy metal environment," he says. Mercury suffocates the cells and they die, so the immune system cultivates fungi and bacteria which are able to bind large amounts of the toxic metal in their respective cell walls, thereby enabling the patient's cells to breathe again.

The downside, of course, is that the body must now feed these otherwise undesirable microbes and deal with their toxic waste. In addition, a person with mercury contamination often becomes zinc deficient, and the functioning of copper and other minerals in the body will be compromised as well. This perspective leads Dr. Klinghardt to the following strong statement: "As soon as anybody has any type of medical illness or symptom, whether medical or emotional, the amalgam fillings should be removed and the mercury residues should be eliminated from the body, especially the brain."

To contact **Dietrich Klinghardt, M.D., Ph.D.:** American Academy of Neural Therapy, 410 East Denny Way, Suite 18, Seattle, WA 98122; tel: 206-749-9967. Dr. Klinghardt regularly instructs physicians in the U.S. and Europe in neural therapy techniques. For information about **cilantro tincture,** contact: Dragon River Herbals, P.O. Box 28, El Rito, NM 87530; tel: 800-813-2118 or 505-581-4441; fax: 505-581-4441. For **chlorella,** contact: Nature's Balance, Inc., 635-A Southwest Street, High Point, NC 27260; tel: 800-858-5198 or 910-882-4102; fax: 910-882-4119.

Neural Therapy and Herbs for Mercury Detoxification

In Dr. Klinghardt's clinical experience, it is common for heavy metals to migrate to and accumulate in nerve ganglia (nerve bundles that are the nervous system's relay stations). Neural therapy is useful in treating mercury-based problems in the ganglia, he says.

As a heavy metal (which means heavier than water), mercury tends to accumulate in the lowest parts of the body, such as the floor of the mouth, the pelvic floor, and the feet. Pelvic symptoms, in both men and women, "are very commonly caused by metal toxicity of Frankenhäuser's ganglion." A mercury accumulation in this nerve plexus can account for premature ejaculation and an enlarged prostate in men, and endometriosis, pelvic pain, and hormonal dysfunction in women, Dr. Klinghardt says.

Neural therapy "cleans up" this area by injecting

Frankenhäuser's ganglion (just above the pubic bone) with a local anesthetic. "This opens up most of the ionic channels in the cell wall; the cell is then able to excrete a high number of its toxic components." This painless injection spurs the body to dump a large amount of mercury into the urine, Dr. Klinghardt says.

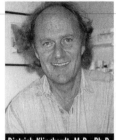

Dietrich Klinghardt, M.D., Ph.D.

"As soon as anybody has any type of medical illness or symptom, whether medical or emotional, the amalgam fillings should be removed and the mercury residues should be eliminated from the body, especially the brain," states Dietrich Klinghardt, M.D., Ph.D.

As an adjunct to neural therapy, Dr. Klinghardt employs botanical substances to assist in removing the mercury. Cilantro and chlorella are particularly effective. The herb cilantro (Chinese parsley) is known to detoxify the brain and central nervous system of heavy metals. Taking it in an alcohol-based tincture guarantees fast delivery of the cilantro to the brain, he says. A typical dose is ten drops of cilantro tincture twice daily.

While cilantro mobilizes mercury or tin stored in the brain and spinal cord and moves it out of those tissues, it does not facilitate the removal of these heavy metals from the body. For this, a natural detoxifying agent such as the algae chlorella is needed to bind up the mercury and carry it out through the feces. Dr. Klinghardt notes that a typical dosage of chlorella for this purpose is 12 capsules daily, with each capsule containing 330 mg.

Getting Mercury *Safely* Out of the Body

Although it eliminates the source of further contamination, mercury amalgam removal alone does not put an end to the mercury poisoning. The mercury which leached from the fillings in the mouth is stored in cells throughout the body and continues to exert its damaging influence. Therefore, amalgam removal should be accompanied by a detoxification program to rid the body of the mercury accumulation. In the following section, **Daniel F. Royal, D.O.**, of Henderson, Nevada, describes his highly successful protocol for mercury detoxification:

A Quick Guide to the Nervous System

Standard anatomy describes two components to the nervous system. The **central nervous system (CNS)** comprises the spinal cord, containing millions of nerve fibers, and the brain, while the **peripheral nervous system (PNS)** is the network of nerves estimated to extend 93,000 miles inside the body. The PNS is the sensory motor branch that pertains to the five senses and to how sensory information from the outside world gets translated into muscle movements.

The **autonomic nervous system (ANS)**, involving elements of both the CNS and PNS, is controlled by the brain's hypothalamus gland, and pertains to the automatic regulation of all body processes, such as breathing, digestion, and heart rate. It can be likened to the body's automatic pilot, keeping you alive without you being aware of it or participating in its activities. Neural therapy focuses its injections of anesthetics into body structures whose nerve supply is linked with the autonomic nervous system. Within the ANS, there are two branches—the parasympathetic and sympathetic branches—which are believed to counterbalance each other.

The **parasympathetic nervous system** slows heart rate, inhibits activity, conserves energy, and calms the body, but stimulates gastric secretion and intestinal activity. The **sympathetic nervous system** involves the expenditure of energy and is associated with arousal and stress. It prepares us physically when we perceive a threat or challenge by increasing our heart rate, blood pressure, and muscle tension. The sympathetic portion links all the cells of the body together; it regulates the contraction and expansion of blood vessels; it regulates the activity of connective tissue necessary for regenerating body systems; and it regulates the voltage (membrane potential) across a cell wall. Neural therapy primarily addresses this system.

A **ganglion** is a bundle, knot, or plexus of nerve cell bodies with many interconnections; it acts as a sorting and relay station for nerve impulses. There are several dozen ganglia throughout the body.

Membrane potential refers to differing electrical charges, which constantly change around a certain baseline, measured in millivolts, inside and outside of a cell. This, in turn, influences how easily (or not) substances (nutrients or toxins) can pass into and out of a cell. Sodium ions are pumped out of the cell (to create the normal resting potential of 80 mV) and potassium ions are pumped in. The three means by which substances are transported across the cell membrane are called ion pumping, ionic channel transport, and carrier-protein transport. Transport is voltage dependent and resembles the ebb and flow of tidal water, with nutrients "washing in" and toxins "washing out" with each pulse of the electrical current every 2-5 milliseconds.

In my medical practice, based on urine samples taken during a 24-hour period, I've documented many cases of mercury poisoning. Even if amalgam fillings are no longer present in a patient's mouth, mercury levels can often still be detected. It is not unusual to see patients who have had their amalgam fillings removed and replaced ten to 15 years prior to testing still having elevated levels of mercury in the body.

Once mercury toxicity has been demonstrated, by tests such as high electrogalvanism (SEE QUICK DEFINITION), high mercury vapor emissions, and/or high mercury body burden (tissue deposits), mercury amalgam removal and replacement with alternate, nontoxic materials is the recommended next step.

While removal of amalgam fillings stops any further source of poisoning from mercury fillings, you still need to detoxify the body to eliminate the residual effect from mercury that remains behind in the body. After all, it has been accumulating for as long as you've had amalgam fillings. First, you "turn off the faucet" by removing the fillings; then you "pull the plug" through oral detoxification; and lastly, you "drain the bathtub" (your body) of all traces of mercury.[10]

Ideally, for those who are about to have amalgams removed and replaced, the detoxifying program detailed below should be initiated at least two weeks before amalgam removal and continued for at least three months after the last amalgams are removed. If you have already had your amalgams removed, then start today. The usual length of time required for elimination of mercury from the body is three to six months.

For more about **chlorella**, see Chapter 10: Ending Nutritional Deficiencies with Supplements, pp. 287-288.

The device used to measure **electrogalvanism** is a Galvanometer which, in this case, was made specifically for Dr. Royal's clinic. They use it to determine the amount of positive or negative charges that the various metals in the patient's teeth are emitting. For measuring mercury vapor emissions from the teeth, Dr. Royal uses the Jerome Mercury Vapor Analyzer, the same device used by the Environmental Protection Agency to check the mercury levels in dental offices.

A Complete Mercury Detoxification Program

In my practice, I use the following substances which, taken together, successfully remove mercury residues from the body:

Chlorella—This medicinal green algae helps move mercury out of connective tissue so that substances such as DMPS can then bind with it and eliminate it from the body. Begin with only one chlorella capsule daily for the first few weeks after amalgam removal, then gradually increase to three daily.

L-glutathione—This natural detoxifying substance (made from the amino acid cysteine) improves liver function and metabolism, thereby helping the body detoxify. Take 150 mg once daily (see Chapter 4: Restoring Immune Vitality, pp. 127-129, for more on glutathione).

Kyolic Garlic—Garlic's high sulfur and cysteine content enable it to bind

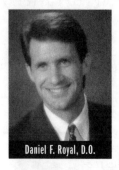

Daniel F. Royal, D.O.

While removal of amalgam fillings stops further poisoning from mercury fillings, you still need to detoxify the body to eliminate the residual effect from mercury that remains behind in the body. After all, it has been accumulating for as long as you've had amalgam fillings.

On the day of amalgam removal, vitamin C should not be taken until after the procedure; otherwise, it may interfere with the anesthesia.

Chelation therapy refers to a method of binding up ("chelating") toxins (e.g. heavy metals) and metabolic wastes and removing them from the body while at the same time increasing blood flow and removing arterial plaque. One type of chelation therapy involves the chelating agent disodium EDTA given as an intravenous infusion over a 3-1/2 hour period. Usually 20 to 30 treatments are administered at the rate of one to three sessions per week. Chelation therapy is especially beneficial for all forms of atherosclerotic cardiovascular disease including angina pectoris and coronary artery disease.

up (chelate—SEE QUICK DEFINITION for chelation) toxic metals and chemicals, and to work against harmful microbes. Take one capsule with meals three times daily.

Silymarin—Also known as milk thistle seed, silymarin has long been used as a liver purifying agent. Take one capsule twice daily.

Vitamin C—Ascorbic acid has a protective effect against free radical (SEE QUICK DEFINITION) damage which can occur as heavy metals are being removed and excreted through the kidneys. On the day before amalgam removal, take your bowel tolerance of vitamin C. This is the amount your system can tolerate before producing diarrhea, usually 8,000-16,000 mg daily, divided into hourly doses of about 2,000 mg for a 150-pound person; decrease the dosage if you get diarrhea. My recommendation is 2,000-8,000 mg daily.

Vitamin B Complex—Take 25-100 mg daily to help replenish nutrients lost when heavy metals are bound up and excreted.

DHEA—(SEE QUICK DEFINITION) This is an adrenal hormone precursor. The adrenal glands of patients with mercury toxicity are often weak, contributing to an inability to handle stress. My recommended daily dosage is 5 mg for men and 2.5 mg for women to be taken daily with pregnenolone.

Pregnenolone—(SEE QUICK DEFINITION) This substance (a steroid building block made from cholesterol, usually extracted from soybeans or wild yam) aids in the formation of key brain chemicals associated with memory and thinking. The recommended daily dosage is 10 mg for men and 30 mg for women. This dosage should initially be taken daily and may be decreased as symptoms improve.

DMSA—DMSA (2,3-dimercaptosuccinic acid) is an effective chelating (binding-up) agent for heavy metals because it crosses the blood-brain barrier and thus helps remove the remaining toxic residues from the central nervous system. On the day of amalgam removal, take three 100 mg capsules both in the morning prior to removal and on the day after removal. Take 30 minutes before or after eating. Once the amalgams have been removed and after you have been on this supplement program for three months, on one occasion only, take two capsules (100 mg each) three times daily for three days.

DMPS–DMPS (2,3-dimercaptopropane-1-sulfonate), is the chelating (binding-up) agent of choice for the removal of elemental mercury from the human body. First developed in China, DMPS then was introduced in Russia where it was used for workers injured by exposure to heavy metals. DMPS has since been researched for over 40 years in Japan, Germany, and the former Soviet Union, and, for the past 25 years, it has been used as a treatment for humans in these countries.

DMPS can be given orally, intravenously, or intramuscularly with a maximum dose of 3 mg/2.2 pounds of body weight, with 250 mg being the typical dose. I recommend a single 250 mg capsule taken once a month, or the same amount by injection, also once monthly. On the day of the last amalgam removal, the first DMPS treatment may be given. People who have had exposure to amalgam through their fillings will usually require 3-5 injections. Those who have never had amalgam fillings, but show evidence or suspicion of heavy metal toxicity through other sources, may require only 1-2 injections. An injection every 4-6 months thereafter is recommended for patient maintenance. Usually, the patient will begin to notice improvement within three to four weeks following the DMPS injections.

Essential Minerals–DMPS and DMSA unavoidably remove vital nutrients from the body, so zinc, copper, magnesium, and manganese should be taken in addition to the other vitamin supplements to replenish the body's supply.

Homeopathic Amalgam Drops—This is a combination of homeopathically prepared elements found in amalgam fillings given for the purpose of enhancing the removal of heavy metals from the body. Beginning one week prior to amalgam removal, take ten drops three times daily; continue this dosage for one week after amalgam removal. Once all the amalgams have been removed, begin taking homeopathic mercury (*Mercurius Solubilis* 30C) at the rate of 30 drops, two to three times weekly for the duration of the oral detoxification program or until you feel improved.

Dr. Royal's Additional Supplements and Guidelines

■ Selenium—Take 50 mcg three times daily between meals and, whenever possible, two hours before or after you have taken vitamin C, to help bind up mercury.

■ *Lactobacillus acidophilus*—This helps to restore the microflora of the intestine which can be adversely affected by the presence of mercury. In my estimation, Torrence Company manufactures the most potent *acidophilus* with 250 billion organisms per teaspoon. Take one teaspoon daily, or more, if diarrhea or constipation are present.

■ Psyllium Husk—This acts as a bulk fiber laxative to absorb toxins and facilitate the removal of fecal debris from the intestines. Drink at least 6-8 glasses of water daily and slowly build up the amount of psyllium consumed. Begin with one teaspoon in liquid once daily and gradually increase to three teaspoons once daily (three times daily if constipation is present). Take psyllium separately from vitamin and mineral supplements as the fiber will reduce their effectiveness.

■ Avoid Fish—This is the largest dietary source of mercury. While some fish have comparatively lower mercury content (e.g., sardines, herring, pollack, mackerel, cod, redfish, and Greenland halibut), most tuna has a fairly high content of mercury.

■ Don't Eat Shellfish—Individuals who are sensitive to mercury usually have some type of adverse reaction to shellfish.

■ Reduce Consumption of Chicken and Eggs—Fish meal has become a major feed for chickens. Depending on the mercury content of the fish products used to make the fish meal, chickens and eggs have the potential of having a significant mercury content.

■ Eat a High Fiber Diet—A high fiber diet, consisting primarily of

Pregnenolone is a hormone produced in the brain and adrenal cortex from cholesterol; in turn, pregnenolone is the "parent" hormone for DHEA and other key hormones. Usually, starting at age 45, pregnenolone production slows down, and by the time one turns 75, the body produces 60% less pregnenolone than in one's youth. As a brain power hormone, pregnenolone enhances memory, improves concentration, reduces mental fatigue, and generally keeps the brain functioning at peak capacity. A typical recommended dose for brainpower enhancement is 50 mg daily, best taken in the morning. Generally, one can expect a "modest improvement" in brainpower within hours after taking pregnenolone, but as this hormone's effect is cumulative, the full beneficial effects will emerge over time.

fruits, vegetables, and legumes, helps decrease fecal transit time, reduces the amount of time that liquids containing heavy metals remain in the colon, and thus cuts back the amount reabsorbed from the colon.

■ Decrease Refined Carbohydrates—These include simple sugars, white flour, and saturated fats which may reduce the availability of essential enzymes and nutrients required for more beneficial purposes.

Use a Sauna to Sweat the Mercury Out of Your Body

Skin is one of the body's detoxification mechanisms and sweating can help draw mercury from the body. Saunas are a useful adjunct to safe mercury removal because they induce copious sweating. Initiate sweating and increased circulation by exercising 20-30 minutes on a stationary bicycle, trampoline, or treadmill. Immediately following the exercise, sit in the sauna for up to 30 minutes, then take a cool (but not cold) shower.

The temperature from a "low heat" sauna should be between 140° F to 180° F in contrast to the 200° F to 210° F for a nontherapeutic standard sauna. The sauna may be repeated again followed by a plunge into a bath or under a shower whose temperature is 65° F. Over a period of three to four days, increase your time in the sauna to a total of up to two hours, divided into 30-minute periods with a short cooling-off period in between. It's important to shower and towel dry because the removal of sweat prevents reabsorption of toxins.

While doing the sauna program, consume adequate amounts of water to avoid dehydration. This is a minimum of two quarts before and after entering the sauna. Replace your electrolytes lost to perspiration with grape or prune juice and take a cultured milk product to compensate for calcium-magnesium loss through the skin. Take a full range of nutritional supplements to help detoxify and minimize nutrient loss, including:

■ Niacin: 400 mg in divided doses; gradually increase to a daily divided dose of 3,000-6,000 mg, depending on your tolerance

■ Vitamin C: 2,000-8,000 mg/day in divided doses

■ Vitamin E: 400-1,200 IU/day

■ Vitamin A: 25,000-50,000 IU (or beta carotene; 15-25 mg) daily

■ Magnesium/calcium: in a 3:1 ratio, with 1,500 mg magnesium and 500 mg calcium daily

CAUTION

Heavy metal-related symptoms, such as joint pains, depression, burning sensations, digestive problems, and fatigue can be temporarily aggravated as DMPS removes toxins from the cells. This is a transient occurrence. The routine use of intravenous DMPS is not advisable for patients who still have mercury amalgam fillings. This is because DMPS may appear in the saliva and act to dissolve the surface of the existing amalgam fillings. The potential outcome is acute toxicity from heavy metal injury to the lining of the gut.

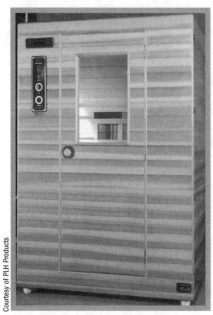

Skin is one of the body's detoxification mechanisms and sweating can help draw mercury from the body. Saunas are a useful adjunct to safe mercury removal because they induce copious sweating.

■ Multivitamin/mineral: take daily for trace minerals and B vitamins (minimum 25 mg)

■ Flaxseed oil: one to two tablespoons daily

■ Lecithin: two tablespoons daily.

This simple program works quickly. You will derive immediate benefits from sauna detoxification, such as mental alertness, a sense of inner cleanliness, and enhanced well-being. ■

The Truth About Quackery in Dentistry

It may surprise you to learn that in 1840, when organized dentistry formed the American Society of Dental Surgeons, members were required to sign "pledges" promising not to use mercury in dental fillings. Several members were suspended from the dental society in New York City in 1848 for "malpractice for using silver mercury fillings."

Mercury was called "quicksilver" in this country and "quacksalver" in some European countries. A "quack" is one who pretends to cure disease, and a "salve" is a substance for application to wounds or sores. The derogatory term "quack" was first used in reference to anyone using mercury preparations on the skin to "cure" diseases. When the skin lesions of syphilis were treated with mercury salves, the skin eruptions would disappear, but their disappearance also resulted in the deeper penetration of the dreaded disease to the organs and nervous system, resulting in a painful death. Thus, mercury has been associated with medical quackery from the beginning.

Internal strife over the use of mercury by 19th-century dentists led to the formation of a new dental organization, the American Dental Association (ADA) in 1859. Its leaders not only did not oppose the use of mercury but now, 137 years later, the ADA condemns dentists who inform their patients that the mercury they are implanting in their teeth is a poison!

Today, dentists in some states believe that the ADA actually sends "undercover agents" into dental offices in which they suspect a dentist is disseminating "negative" (read, truthful) information about mercury. Hence, dentists who attempt to practice "mercury-free" dentistry do so at the peril of losing their licenses.

If mercury is "safe," then why has Sweden banned it and offered to pay for its citizenry to have their fillings replaced? Why is Germany imposing severe restrictions on its use? Why has the world's largest manufacturer of dentistry metals stopped producing amalgam? If we ban mercury in paint and we disallow it in batteries, then why are we still leaving it inside our mouths as a lifetime implant?

To date, the ADA has never scientifically proven its position that mercury in dental fillings is "safe." At best, the ADA's official position is simply a political opinion. Their argument can be summed up in a few words: "We've been using it for over 160 years, so it must be safe." Fortunately for the American public, real scientific evidence refuting the notion that mercury amalgam fillings are safe is mounting every day in opposition to dentistry's politicians.

To contact **Daniel F. Royal, D.O.**: 2501 North Green Valley Parkway, Suite D-132, Henderson, NV, 89014; tel: 702-433-8800; fax: 702-433-8823. Dr. Royal's book, *The Royal Treatment*, discusses numerous innovative alternative medicine approaches and is available from the Nevada Clinic. **Homeopathic amalgam drops** are available from the Nevada clinic or contact: Bio-Energetics, P.O. Box 127, Sandy, OR 97055; tel: 800-334-4043. For **chlorella**, contact: Nature's Balance, 10705 North Main Street, Archdale, NC 27263; tel: 910-434-4102; fax: 910-434-4119. For **Kyolic garlic**, contact: Wakunaga of America, 23501 Madero, Mission Viejo, CA 92691; tel: 800-421-2998; fax: 714-588-0876. For **Silymarin**, contact: Threshold Enterprises, 23 Janis Way, Scotts Valley, CA 95066; tel: 800-777-5677; fax: 408-438-7410. For **pregnenolone**, contact: Kenogen, P.O. Box 3427, Eugene, OR 97403; tel: 503-345-9855; fax: 503-683-4279. **DMPS** is available from any reputable compounding pharmacy. For Apothe'Cure DMPS injectables and capsules (with a doctor's prescription), contact: College Pharmacy, 833 North Tajone, Colorado Springs, CO 80903; tel: 800-888-9358; fax: 800-556-5893. *Mercurius Solubilis* **30C** requires a homeopath's prescription. For *acidophilus*, contact: The Torrence Company, 800 Lenox Avenue, Portage, MI 49002; tel: 800-327-0722.

8 Replenishing Enzyme Deficiencies

Enzyme deficiencies can play a prominent role in chronic fatigue syndrome. This fact was vividly illustrated in several of the cases discussed earlier in the book. The digestive disorders which are common in CFS may stem from an enzyme deficiency. This shouldn't be surprising, because as enzymes are necessary for every chemical reaction which takes place in the body, a deficiency in these vital proteins affects every system, organ, and cell. The impact of this deficiency on digestive function alone sets up a reverberation throughout the body.

The poor digestion and intestinal dysfunction which result from enzyme deficiencies deplete the immune system by not providing the body with necessary nutrients and by allowing toxins to leak from the intestines into the bloodstream. Then the immune system has to expend energy trying to eliminate them.

When immunity is already compromised by the presence of multiple viruses or infections, an enzyme deficiency adds another load which can tip the balance into creating chronic fatigue syndrome.

As more enzymes are needed to help deal with the overload of toxins circulating in the blood, less enzymes are available to break down food, so digestive function worsens and more toxins end up in the blood, creating a further burden on the immune system. When immunity is already compromised by the presence of multiple viruses or infections, this deficit adds another load which can tip the balance into creating chronic fatigue syndrome. An enzyme deficiency is yet another factor in what, in Chapter 5, Dr. Serafina Corsello called the "loading theory" of toxicity and illness.

Again, as with the viruses associated with CFS, it is unclear which comes first—the weakened immune system or the enzyme deficiencies. In either case, supplementing with plant enzymes can correct the enzyme imbalance and break the cycle of ill health, with dysfunction in one system worsening dysfunction in another. In addition, as explained in Chapter 3, enzymes are antiviral agents, capable of digesting the protective protein coating of numerous viruses, leaving the microorganisms open to destruction. Enzymes also help get rid of toxins in the bloodstream. Obviously, enzyme therapy, the precise supplementation with enzymes and other nutrients, can be an important component in a CFS treatment plan.

Being precise means developing a personalized program of recovery for the individual patient. **Maile Pouls, Ph.D.,** a clinical nutritionist, health educator, and cofounder of the Health Enhancement Center in Santa Cruz, California, explains the importance of gathering information on digestive function as a basis for designing a precise treatment program. Dr. Pouls shows the success of this approach in three cases of patients who had typical CFS symptoms:

Digestion is the Key

We're born with a "bank account" of pancreatic

Conditions Associated with an Enzyme Deficiency

allergies

anxiety

bacterial and viral infections

bronchial and respiratory conditions

candidiasis

chronic fatigue syndrome

depressed immunity

depression

environmental illness

frequent sore throats

gastrointestinal problems

hypothyroidism

indigestion

insomnia

irritability

lack of concentration

lymphatic congestion with swollen glands

memory loss

mental sluggishness

mood swings

sinusitis and sinus infections

enzymes necessary for digestion, but if over a lifetime we eat too many cooked and processed foods (known to be enzyme deficient), this pancreatic enzyme reserve gets depleted. Then the pancreas has to make more enzymes, but it does this at the expense of the enzymes in your white blood cells. Some people report feeling very tired, run down, and even a little shaky after eating and this is because their system is pulling enzymes from the immune system. With the immune system taxed in this way, you can become more susceptible to illness.

In an illness as complex as chronic fatigue syndrome, it is crucial to look at as many factors which may be involved in the health problem as possible. For this, a 24-hour urine analysis is indispensable. A standard blood test can often read "normal," even if a patient is becoming sick or is already ill; it doesn't always reveal the true biochemical status. A 24-hour urinalysis can indicate predispositions to diseases long before they manifest and show why a person has multiple, even confusing symptoms, many of them founded on digestive problems.

With my patients, the first thing I check is digestive competence, because over 90% of the patients I treat either have digestive problems or digest less than optimally. If your digestion is not functioning well, it doesn't matter how healthy the food is that you eat, or how high the quality of supplements you take. If you can't assimilate nutrients from food and/or supplements, the body becomes deficient, not to mention toxic, as a result of this poor digestion.

There are three factors the body needs for optimal digestion: enzymes, *Lactobacillus acidophilus* (SEE QUICK DEFINITION), and the correct pH (SEE QUICK DEFINITION). If you lack any of these, the foods you eat are prone to ferment and putrefy, and create acid indigestion, gas, bloating, diarrhea, or constipation. Even worse, the toxins from poorly digested food can migrate into your bloodstream, creating a bodywide state of toxicity. To address digestive problems, it is important not to treat symptoms, but rather to focus on what is setting the person up for poor digestion and bowel toxicity.

Once you know how a person is digesting food, then precise supplementation with enzymes and nutrients can bring about rapid and permanent beneficial changes in a

A Glossary of Urine Analysis Terms

The following are specific values measured in a 24-hour urine analysis:

Volume—The total urine output, either excessive (polyuri) or minimal (oliguria), in relationship to the specific gravity indicates how well the kidneys are functioning.

Indican—This indicates the degree of toxicity, putrefaction, gas, and fermentation in the intestines. Indican comes from putrefying proteins in the large intestine which are kicked back into the blood and excreted through the kidneys. Indican is extremely toxic and causes many symptoms; the higher the level, the greater the intestinal toxemia or inflammation in the digestive tract. Readings as close to zero as possible are desirable.

pH—Based on hydrogen ion concentration, this value indicates the degree of urine acidity versus alkalinity on a scale of zero to 14, with urine pH usually ranging from 4.5 to 8.0 and with 7.0 being neutral.

Chlorides—These are salt residues in the urine and the values here give information on salt intake and assimilation.

Specific gravity—This value measures the weight of total dissolved substances (solutes) in the urine against an equal amount of water, such that a normal reading of 1.020 means the urine is 20% heavier than water. Specific gravity shows the general water content (hydration) of the body. Values can typically range from 1.005 to 1.030; a high reading indicates solute concentration and kidney stress.

Total sediment analysis—This indicates the amount of dissolved organic and mineral substances remaining in the urine after digestion; an optimal total reading for the three sediment categories is 0.5.

Calcium phosphate—A reading here indicates the status of carbohydrate digestion; a level of 0.5 signifies normal carbohydrate digestion.

Uric acid—Levels of uric acid signify the status of protein digestion; optimal digestion yields a reading of zero.

Calcium oxalate—This value indicates the status of fat digestion; a reading of zero signifies optimal fat digestion.

Vitamin C—Levels of vitamin C indicate body reserves of this key nutrient; a reading of 1 is high, 2-5 normal, and 6-10 deficient.

wide range of symptoms seemingly unrelated to digestion, as is true of many CFS symptoms such as headaches, depression, and yeast infections. It may seem paradoxical, but the more extreme the patient's condition, the faster their response to treatment. They may have such a serious imbalance that as soon as you start providing the missing essential nutrients, combined with enzymes, they feel the changes almost *immediately*. This was the case with Holden, as you will see.

Success Story: Ten Years of Fatigue and Indigestion Reversed with Enzymes

Holden, 41, came to me with long-standing symptoms of fatigue and

"If your digestion is not functioning well, it doesn't matter how healthy the food that you eat is, or how high the quality of supplements you take. If you can't assimilate the nutrients, the body becomes deficient, not to mention toxic, as a result of this poor digestion," states Dr. Pouls.

very low energy, a lingering viral infection, chronic indigestion, stomach and kidney pain, and headaches. His indigestion was so severe that he had been taking six to ten Rolaids every day for ten years in an attempt to relieve it.

A 24-hour urine test gave me the following information about Holden's problem: 1) both his liver and kidneys were distressed, indicated by his urine's high specific gravity and its protein and ketone acid content; 2) his organs were malfunctioning without the proper amount of water, which led to severe bowel toxicity; 3) at 5.9, his pH was highly acidic; and 4) his protein, carbohydrate, and fat digestion were poor. Before laying out his treatment plan, I had Holden checked for ulcers and gastritis because certain enzyme formulas can aggravate an irritated stomach; he had neither condition.

Holden began taking four different enzyme formulations from the Ness line of enzymes: #18 would optimize fat digestion and address his acidic pH and the high levels of calcium oxalates (indication of how fats are being digested; in this case, poorly); #6 was to increase protein utilization and reduce the amount of uric acid crystals in his urine (signifying the status of protein digestion); #301 would support his kidneys and lymphatic system; and #416 would help detoxify his system and bolster his immune response. The effect of taking the #416 formula is like getting a second set of white blood cells. After so many years on Rolaids, antibiotics, and other drugs, Holden's natural resistance was low and, as a result, he tended to go from one infection to the next.

Enzymes are an energy source, a kind of "work horse" for the body. If you take them with food, the first thing that any enzyme supplement will do is to begin predigesting this food in the upper stomach. However, when enzymes are taken on an empty stomach, they enter the bloodstream and the targeted tissues often in as fast as 15 minutes.

You might think of enzymes as little "Pac men"—they can eat up undigested protein, cellular debris, chemicals, toxins, free radicals, and antigen-antibody (SEE QUICK DEFINITION) complexes resulting from allergic reactions. This spares the immune system these tasks, and it is then free to concentrate its full action on the bacterial or viral problems.

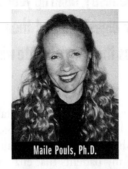

Maile Pouls, Ph.D.

You might think of enzymes as little "Pac men"—they can eat up undigested protein, cellular debris, chemicals, toxins, free radicals, and antigen-antibody complexes resulting from allergic reactions.

Holden took these enzymes daily for a month, reduced his dietary salt intake, ate more alkaline foods (some examples are salad greens, raw vegetables, potatoes, and fresh fruits), and drank more water. His system's response was quick and decisive. Within a week, he no longer needed Rolaids; after a month, his energy level was much improved; he no longer had indigestion or stomach and kidney pains; and instead of daily headaches, he had only one in 30 days. His pH measured 6.7, which is acceptably close to a healthy alkaline level. His levels of chloride and sediment ratios (indicating how well he was handling fats, proteins, and carbohydrates) dropped to normal and his digestion was greatly improved. Now it was time to shift his enzyme formulas.

I started Holden on two products, UltraFiber and Ness #401 with *acidophilus*, to detoxify his intestines. He took two scoops of UltraFiber in water, two times daily, on an empty stomach. Within two months of taking these, Holden's intestinal toxicity (measured by the level of indican) dropped from 3 to 1, an excellent improvement, though not yet optimal, which would be a value of zero.

To accomplish this, three months after beginning the enzyme program, Holden started a more extensive colon cleanse program called Cleanse Thyself™ by Arise and Shine, which included a specific *acidophilus* formula (Flora Grow), a psyllium product, bentonite clay, and two herbal mixtures for clearing the deposits from the colon wall and for healing the intestinal lining. I also shifted a few of his

QUICK DEFINITION

An **antigen** is any biological substance (a toxin, virus, fungus, bacterium, amoeba, or other protein) that the body comes to regard as foreign and dangerous to itself. As such, an antigen induces a state of cellular sensitivity or immune reaction that seeks to neutralize, remove, or destroy the antigen by dispatching antibodies against it.

An **antibody** is a protein molecule containing about 20,000 atoms, made from amino acids by B lymphocyte cells in the lymph tissue and set in motion by the immune system against a specific foreign protein, or antigen. An antibody is also referred to as an immunoglobulin and may be found in the blood, lymph, colostrum, saliva, and the gastrointestinal and urinary tracts, usually within three days after the first encounter with an antigen. The antibody binds tightly with the antigen as a preliminary to removing it from the system or destroying it.

We will balance your chemistry, build up your enzyme and nutrient reserve, improve your digestion, and then watch many of the symptoms disappear as the body's innate wisdom takes charge, says Dr. Pouls.

enzyme mixtures to combinations more suitable for maintenance.

Holden continued to improve, his symptoms gradually disappearing. After three months, his urine analysis values had shifted to normal readings. I never tell my patients that enzymes are a magic bullet or that we're going to "cure" anything. Rather, I say we will balance your chemistry, build up your enzyme and nutrient reserve, improve your digestion, and then watch many of the symptoms disappear as the body's innate wisdom takes charge.

The urine analysis enables me to continually monitor progress and play detective with the patient's biochemistry. I do expect many positive improvements, but I never know how long it will take to achieve these changes; it might take another person with similar conditions four months to get the results Holden started having in the first month.

Success Story: Getting to the Root of Fatigue

Muriel, 47, came to me with a lengthy list of problems, including severe fatigue, low stamina, low blood sugar (hypoglycemia), nervousness, irritability, premenstrual syndrome (PMS—SEE QUICK DEFINITION), muscle cramping, heart palpitations, insomnia, stress, constipation, a vaginal yeast infection, an inability to gain weight, bleeding gums, and a tendency to bruise easily. Whenever she exercised, Muriel felt exhausted and sick afterwards; she had virtually no muscle strength. If you recall, post-exercise exhaustion is one of the symptoms of chronic fatigue syndrome.

A Guide to Ness Enzyme Formulas

#6: Marshmallow root, rosehips, amylase, protease

#11: Citrus bioflavonoids, rosehips, acerola cherries, amylase

#14: Kelp, Irish moss protease

#17: Pau d'arco, yellowdock, echinacea, mullein leaf, amylase, organic germanium

#18: Lipase, amylase, protease, cellulase

#301: Rosehips, alfalfa juice concentrate, echinacea, lipase, protease, mullein

#401: Horsetail, *L. acidophilus*, lipase

#416: Protease, calcium lactate, amylase, lipase

#801: Cellulase, *L. acidophilus*, *L. bifidus* (non-dairy source)

Muriel's urine analysis indicated she had severe bowel toxicity and poor nutrient assimilation. A serious calcium and magnesium deficiency accounted for her inability to relax her muscles or feel calm. Her overly alkaline pH contributed to her poor digestion of proteins, causing an amino acid (SEE QUICK DEFINITION) shortage which, in turn, affected the amino acid levels needed to transport calcium and magnesium into the tissues.

After two months on these supplements, Muriel's urine sediment level was almost normal, her bowel toxicity was much reduced, and many of her other symptoms had abated as her urine test measures improved, says Dr. Pouls.

Muriel was radically deficient in vitamin C, showing the lowest possible reading on the scale (a reading of 6 to 10 is deficient); this accounted for her bleeding gums and the tendency to bruise easily. Her total urine sediment was very low which means she was starving for nutrients and severely deficient in enzymes. Muriel's low levels of calcium phosphate (indicating problems with carbohydrate digestion) contributed to her low blood sugar level.

At the top of Muriel's supplement program, I used Ness #21 to address her chronic low blood sugar and intolerance for dairy products and sugar. To rebuild her amino acid reserves, speed up muscle repair (addressing the exhaustion after exercise), and improve her stamina, I put her on an amino acid formula called Aminoplex. This would also help correct Muriel's hypoglycemia. Approximately 70% of the amino acids in this mixture are digested in about 15 minutes after consumption and start forming glucose which, in turn, restores normal blood sugar levels and reduces sugar cravings.

Muriel also started taking Calcium+ (containing "nutrient partners" such as magnesium, manganese, iron, and vitamins) to ease her nervous system, reduce constipation, and enhance her ability to sleep restfully at night. In addition, she took a product called Trace Minerals (20 drops in a quart of water) which contains plant-based minerals derived from ancient sea beds in Utah. This supplement would replenish electrolytes (SEE QUICK

QUICK DEFINITION

Premenstrual syndrome (PMS) symptoms include bloating, cramping, achiness, irregular bleeding, headaches, short temper, irritability, sudden mood swings, depression, frustration, breast tenderness, weepiness, and abdominal discomfort. An estimated 5% of American women have such severe PMS symptoms that they are incapacitated for a few days every month.

Amino acids are the basic building blocks of the 40,000 different proteins in the body, including enzymes, hormones, and the key brain chemical messenger molecules called neurotransmitters. Eight amino acids cannot be made by the body and must be obtained through the diet; others are produced in the body but not always in sufficient amounts. The body's main "amino acid pool" consists of: alanine, arginine, asparagine, aspartic acid, carnitine, citrulline, cysteine, cystine, GABA, glutamic acid, glutamine, glycine, histidine, isoleucine, leucine, lysine, methionine, ornithine, phenylalanine, proline, serine, taurine, threonine, tryptophan, tyrosine, and valine.

QUICK DEFINITION

Electrolytes are substances in the blood, tissue fluids, intracellular fluids, or urine which conduct an electrical charge, either plus or minus. Examples include acids, bases, and salts, such as potassium, magnesium, phosphate, sulfate, bicarbonate, sodium, chloride, and calcium. Electrolytes provide inorganic chemicals for cellular reactions and control mechanisms, such as the conduction of electrochemical impulses to nerves and muscles. Electrolytes are also needed for key enzymatic reactions involved in metabolism, or the release of energy from food.

An **antioxidant** (meaning "against oxidation") is a natural biochemical substance that protects living cells against damage from harmful free radicals. Antioxidants work against the process of oxidation—the robbing of electrons from substances. If unblocked or left uncontrolled, oxidation can lead to cellular aging, degeneration, arthritis, heart disease, cancer, and other illnesses. Antioxidants in the body react readily with oxygen breakdown products and free radicals, and neutralize them before they can damage the body. Antioxidant nutrients include vitamins A, C, and E, beta carotene, selenium, coenzyme Q10, pycnogenol (grape seed extract), L-glutathione, superoxide dismutase, and bioflavonoids. Plant antioxidants include *Ginkgo biloba* and garlic. When antioxidants are taken in combination, the effect is stronger than when they are used individually.

DEFINITION), as Muriel's urine test showed her electrolyte levels were deficient.

To improve her vitamin C levels, Muriel took Ness #11; in two months, this brought them back up to a 3, within the normal range. Ness #801 uses *acidophilus* and cellulase enzymes to kill yeast and eliminate vaginal yeast infections. I had her take this supplement orally ($\frac{1}{2}$ teaspoon with each meal) and internally, in the form of a douche or a vaginal suppository at night. She made a paste from the powder and inserted it into her vagina. In three days, her yeast infection cleared up.

After two months on these supplements, Muriel's pH shifted to a more appropriate 6.8. Her urine sediment level was almost normal, her bowel toxicity was much reduced, and many of her other symptoms had abated as her urine test measures improved. As her problem with low blood sugar started to ease off and Muriel began a more intensive weight-lifting and exercise program, I switched her amino acid formula to Amino-Stasis, which contains a different balance of specific amino acids more suited to muscle repair.

To complement her vitamin C intake at this point, I put Muriel on Pycnogenol C, a supplement made from grape seed and pine bark that is many times more potent as an antioxidant (SEE QUICK DEFINITION) than vitamin C alone. As her calcium levels were approaching normal, I switched her from Calcium+ to Osteoprime Forte; this would work as a longtime preventive strategy against osteoporosis, a condition towards which her extreme calcium deficiency had been leading her. After another two months, most of Muriel's key biochemical factors (including her electrolyte levels) became normal and nearly all of her multiple symptoms disappeared.

Success Story:
Ending Maryann's Fatigue and Depression

Like Holden and Muriel, Maryann, 31, complained of many symptoms typical of CFS, beginning with great fatigue. She also had constant headaches, anemia, constipation, PMS, kidney and intestinal pain, dry skin, and low body temperature along with cold hands and feet which can be a sign of hypothyroidism.

She was unable to lose weight and was taking the antidepressant Prozac for serious depression. More seriously, she had all the signs of irritable bowel syndrome, which in her case, exhibited as bleeding and inflammation of the intestines; she also had symptoms suggesting an ulcer in the small intestine. She was on Tagamet for stomach ulcers and an iron supplement for her anemia.

This case demonstrates another aspect of biochemical functioning revealed by a urine analysis. In Maryann's case, she had high values for specific gravity and total sediment, indicating a heavy concentration of substances in her urine. It turns out Maryann drank very little water and, as a result, passed very little urine, a condition clinically called oliguria, or underproduction of urine. Her low level of water intake created considerable problems for her. She was becoming toxic from lack of water, as water is needed to flush waste products out of the tissues and to absorb nutrients. Water also acts as an intestinal lubricant; Maryann's constipation and high level of bowel toxicity were partly due to this deficiency.

In treating Maryann, I had to keep in mind the fact that a strong enzyme formula, especially one containing higher amounts of protease (which digests proteins), could irritate her inflamed stomach wall. I started her on Gastritis Complex which is a plant enzyme formula

Maryann's low level of water intake created considerable problems for her. She was becoming toxic from lack of water, as water is needed to flush waste products out of the tissues and to absorb nutrients.

containing gamma oryzanol, marshmallow root, and slippery elm. I also prescribed Chlorophyll Perles for her intestinal ulcer. In this form, the chlorophyll is fat soluble which means it does not get digested in the stomach but moves on to the intestines, where it literally adheres to the gut wall forming a kind of lubricating film and healing ointment.

To address Maryann's depression and to provide an alternative to Prozac, Maryann started taking Stabilium, a form of essential fatty acids (EFAs). With this product, I have been able to assist over 40 patients in getting off Prozac, with their physician's supervision. Stabilium helps boost physical energy and stamina, decrease mood swings, lessen anxiety, agitation, and melancholia, and improve the quality of sleep. For the continuing fatigue, I put her on Adaptogen which contains a variety of energy-balancing Chinese herbs. To eliminate the PMS, Maryann took natural progesterone (SEE QUICK DEFINITION) in the form of a cream called ProGest.

Maryann took Ness #17 to address her headaches and anemia, as she was not absorbing the iron from the conventional supplement she had been taking. Ness #17 contains the herb yellowdock as an easily assimilated form of plant-based iron. It also contains germanium, which gets oxygen into the cells including those in the brain, thereby helping to relieve tension-type headaches which result from too little oxygen being available in the brain.

Maryann had low body temperature, especially in her hands and feet. To rebalance this, I put her on Omega EFA (containing both omega-3 and omega-6 essential fatty acids [SEE QUICK DEFINITION], plus borage oil and vitamin E), two capsules twice daily with meals. Since EFAs bind oxygen to hemoglobin (made of iron and amino acids, its job is to transport oxygen in the blood), getting more EFAs into the body will improve circulation and thus bring warmth to the hands and feet. To address Maryann's underactive thyroid and still deficient electrolyte levels, I gave her Ness #14.

Within two months on this program, Maryann was no longer tired and depressed, nor was she taking Prozac or Tagamet. She passed a normal volume of urine after increasing her water intake; in fact, her urine output more than doubled. Marked changes also occurred in her readings for specific gravity, which dropped from 1.033 to 1.018 (normal is 1.020), and in her total sediment, which went down from 1.1 to 0.60 (normal is 0.5). Even the color of Maryann's urine showed the change: before it had been a hazy yellow brown; now it was a more normal yellow. Her constipation disappeared, her skin was less dry, her extremities were not cold all the time, and she lost five pounds.

As a result of taking Prozac, Tagamet, and other drugs, which can tax the liver, Maryann needed nutritional support, so I put her on a product called Liverguard. After four months on the program (the components of which I shifted as she progressed), most of Maryann's urine readings fell within the normal range and nearly all of her symptoms disappeared.

These three cases give a clear idea of what nutrients and enzymes can do in shifting body chemistry to relieve health problems.

By getting a complete picture of exactly what is happening in the body, as can be obtained through a 24-hour urine analysis, the specific components of even a complex, multilayered disorder such as chronic fatigue syndrome can systematically be addressed and the body restored to health. ■

By getting a complete picture of exactly what is happening in the body, as can be obtained through a 24-hour urine analysis, the specific components of even a complex, multilayered disorder such as chronic fatigue syndrome can systematically be addressed and the body restored to health, Dr. Pouls says.

For more information about **UltraFiber**, contact: Metagenics West, Inc., 12445 East 39th Avenue, Suite 402, Denver, CO 80239; tel: 800-321-META or 303-371-6848; fax: 303-371-9303. For **Ness enzymes**, contact: Ness, 100 Business Park Lane NW, Riverside, MO 64150; tel: 800-637-7893 or 816-746-0110. For **Aminoplex** and **Amino-Stasis**, contact: Tyson & Associates, 12832 Chadron Avenue, Hawthorne, CA 90250; tel: 800-318-9766 or 310-675-1080; fax: 310-675-4187. For **Cleanse Thyself™**, contact: Arise & Shine, 401 Berry Street, P.O. Box 1439, Mt. Shasta, CA 96067; tel: 916-926-0891 or 800-688-2444; fax: 916-926-8866. For **Calcium Plus** and **Adaptogen**, contact: Rainbow Light, P.O. Box 600, Santa Cruz, CA 95061; tel: 800-635-1233 or 408-429-9089; fax: 408-429-0189. For **Pycnogenol C**, contact: Health Products Distributors, Inc., 23847 Peaceful Ridge Road, Smithsburg, MD 21783; tel: 800-228-4265 or 520-398-9000; fax: 520-398-9756. For **Gastritis Complex**, contact: Tyler Encapsulations, 2204-8 NW Birdsdale, Gresham, OR 97030; tel: 800-869-9705 or 503-661-5401; fax: 503-661-4913. For **Chlorophyll Perles**, contact: Standard Process, P.O. Box 1289, Alameda, CA 94501; tel: 800-662-9134 or 510-865-4322; fax: 510-865-4335. For **Stabilium**, contact: Allergy Research, 400 Preda Street, San Leandro, CA 94577; tel: 800-545-9960 or 510-639-4572; fax: 510-635-6730. For **Liverguard**, contact: Source Naturals, 23 Janis Way, Scotts Valley, CA 95066; tel: 800-777-5677 or 408-438-6851; fax: 408-438-7410. For **ProGest**, contact: Health Products, Inc., 23847 Peaceful Ridge Road, Smithsburg, MD 21783; tel: 800-228-4265. For **urine analysis**, patients may call Dr. Pouls; they may also contact her for a referral to a licensed practitioner in their area who provides these services. Many of the products listed above are only available to licensed health-care professionals.

Recently, Dr. Pouls has formulated new products combining ingredients that better accommodate the needs of the patients she is encountering in her practice. She now uses Digestion & Stomach Upset Support System or Ness #21; Athletic Enzyme Support System or Aminoplex; *Acidophilus/Candida* Support System or Ness #801; Allergy Enzyme Support System or Ness #301; Digestion Enzyme Support System or Ness #18; Digestion and Stomach Upset Support System or Gastric Complex; Anti-Aging/Antioxidant Enzyme Support System or Liverguard; and Stress Relief & Energy Support System or Adaptogen. For information regarding these new products, contact the sources listed above or: Alternative Therapy, Inc., 222 East Cliff Drive, Suite 5B, Santa Cruz, CA 95062; tel: 408-477-1040. For a personalized nutritional program, a urine analysis to evaluate your individual nutritional needs, and specific nutrients and plant enzymes to optimize your body chemistry (via phone consultation), contact **Dr. Maile Pouls**: 517 Liberty Street, Santa Cruz, CA 95060; tel/fax: 408-425-2222.

Signs and Symptoms of Enzyme Deficiency

"Depletions of plant enzymes lead to a host of chronic diseases that could in part be avoided if we provided the body with the enzymes it needs," says Lita Lee, Ph.D., an enzyme therapist based in Lowell, Oregon. "As it is, we are not aware of enzyme deficiencies because they take so long to manifest. When there are signs, the body is already in a state of exhaustion." If you are wondering whether a shortage of enzymes may be contributing to your CFS, Dr. Lee states, "If you have fatigue, allergies, bloating, gas, constipation, indigestion, or any symptom of undigested food, then you most likely have an enzyme deficiency."

As mentioned above, a simple urine analysis can precisely pinpoint your deficiencies, but here, in the following section, **Lita Lee, Ph.D.**, explains the signs and symptoms associated with deficiencies of the main digestive enzymes: protease, amylase, lipase, cellulase, and disaccharidase:

Protease (digests protein)

Protease digests protein; not only protein from food, but also other organisms which are composed of protein, such as the protein coating on certain viruses, toxins from dead bacteria and other organisms, and certain harmful substances produced at sites of injury or inflammation.

Protease is especially effective during inflammatory processes to control swelling, redness, heat, fever, and pain. Due its ability to bolster immunity, protease is an important line of defense in the immune system. Consequently, immune system disorders are among the most common symptoms of protease deficiency. Additionally, since about half the protein you eat is converted to sugar, protease deficiency and inadequate protein digestion lead to hypoglycemia (low blood sugar), with such symptoms as moodiness, depression, anxiety, irritability, and attention deficit disorder (ADD).

Toxic colon syndrome, also called indicanuria or intestinal toxemia, is anoth-

Conditions Associated with Protease Deficiency

anxiety

cold hands and feet

water retention (edema)

frequent bacterial/viral infections

colon problems

kidney disease

bone problems (osteoporosis, spurs)

blood clots

low blood sugar (hypoglycemia)

er result of protease deficiency and the inability to digest protein. Undigested protein decomposes at the intestinal level. The products of this putrefaction (called indican) leak into the blood from the intestines. From there, they reach the liver. The liver can

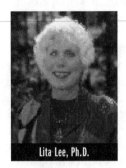

Lita Lee, Ph.D.

"We are not aware of enzyme deficiencies because they take so long to manifest," says Dr. Lee. "When there are signs, the body is already in a state of exhaustion."

detoxify only some of these products, and in doing so, becomes stressed. Those substances that cannot be processed are excreted through the urine.

Indicanuria is identified by elevated levels of indican in the urine, as determined by a 24-hour urine analysis. Research has found that numerous inflammatory or pathological conditions can result from elevated indican. In fact, indicanuria can cause more than 100 symptoms or conditions. The following (all are associated with CFS) are among those which have been linked to high indican levels: fatigue, allergies, gastrointestinal problems, hypothyroidism, lack of concentration, memory loss, and sinusitis and sinus infections.

Amylase (digests carbohydrates)

Amylase digests carbohydrates, breaking them down into smaller units which are later converted into monosaccharides (simple sugars) such as glucose and fructose. People who can't digest fats often eat large amounts of sugar and carbohydrates to make up for the lack of fat in their diet. If their diet is excessive in carbohydrates, they can develop an amylase deficiency. Amylase is important in preventing the proliferation of dead leukocytes, or white blood cells, which manifests as pus.

Amylase is used in combination with lipase, fatty acids, and herbs to reduce certain viral problems, including all types of

Conditions Associated with Amylase Deficiency

skin problems (hives, rashes)

eczema

psoriasis

herpes

allergies to bee stings and insect bites

muscle soreness and pain

joint stiffness

thick blood

herpes, and to remove the pus from inflamed areas. Additionally, amylase aids in clearing the lungs.

Lipase (digests fats)

Lipase is the enzyme responsible for digesting fats. This includes fat in foods and the fat-based coatings of certain viruses—lipase can effectively destroy some viruses by digesting their outer coating. Certain viral infections may accompany a lipase deficiency, and are characterized by symptoms including fatigue, sore throat, and swollen glands. People who are diagnosed with chronic fatigue syndrome fall into this category. A prominent indicator of lipase deficiency is chronic fatigue syndrome or "hidden" viruses. A lipase-deficient person is also likely to have irritable bowel symptoms.

Here is a classic case of chronic fatigue and lipase deficiency: A frail, 47-year-old woman came to me with chronic fatigue, allergies, and abdominal pain of 20 years duration. She had been to countless doctors and health clinics, all to no avail. She had been trying to gain weight for years, and she was so painfully thin and listless, I wondered how she mustered up enough energy to come to my office. Her diet was mainly liquefied greens, sprouted seeds, salad, potatoes, yams, corn, fresh vegetables, and raw juices. Her tests indicated a toxic colon, poor digestion, and extreme lipase deficiency.

A prominent indicator of lipase deficiency is chronic fatigue syndrome or "hidden" viruses.

I recommended a high lipase formula required in cases of fiber-intolerant, lipase-deficient clients. When she started taking the high-lipase multiple-digestive formula, she began to gain weight and her abdominal pains diminished.

Conditions Associated with Lipase Deficiency

cardiovascular problems
diabetes
dizziness
high blood pressure
high cholesterol
obesity
difficulty losing weight

Cellulase (digests fiber)

Cellulase digests fiber. It also "eats" pathogenic yeast, so candidiasis from a *Candida* overgrowth is often the result of inadequate "friendly" bowel bacteria coupled with a cellulase deficiency. Sudden, acute allergies can also be an outcome of cellulase deficiency. Candidiasis sets the stage for leaky gut syndrome which in turn can lead to the development of food allergies, as undigested food particles make their way into the bloodstream and trigger an immune response. Once these food particles have passed from the digestive system to the circulatory system, the brain no longer interprets them as "food." Instead, they are considered foreign substances which must be eliminated from the body.

For more on **candidiasis and allergies,** see Chapter 9: Addressing the Allergy Connection, pp. 232-258.

Disaccharidase (digests sugars)

Disaccharidases digest sugars. The sugar intolerance which results from a deficiency in these enzymes can lead to various health conditions. The inability to digest complex sugars (sucrose, lactose, and maltose) and convert them into the simple sugars (glucose and fructose) lowers the blood sugar level and starts starving the brain of nourishment. The end result can be a range of problems, including depression, attention deficit disorder (ADD), and even seizures. Disaccharidase deficiency is also associated with environmental illness, asthma, and diarrhea.

The Essentials of Enzyme Therapy

The human body makes approximately 22 different digestive enzymes, capable of digesting protein, carbohydrates, sugars, and fats. The body digests food in stages: beginning in the mouth, moving to the stomach, and finally through the small intestine. At each step, specific enzymes break down different types of food. An enzyme designed to digest protein, for example, has no effect on starch, and an enzyme active in the mouth will not be active in the stomach. This process is balanced through acidity; each site along the digestive track has a different degree of acidity that allows certain enzymes to function while inhibiting others.

Conditions Associated with Cellulase Deficiency

acute food allergies

candidiasis

facial pain or paralysis

gas and bloating

Conditions Associated with Disaccharidase Deficiency

asthma

bronchitis and other lung problems

chronic diarrhea

dizziness

environmental illness

hyperactivity

insomnia

mood swings

seizures

Metabolism and the Life of Enzymes

Metabolism is the biological process by which energy is extracted from the foods consumed, producing carbon dioxide and water as by-products for elimination. Biochemically, metabolism involves hundreds of different chemical reactions, necessitating the involvement of hundreds of different enzymes, each of which handles a specific reaction. There are two kinds of metabolism constantly under way in the cells: anabolic and catabolic.

In anabolic metabolism, the upbuilding phase, larger molecules are constructed by joining smaller ones together; in catabolic metabolism, the deconstructing phase, larger molecules are broken down into smaller ones. The anabolic function produces substances for cell growth and repair, while the catabolic function controls digestion (called hydrolysis), disassembling food into forms the body can use for energy.

Circulating immune complexes (CICs) form in the body when poor digestion results in undigested food proteins "leaking" through the intestinal wall and into the bloodstream. The immune system treats these foreign substances or antigens as invaders, causing antibodies to form and couple with them. This antigen and antibody combination is known as a CIC. In a healthy person, CICs are neutralized, but in someone with a compromised immune system, they tend to accumulate in the blood where they burden the detoxification pathways or initiate an allergic reaction.

If too many CICs accumulate, the kidneys cannot excrete enough of them via the urine. The CICs are then stored in soft tissues, causing inflammation and bringing stress to the immune system. The overload can lead to a variety of chronic health conditions.

As enzymes begin digesting food in the mouth and continue their work in the stomach, plant enzymes (derived from food itself or taken as a supplement) become active. The food then enters the upper portion of the small intestine where the pancreatic enzymes supplied by the pancreas (a digestive organ that feeds enzymes into the gut) further break down the food. Final breakdown of remaining small molecules of food occurs in the lower small intestine.

Ideally, plant and pancreatic enzymes work together, digesting food and delivering nutrients to cells to maintain their health. Protocols for enzyme therapy are based on this sequence of events. "One of the most important processes in the metabolism of food is the chain of reactions that convert glucose to energy," states Dr. Lee.

"Several vitamin and mineral coenzymes are necessary for these reactions. Coenzymes are consumed in the process. Our bodies need a continuing supply. All the food we eat, that eventually becomes energy, passes through this same set of reactions, whether the food is a fast-food hamburger or a raw carrot. Coenzymes are always needed, and when the food doesn't provide these, we use the vitamins and minerals stored in our body until these reserves are used up. Only when we eat whole and raw foods can we maintain a good supply of the parts that keep the metabolic machinery going."

When the body receives plentiful supplies of enzymes, says Edward Howell, M.D., an accomplished author and pioneer in the field of enzyme therapy in the United States, "its internal enzyme supplies are preserved for the important work of maintaining metabolic harmony." As a result, many body systems are strengthened.[1]

The importance of raw foods becomes clear once you understand that plant enzymes, more heat-sensitive than vitamins, are destroyed in the process of cooking food at temperatures above 118° F[2] and, as Dr. Lee points out, "are deactivated or destroyed by pasteurizing, canning, and microwaving." Given the predominance in our diet of these methods of food preserving and preparation, you can see how enzyme deficiency can easily develop.

The importance of raw foods becomes clear once you understand that plant enzymes, more heat-sensitive than vitamins, are destroyed in the process of cooking food at temperatures above 118° F, and, as Dr. Lee points out, "deactivated or destroyed by pasteurizing, canning, and microwaving."

However, while raw foods are recommended, a 100% raw foods diet is not necessary. Some people may have problems digesting uncooked food because of a lack of cellulase in their bodies (an enzyme that breaks down cellulose, part of the plant's cell wall) which can be liberated from raw foods, but only if chewed slowly.

To contact **Lita Lee, Ph.D.**: Enzyme Therapy, P.O. Box 516, Lowell, OR 97452; tel: 541-937-1123; fax: 541-937-1132.

According to Dr. Lee, when a patient's plant enzyme deficiencies are addressed many other conditions can be resolved, from digestive ailments and common sore throats to candidiasis, which is a common complaint of chronic fatigue syndrome sufferers. Howard F. Loomis Jr., D.C., founder and president of 21st Century Nutrition in Madison, Wisconsin, agrees. "It cannot be said that a *particular* enzyme can help a *particular* illness, but by clearing up digestive prob-

Dr. Loomis developed a line of plant enzyme formulas after a personal experience with the healing abilities of enzymes. He finally treated himself with massive doses of protease enzymes and his 43-year-old ear infection cleared up within 36 hours.

To contact **Howard F. Loomis Jr., D.C.:** 21st Century Nutrition, 6421 Enterprise Lane, Madison, WI 53719; tel: 800-662-2630. His first line of enzymes was marketed under the brand name of Ness. His second generation line of 29 enzyme formulas is called Chirozyme or Therazyme and is available from 21st Century Nutrition.

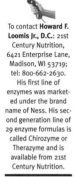

For more on **enzymes and allergies**, see Chapter 9: Addressing the Allergy Connection, pp. 232-258.

Further research into the benefits of enzyme therapy is necessary as it has been clinically proven to alleviate a wide range of conditions, including chronic fatigue syndrome.

lems, we've found that many other problems seem to go away and new ailments may be prevented, " he says.

Dr. Loomis developed a line of plant enzyme formulas after a personal experience with the healing abilities of enzymes. He had been searching for years for a solution to his chronic ear problems—hearing loss and continual ear infections which had plagued him since infancy when he had severe whooping cough. Medications had proven ineffective against the infection and he was unable to wear hearing aids because his ears were constantly draining. He finally treated himself with massive doses of protease enzymes and his 43-year-old ear infection cleared up within 36 hours.

As discussed previously, in addition to their crucial role in digestion, enzymes directly assist the defense mechanisms of the immune system.[3] Enzymes produced by the pancreas or from supplements of plant or pancreatic (animal-derived) enzymes taken between meals act, as Dr. Pouls says, like "little Pac men" in the bloodstream, getting rid of unwanted material. With their ability to digest foreign proteins, enzymes are useful in clearing out infecting organisms, scar tissue, and the products of inflammation.

For example, CFS sufferers characteristically have high Epstein-Barr virus (EBV) antibody levels. Enzymes can digest the protective protein coat of EBV so the virus can be destroyed. Enzymes are also helpful in the removal of circulating immune complexes (CICs) that are abundant in viral disease and, in particular, in patients with immune deficiencies.[4] Supplemental enzymes share the workload of the body's own pancreatic enzymes and therefore ease the burden of that organ's production of enzymes needed for digestion, immune function, and all other chemical reactions in the body.

The poor digestion and
intestinal dysfunction which result from enzyme
deficiencies deplete the immune system
by not providing the body with necessary nutrients
and by allowing toxins to leak from
the intestines into the bloodstream.
Then the immune system has to expend energy
trying to eliminate them.
When immunity is already compromised by the
presence of multiple viruses or infections,
this deficit adds another load
which can tip the balance into creating
chronic fatigue syndrome.

CHAPTER

9

Addressing the Allergy Connection

ALLERGIES ARE A COMMON complaint of people who suffer from chronic fatigue syndrome and fibromyalgia and they are the defining feature of environmental illness. Characterized by multiple and extensive allergies, environmental illness could be called the "ultimate allergy." Allergies in all three syndromes contribute to an already taxed immune system. Allergies and the immune response they generate can be a factor in up to 80% of patients with chronic fatigue.[1] As a contributor to immune overload, ongoing allergic reaction is an essential condition to address in the treatment of CFS.

Previous chapters in this book have shown how immune dysfunction and enzyme deficiencies are related to intestinal problems. Allergies are closely linked to intestinal disorders as

"Dysbiosis [imbalance in intestinal flora] and delayed food allergies are almost universally present in people with autoimmune disorders," observes Serafina Corsello, M.D.

well. For example, candidiasis (overgrowth of the intestinal fungus *Candida albicans*) and allergies are often paired. As in the domino effect of mercury toxicity (see Chapter 7: Eliminating Heavy Metal Toxicity, pp. 190-211), the intestinal dysfunction created by candidiasis can lead to "leaky gut" syndrome.

Here, undigested food particles pass through the intestinal walls into the bloodstream where the body launches an allergic reaction against these foreign substances. When the condition is chronic, the development of an allergy to that food may be the result. A delayed

A Primer on Allergies

Allergy—This is an adverse immune system reaction—sometimes mild, sometimes severe—to a substance that other people may find harmless. Quite often, an allergen (a substance provoking an allergy symptom) is a protein that the body judges to be foreign and dangerous. The adverse reaction that follows is called an allergic response.

Common manifestations of this allergic response include fatigue, headaches, sneezing, watery eyes, and stuffy sinuses following exposure to an allergen. Allergies fall into two categories, those caused by environmental factors and those caused by food. The most common source of environmental allergies is the pollen of plants, particularly trees, weeds, and grass. The most common culprits in food allergies are wheat, corn, milk and other dairy products, egg whites, tomatoes, soy, shellfish, peanuts, chocolate, and food dyes and additives.

Common Symptoms of an Allergic Reaction—Breathing congestion, inflamed, bloodshot, or scratchy eyes, watery eyes, tears, sneezing, coughing, itching, nosebleeds, puffy face, flushing of the cheeks, dark circles under the eyes, runny nose, swelling, hives, vomiting, stomachache, intestinal irritation or swelling.

Common Health Problems Partly Caused by Allergens—Acne, allergic rhinitis (inflammation of mucous lining of nose), bedwetting, diarrhea, asthma, ear infections, eczema, fatigue, chronic runny nose, headache, irritability, hay fever, concentration problems, hyperactivity, attention deficit disorder.

The Cycle of Food Allergies—With food allergies there is a strange situation: often a person becomes addicted to a food that produces an allergic response. When a person stops eating an allergy-producing food to which their body is "addicted," such as coffee or chocolate, there is a three-day period in which they experience unpleasant withdrawal symptoms, such as fatigue; eating more of this addictive substance can actually improve the situation by suppressing these withdrawal symptoms. This of course becomes an unhealthy cycle of addiction, craving, and fulfillment that eventually leads to more serious health problems. Allergy experts call this suppression of symptoms by an allergy-producing (allergenic) food "masking," because it masks or disguises the true allergic symptoms.

What Happens in an Allergic Response—The typical allergic reactions many people have to foods, dust, pollen, and other substances are the body's way of fending off the intrusion of toxins that disrupt the body's equilibrium. Allergens, or foreign substances judged by the body to be harmful, enter the body through breathing, the skin, through eating or drinking, or by injection, such as insect bites or vaccinations.

Because the body judges the allergens to be dangerous to its health, the immune system identifies them as *antigens*. Antigens trigger an allergic inflammatory response. The immune system then releases specific forms of protein called *antibodies* to deactivate the allergenic antigens, setting in motion a complex series of events involving up to 12 different biochemicals. These chemicals then produce the inflammation or other typical symptoms of an allergy response.

An antibody known as IgE is most

continued on page 234

commonly involved in the allergic response to pollens and foods. IgE is one of five immunoglobulins, or antibodies, involved with allergic responses. An immunoglobulin is one of a class of five specially designed antibody proteins produced in the spleen, bone marrow, or lymph tissue and involved in the immune system's defense response to foreign substances. The main types of immunoglobulins, grouped according to their concentration in the blood, are: IgG (80%), IgA (10% to 15%), IgM (5% to 10%), IgD (less than 0.1%), IgE (less than 0.01%). Technically, all antibodies are immunoglobulins.

Mast cells, which produce the allergic response and are found throughout the body's tissues, next come into play; they tend to be concentrated in the skin, nose and lung linings, gastrointestinal tract, and reproductive organs. A single mast cell, for example, contains between 100,000 and 1 million receptor sites on its surface for the IgE antibody; it also has about 1,000 granules containing a substance called histamine.

When the IgE antibody senses an allergen, it triggers the mast cells to release histamine and 28 other chemicals and the allergic response flares into action. The IgE molecules also attach themselves, like a key fitting a lock, to the allergens.

Histamine—This is the substance that causes the blood vessels to widen enabling more fluid to pass into body tissues, resulting in swelling; it also triggers the smooth involuntary muscles in the lungs, blood vessels, heart, stomach, intestines, and bladder to contract. Histamine gives us runny noses, red itchy eyes, hot, tender, or swollen body parts, flushing, and the other symptoms associated with allergic reactions.

In general, the allergic response, in the form of an inflammation, swelling, heat, redness, or tenderness, is the body's attempt to heal itself from the effect of the allergen. In other words, these responses are normal ways the body takes care of itself, albeit in the process they can make us feel miserable. They may be the body's protective mechanism, but if they continue unchecked for too long your health will suffer.

The allergic response can happen as quickly as 15 minutes after your initial exposure to an allergenic substance. If the histamine and related biochemicals are released in the chest you may experience coughing or asthma-like symptoms; if they come out through the skin, the symptoms may be hives or eczema; if in the intestines, the allergic response may show up as diarrhea; and if in the brain, it may result in a migraine headache.

Other Chemicals Released During an Allergic Response—

■ Heparin: Increases blood flow to the site of inflammation or swelling.

■ Platelet Activating Factor: Causes blood platelets to group together so that they release chemicals to change the diameter of blood vessels, thereby affecting blood pressure.

■ Serotonin: A brain chemical known as a neurotransmitter, found mostly in the mucous membrane cells of the gastrointestinal tract, and involved in the allergic response to foods.

■ Lymphokines: Produced by white

blood cells (lymphocytes) and involved in communications among cells.

■ **Leukotrienes:** Found in cell membranes and involved in making the lung muscles contract and the lungs retain more air, as in the bronchial spasm of asthma.

■ **Prostaglandins:** Hormone-like substances that help dilate blood vessels, affect smooth muscle contraction, increase pain in affected areas, and heat up inflamed tissues.

■ **Thrombaxanes:** Chemicals which cause the blood vessels and bronchial tubes to contract .

■ **Bradykinin:** Support the cascade of inflammatory symptoms set in motion by the mast cells.

■ **Interleukins:** Antigens involved in the activity of lymphocytes, including the irritation of tissues.

■ **Interferons:** Produced by lymphocytes to regulate the speed of immune responses.

---

allergic reaction (hours to days after eating a food) is common and means you can have food allergies and not know it. Continued dysbiosis (SEE QUICK DEFINITION) leads to more allergies and serious health disorders such as chronic fatigue syndrome. "Dysbiosis and delayed food allergies are almost universally present in people with autoimmune disorders," observes Serafina Corsello, M.D., director of the Corsello Centers for Nutritional Complementary Medicine in New York City and Huntington, New York.

In this chapter, you will learn about a highly effective technique for permanently getting rid of your allergies. Developed by Devi Nambudripad, D.C., L.Ac., R.N., Ph.D., this innovative method is called the Nambudripad Allergy Elimination Technique (NAET—SEE QUICK DEFINITION). You will also learn how other alternative medicine physicians treat the underlying causes that go into creating allergies and the attendant CFS. One of these physicians, Susan Lange, O.M.D., L.Ac., explains the "sick building syndrome" as a contributing factor in environmental illness and describes how she healed herself of this debilitating condition.

We begin with the case of Elinor, whose story is a vivid illustration of how unidentified allergies and their companion, untreated candidiasis, can prevent recovery from chronic fatigue syndrome.

Intestinal **dysbiosis** refers to an imbalance of intestinal flora. Specifically, these flora are friendly, beneficial bacteria, called probiotics, such as Lactobacillus acidophilus and Bifidobacterium bifidum, and unfriendly bacteria in the intestines such as Escherichia coli and Clostridium perfringens. In dysbiosis, the unfriendly bacteria predominate; they begin fermentation producing toxic by-products such as ammonia, amines, nitrosamines, phenols, cresols, indole, and skatole, which interfere with the normal elimination cycle. Dysbiosis is considered a primary cause or major cofactor in the development of many health problems, such as acne, yeast overgrowth, chronic fatigue, depression, digestive disorders, bloating, food allergies, PMS, rheumatoid arthritis, and cancer.

The Nambudripad Allergy Elimination Technique (NAET) is used for the detection and elimination of allergies. Developed by Devi Nambudripad, D.C., L.Ac., Ph.D., R.N., this noninvasive method combines kinesiology's muscle response testing, acupuncture, and chiropractic. After identifying allergenic substances through muscle response testing, the NAET practitioner uses acupuncture (or acupressure if the patient dislikes needles) to retrain the brain and nervous system to no longer respond allergically to those substances. For the treatment to become permanent, the patient must stay away from the offending substance for at least 24 hours, and sometimes more than one treatment is necessary.

Success Story: Uncovering Hidden Allergies to Reverse Chronic Fatigue

When Elinor, 45, came to see Milton Hammerly, M.D., medical director of the American Whole Health Clinic in Littleton, Colorado, she had been suffering from a long list of symptoms for 18 years. They included severe fatigue, depression, brain fog, concentration troubles, muscle spasms and aches, night sweats, premenstrual syndrome (PMS—SEE QUICK DEFINITION), frequent infections including bronchitis and sore throats, "migratory" rashes that sprang up on different areas of her body, and not feeling refreshed after sleeping. Elinor also had digestive problems, including frequent constipation and bloating, indicating a probable imbalance in the microfloral population of her intestines (called dysbiosis).

She had been taking Synthroid, a synthetic thyroid drug for an underactive thyroid (a condition called hypothyroidism—SEE QUICK DEFINITION) for 12 years. Elinor was also taking a battery of standard drugs to address her other symptoms, including prescription synthetic progesterone for her PMS, and had become dependent on many of them. Elinor was generally unable to function; she couldn't hold a job or engage in normal social interactions. Elinor's husband had to drive her around and handle most of the domestic chores. Over the years, Elinor had seen many specialists and experimented with many drugs, but nothing had really helped. "Her symptoms were typical of CFS and fibromyalgia, both of which have come to be umbrella-like terms for this type of condition," observes Dr. Hammerly.

A blood test revealed that Elinor was deficient in DHEA, a hormone produced by the adrenal glands. While the range for DHEA is 130 to 980, Elinor's 136 was characteristic of a woman of 80, not 45, notes Dr. Hammerly. To start off her treatment, he put her on 25 mg once daily of DHEA. After a month of supplementation, a follow-up blood test showed her levels had climbed to a more acceptable 522.

With the raising of her DHEA levels, Elinor observed

that her sleeping was improved and she had less aches and pains, but she was still very tired. At the same time as Dr. Hammerly had Elinor taking DHEA, he started her on digestive enzymes, taken with meals, to address her gastrointestinal disorders. He also gave her a product called Bioflora (containing beneficial bacteria needed by her intestines for better digestion and absorption); and 500 mg twice daily of chelated magnesium citrate (to help reduce muscle spasms). To complete his nutritional recommendations, Dr. Hammerly suggested a variety of key antioxidants; such as vitamin A (15,000-25,000 IU daily), vitamin C (2,000 mg daily), vitamin E (400-800 IU daily), and grapeseed extract (100 mg daily).

Dr. Hammerly taught Elinor a pain relief healing technique called electrostatic massage (SEE QUICK DEFINITION). He also suggested an energy therapy in the form of magnets (SEE QUICK DEFINITION) which he had Elinor apply to the pained muscles. A negative magnetic field has been found to be therapeutic for a range of conditions, including chronic pain and sleep disorders. Dr. Hammerly also recommended that Elinor get a magnetic mattress pad so that the energy of the magnets could gently work on her physiology (organs, tissues, and cells) during sleep. After using this mattress for only a week, she reported sleeping better, and decided to continue using it regularly.

Yet, Elinor was still very tired. At this point, two months into Dr. Hammerly's program, a registered nurse at the center treated Elinor with therapeutic touch, which is a way of delivering subtle healing energy through the hands. "Due to her degree of soreness, Elinor would not have responded well to massage, but needed a gentler 'hands off' approach, such as therapeutic touch which works with the body's energy fields rather than muscles." Dr. Hammerly notes that after the healing touch session, Elinor reported having a lot more energy and for the first time in 18 years she felt ready and able to start an exercise program.

The healing benefits of therapeutic touch were, of course, working synergistically with the other components of the program. Elinor continued with this program, but three months later, her fatigue returned, accompanied by pressure in her head, sores in her nose and mouth, upper respiratory

For more on **hormone testing**, see Chapter 2: Testing, pp. 34-72. For more on **the role of the thyroid and CFS**, see Chapter 6, Reversing Hidden Thyroid Problems, pp. 164-189.

Electrostatic massage (EM) is a therapeutic technique which uses static electricity to relieve pain by normalizing the malfunctioning nervous system, organs, and cells. A negatively charged PVC pipe is moved over the painful area of the body; this pushes electrons to the symptomatic area where they facilitate the normal healing process, stimulating the metabolism and increasing the amount of oxygen to the cells. EM can reduce swelling due to water retention or edema by moving the water that accumulates in an area of inflammation. EM is used on patients suffering from general muscular pain, arthritis, fibromyalgia, headaches (tension and sinus), and tendinitis.

Magnet therapy works with the body's own electromagnetic fields to effect important metabolic changes in the body. Commonly, small, simple magnets are employed, providing a "calming" negative charge which helps to normalize pH, oxygenate the blood, reduce swelling, and cancel out free radicals, among other things.

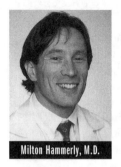

"Due to her degree of soreness, Elinor would not have responded well to massage, but needed a gentler 'hands off' approach, such as therapeutic touch which works with the body's energy fields rather than muscles," Dr. Hammerly notes.

For more on **candidiasis testing**, see Chapter 2: Testing, pp. 34-72. For more on **treating candidiasis**, see Chapter 3: Eliminating Viruses, Infections, Candidiasis, and Parasites, pp. 74-106.

To contact **Milton Hammerly, M.D.:** American Whole Health, 5161 East Arapahoe Road, Suite 290, Littleton, CO 80122; tel: 303-694-2626; fax: 303-796-8174. For **Bioflora®**, contact: PhysioLogics, 6565 Odell Place, Boulder, CO 80301; tel: 800-765-6775 or 303-530-4554; fax: 303-516-5233 or 303-530-2592. Bioflora contains five principal beneficial or "friendly" bacteria in capsule form, including *Lactobacillus acidophilus, L. bulgaricus, Bifidobacterium bifidum, B. longuim*, and *Streptococcus thermophilus*. For the **Candida Antibodies Panel**, contact: National BioTech Laboratory, 13758 Lake City Way NE, Seattle, WA 98125; tel: 206-363-6606 or 800-846-6285; fax: 206-363-2025.

problems, and hair loss. When he examined her, Dr. Hammerly found swollen lymph nodes and muscle tenderness. A food allergy test, called the IgG-Antibody, which shows a patient's delayed reaction (hours to days after exposure) to allergenic substances and screens for reactions to 96 foods and 24 spices, indicated she was allergic to dairy products, eggs, gluten, and wheat.

Another test called Candida Antibodies Panel, which checks *Candida albicans* levels, showed that there was a yeast overgrowth in Elinor's mucosal cells lining the intestines, lungs, and mouth. As discussed previously, candidiasis can create leaky gut syndrome which can, in turn, lead to the development of allergies, as undigested food particles find their way from the intestines into the bloodstream where the immune system launches an allergic reaction against them. *Candida* infestation was also robbing Elinor's system of needed energy.

Here, Dr. Hammerly's approach was twofold, using a technique from both camps of medicine. From the conventional field, he prescribed Nystatin, an antifungal drug commonly given for *Candida*; his recommendation from an alternative approach was for Elinor to stop eating sugar as well as the foods to which she was allergic. In addition, Dr. Hammerly wanted to build her nutrient status, as it is the foundation for energy and was depleted by the candidiasis and continual allergic reaction. He started Elinor on a series of Meyer's Cocktails (SEE QUICK DEFINITION), which involve a slow injection (lasting ten minutes) of mainly B-complex and C vitamins and magnesium. After four "cocktails" given over a four-week period, "her energy was significantly better." Elinor's *Candida* symptoms had also cleared up.

At this point, Elinor's psychiatrist started to reduce her antidepressants, telling Dr. Hammerly this was the first time in many years that Elinor had not seemed depressed to him. Her husband called Dr. Hammerly to exclaim, "I have my wife back for the first time in 18 years!" Two months later, Elinor had a slight relapse, feeling tired again, so Dr. Hammerly put her through a series of six Meyer's Cocktails, one per week; after this, she was fine. "She is out in the world, doing things. She's exercising. Her aches and pains are gone and her energy is good. Her husband is having a hard time keeping up with her," says Dr. Hammerly.

Elinor is one of many chronically ill patients Dr. Hammerly has successfully helped. However, his results weren't always so promising. Before he joined the world of alternative medicine, Dr. Hammerly endured great frustration in his conventional medical practice at not being able to offer many of his patients lasting relief. Typically, Dr. Hammerly would see 25 patients a day and routinely prescribe at least 30 drugs. Many patients had chronic problems and didn't respond to conventional treatments.

"These were people who had already been through the mill of specialists, had tried everything. They were frustrated. I was frustrated. I would roll my eyes and ask myself, 'What am I going to do for this person?'" But now, after becoming versed in alternative medicine, "I actually have something to offer them," says Dr. Hammerly with pleasure, and most of his chronic illness patient —he estimates 70% to 80%—get a good response and heal.

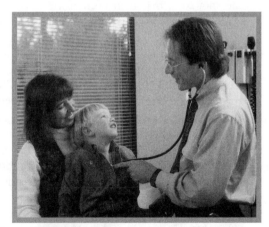

"With alternative medicine, I actually have something to offer my patients," says Milton Hammerly, M.D.

As with other body systems, allergic reaction and immune impairment are interlocking and form a vicious cycle of each worsening the other. As the immune system falters further, more allergies develop.

What Causes Allergies?

One of the primary causes of allergies is an impaired immune system, which substantially increases the risk of allergic reactions. "This occurs when the immune system becomes stressed due to an overload of toxins," says Charles Gableman, M.D., a former practitioner of environmental medicine, now living in Lake Forest, California. Many alternative practitioners agree.

In researching allergies, Leon Chaitow, M.D., D.O., based in London, England, has found that a number of factors have a negative impact on the immune system, including pollution in all its forms, vaccinations and immunizations, and an over-reliance on steroids, birth control pills, and antibiotics. "Antibiotics further add to the confusion the immune system is facing," states Fuller Royal, M.D., of Las Vegas, Nevada, "until the immune system is no longer able to tell friend from foe. When that happens, it starts reacting to all sorts of things which are not foes, that then become treated as allergens. This leads to fatigue and allows viruses, bacteria, and so forth to come in and wreak havoc."

Dr. Royal also believes that the immune system may be weakened by hereditary problems. "Usually this will be reflected in the gastrointestinal tract. The nutrients are not able to be absorbed and utilized properly and this sets you up for food allergies." As with other body systems, allergic reaction and immune impairment are interlocking and form a vicious cycle of each worsening the other. Histamine, which is released during an allergic reaction, is an immune suppressant. As the immune sysem falters further, more allergies develop.

"A repetitive diet can contribute greatly to the development of allergies," says Marshall Mandell, M.D., medical director of the New England Foundation for Allergies and Environmental Diseases. Theron Randolph, M.D., an allergy specialist and founder of environmental medicine (SEE QUICK DEFINITION), found that the diets of allergy patients normally consist of 30 foods or less, which they eat repeatedly. "These 30 foods then become the basis for the most common food intolerances," says Dr. Mandell. "If someone eats bread every day, for instance, he could easily develop a wheat allergy due to the immune system's continuous exposure to it."

As mentioned earlier, leaky gut syndrome, or excessive permeability in the digestive tract, is another major factor that can lead to allergies. Among the causes of leaky gut syndrome, James Braly, M.D., of Fort Lauderdale, Florida, cites poor digestion, viral and bacterial infections, parasitic infestation, vitamin, mineral, amino acid and/or essential fatty acid deficiencies, excessive stress, antibiotics, and candidiasis, all of which can be factors in CFS.

Treating Allergies in Chronic Fatigue and Related Disorders

There are a range of alternative medicine techniques for treating allergies and thus reducing the immune load of a person with CFS or similar illness. Here, we focus on: the Nambudripad Allergy Elimination Technique, nutritional supplements to address the deficiencies which help to create allergies, and Ayurvedic medicine treating digestive dysfunction as the source of allergies. Finally, we hear from Susan Lange, O.M.D., L.Ac., on the "sick building syndrome" and a multifaceted approach to treating environmental illness.

Environmental medicine (formerly called clinical ecology) explores the role of dietary and environmental allergens in health and illness. Dust, molds, chemicals, certain foods, and many other substances can cause allergic reactions which can be linked to disorders such as chronic fatigue, asthma, arthritis, headaches, depression, gastrointestinal problems, and environmental illness. Environmental medicine physicians identify and treat patients' allergies as a means to resolve their health condition. Environmental medicine also addresses "sick building syndrome" which is when the physical environment of a building— its construction materials, furnishings, paints, lighting, ventilation— directly contributes to the ill health of those living or working in it.

The Nambudripad Allergy Elimination Technique

To immediately alleviate the burden on the immune system created by allergies, it is necessary to eliminate the allergic reaction. Many practitioners accomplish this first through an often laborious process of identifying the offending substances and then by advising the patient to avoid these allergens. The Nambudripad Allergy Elimination Technique (NAET), developed by Dr. Nambudripad, takes the laboriousness out of the first step and gets rid of the need for the second step by permanently clearing the body of its allergic reaction to a substance.

Interestingly, NAET was discovered by chance when Dr. Nambudripad, formerly food sensitive herself, accidentally kept a trigger substance in her hand as she gave herself acupuncture in the middle of an intense reaction. To her astonishment, she recovered so

Allergic reaction to foods, chemicals, or environmental substances is often the cause of chronic fatigue syndrome, says Devi Nambudripad, D.C., L.Ac., R.N., Ph.D.

For more on **Devi Nambudripad, M.D., and NAET**, see "The Allergy-Free Body," *Digest* #6, pp. 8-13.

For more information about **NAET testing**, see Chapter 2: Testing, pp. 34-72.

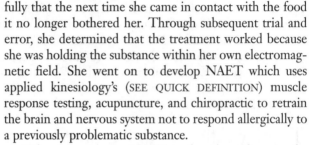

To contact **Devi Nambudripad, D.C., L.Ac., R.N., Ph.D.** (for appointments or referrals for other doctors using NAET): Pain Clinic, 6714 Beach Boulevard, Buena Park, CA 90621; tel: 714-523-0800. Dr. Nambudripad's book about NAET, *Say Goodbye to Illness*, is available from her clinic.

fully that the next time she came in contact with the food it no longer bothered her. Through subsequent trial and error, she determined that the treatment worked because she was holding the substance within her own electromagnetic field. She went on to develop NAET which uses applied kinesiology's (SEE QUICK DEFINITION) muscle response testing, acupuncture, and chiropractic to retrain the brain and nervous system not to respond allergically to a previously problematic substance.

What is unique to NAET is that through a simple, noninvasive procedure allergies can be permanently eliminated. Here's how it works. The practitioner using NAET has the patient lie down on the table, then tests the muscle strength in the patient's arm or leg as they hold a substance in a vial in one hand. Once an allergy-causing substance has been identified, the patient again holds it in one hand while the practitioner uses acupuncture (SEE QUICK DEFINITION), or acupressure if the patient prefers, on specific acupoints to "clear" the charge on that substance. For the treatment to become permanent, the patient must stay away from the offending item for at least 24 hours. Usually, a single treatment is enough to eliminate the allergy, but occasionally it takes more than one.

For the last 15 years, Dr. Nambudripad has used her technique to permanently eliminate the allergies of between 80% and 90% of her patients. Today, over 600 practitioners—including M.D.s, acupuncturists, and chiropractors—have joined her and are using NAET with equal success. They have seen numerous cases of CFS reversed by getting rid of the person's allergies; many of these patients had been going to CFS clinics for years with little result.

Dr. Nambudripad points to genetic susceptibility and the toxic environment in which we live as the sources behind the current epidemic of allergies in the United States. "We are living today in an environment of electromagnetic pollution," she states. "All types of energies are bombarding our bodies from all directions and causing a wide range of psychological and physiological disorders, resulting in a weakening of the immune system that leaves people prey to debilitating illnesses," she says.

Allergic reaction to foods, chemicals, or environmental substances is often the cause of one such illness, chronic fatigue syndrome, says Dr. Nambudripad. Although the role of allergies in CFS has long been overlooked in the medical profession, "the connection between allergies and chronic fatigue syndrome is beginning to get the attention it deserves," she observes.

Frequently, offending substances are seemingly innocuous ones used in everyday life. For example, allergies to acetic acid and formic acid, present in most rubber goods including the erasers on pencils, as well as office correction fluid can trigger extreme fatigue and chronic fatigue syndrome. Some people with CFS are allergic to their own body secretions (saliva, blood, urine, mucus), Dr. Nambudripad reports.

Clearly, the allergies involved in cases of chronic fatigue can be to nearly anything and, as CFS is a serious disorder which has progressed over a long period, are often to many substances. The following brief case histories demonstrate the effectiveness of NAET in reversing CFS and related illnesses, despite the severity of the allergies:

■ A woman, 35, had been treated for CFS for three years. In spite of this and a healthy diet, she was getting progressively worse and had already been on disability for three years when she came to Dr. Nambudripad. A thorough evaluation determined that she was allergic to almost all foods and fabrics. However, she was relieved to learn that she was suffering from allergies rather than some incurable illness. Within a couple of months of beginning NAET treatment, she started showing marked improvement. In all, it took six months (three to four visits per week) to clear all of her allergies. At the end of that period, she felt almost normal and began to work at a regular job.

■ Another woman, a 28-year-old teacher, had been disabled by Epstein-Barr for seven years. She was also found to be allergic to a great many substances—foods, physical agents, fabrics, and especially tap water. It took

QUICK DEFINITION

Applied kinesiology, first developed by George Goodheart, D.C., of Detroit, Michigan, is the study of the relationship between muscle dysfunction (weak muscles) and related organ or gland dysfunction. Applied kinesiology employs a simple strength resistance test on a specific indicator muscle that is related to the organ or part of the body that is being tested. If the muscle tests strong, maintaining its resistance, it indicates health. If it tests weak, it can mean infection or dysfunction. For example, the deltoid muscle in the shoulder shares a relationship to the lungs and therefore is a good indicator of any problems there.

Acupuncture is an integrated healing system developed by the Chinese over 5,000 years ago and introduced in the United States in the mid-1800s. The treatment is administered by an acupuncturist using hair-thin, stainless-steel needles, generally pre-sterilized and disposable; these are lightly inserted into the skin at any of over 1,000 locations on the body's surface, known as acupoints. Acupoints are places where vital energy, or *qi* (pronounced CHEE), can be accessed by acupuncturists to reduce, enhance, or redirect its flow. These acupoints exist on meridians, which are the body's specific pathways for the flow of energy. In most cases, these energy pathways relate to individual organs or organ systems, designated as Lung, Small Intestine, Heart, and others. There are 12 principal meridians and eight secondary channels. Acupuncture is employed for a wide variety of conditions (the World Health Organization counts 104), among them, pain relief, asthma, migraines, and arthritis.

> "We are living today in an environment of electromagnetic pollution. All types of energies are bombarding our bodies from all directions and causing a wide range of psychological and physiological disorders, resulting in a weakening of the immune system that leaves people prey to debilitating illnesses," says Dr. Devi Nambudripad.

A Patient Speaks: No More Allergies

Jill Thompson, of Anaheim, California, says, "I was diagnosed as having Epstein-Barr virus/chronic fatigue syndrome, for which there is no cure. Medical doctors were unable to offer me any hope. Some specialists believe that the root of CFS has something to do with allergies, and my experience with NAET confirms that. Since being treated, my CFS symptoms have ceased."

almost a year of continuous treatment to eliminate her allergies. She was then able to return to teaching full-time.

■ A 48-year-old computer programmer complained of extreme fatigue, frequent headaches, insomnia, and irritable bowel syndrome—conditions he had had since the age of eight. In addition to uncovering various environmental allergies, NAET found this patient to be allergic to the electromagnetic emissions of the computer. All 12 acupuncture meridians were implicated in his disability, meaning that his allergies were so extensive that all the energy channels in his body showed an imbalance. When he was treated with NAET for allergies to radiation and the other substances, he was able to lead a normal life again.

Success Story: Enzymes and NAET Cleared Up Chronic Fatigue and Candidiasis—Elizabeth, 35, had been struggling with chronic fatigue, recurrent candidiasis, and a weight problem for a period of years when she finally went to see Ellen Cutler, D.C., a chiropractor, enzyme therapist, and NAET practitioner at the Tamalpais Pain Clinic in Corte Madera, California. In recent months, Elizabeth had also developed a bladder infection for which she had been taking antibiotics. Soon after beginning the medication, her symptoms disappeared, but the infection returned a few weeks later. This time, she wanted a permanent solution to her chronic problems.

Dr. Cutler was not surprised to hear of Elizabeth's bladder infections. "Women who suffer from chronic candidiasis eventually develop infections of the bladder," says Dr. Cutler. "The one causes the other. If you cure the bladder symptoms without addressing the candidiasis, the bladder infection will simply come back."

Similarly, treating Elizabeth's chronic fatigue and candidiasis without addressing the underlying causes of these ailments would relieve them only temporarily as well. To pinpoint these causes, Dr. Cutler performed an enzyme evaluation and a urine analysis. The tests revealed that Elizabeth's diet might be a key factor in her medical problems; specifically, she was not digesting fats, proteins, and sugars well and she was eating a lot of sugar-rich carbohydrates. Poor absorption of sugars is common in women suffering from candidiasis.

To address Elizabeth's digestive problems, Dr. Cutler put her on a special "sugar-intolerant diet." Elizabeth began eating less sugar and fewer starchy sugar-containing vegetables, such as potatoes, corn, and peas; emphasized protein over carbohydrates; and limited her intake of complex carbohydrates (such as breads and grains) and fruit to two daily servings each. To help break down food, Dr. Cutler recommended an enzyme formula containing amylase (digests carbohydrates), protease (digests proteins), and lipase (digests fats). After a few weeks, the dietary changes and enzyme supplementation noticeably improved Elizabeth's condition. Now her system was strong enough to begin addressing the fatigue and candidiasis.

What is unique to NAET is that through a simple, noninvasive procedure allergies can be permanently eliminated.

Dr. Cutler treated Elizabeth's candidiasis by prescribing two enzyme formulas: *L. acidophilus* cellulase magnesium enzyme and an antifungal called Combat Fung. Elizabeth continued to improve, but Dr. Cutler suspected her problem might have causes other than the *Candida* yeast. "A lot of times the reason people don't succeed in treating *Candida* is that they're just looking at one type of fungus," Dr. Cutler notes. "There are ways of testing that can identify all the different fungi that might be causing an infection."

For this, Dr. Cutler relies on the Nambudripad Allergy Elimination Technique (NAET). Using NAET, Dr. Cutler identified and desensitized Elizabeth to over 50 different kinds of fungus and mold. "I've been in practice 20 years," says Dr. Cutler, "and I've never found any other way to get rid of fungus permanently." After the

NAET treatment, Elizabeth never had another yeast infection. During the course of the NAET, Dr. Cutler also discovered that Elizabeth was allergic to B vitamins. NAET cleared her of this allergy as well.

Elizabeth now reported feeling less tired all the time. To supplement the probable nutritional deficiencies Elizabeth had developed as a result of her faulty digestion and allergy to B vitamins, Dr. Cutler prescribed a multivitamin (two capsules daily). To give her energy a boost by supporting her adrenal glands, Dr. Cutler recommended an enzyme formula called Chirozyme Adrenal (two capsules per dose, to be taken as needed). Soon, Elizabeth's symptoms of chronic fatigue disappeared entirely. "I've run into her a couple of times since we finished the treatment," says Dr. Cutler. "Elizabeth tells me that her fatigue is no longer a problem, and that she's 'religious' about staying on her enzymes."

Success Story: Environmental Illness Reversed with NAET—When Marilyn, 42, consulted Helen Thomas, D.C., a chiropractor and NAET specialist practicing in Santa Rosa, California, she had been enduring the serious symptoms of environmental illness for five years. After the birth of her child five years previously, she had became nauseous, developed chronic fatigue syndrome, her hands and feet swelled, and she experienced severe dizziness and headaches.

Marilyn had also suffered toxemia during her pregnancy and two days before delivery had slipped into a coma and almost died. Her conventional physicians kept her on numerous medications in an attempt to reduce her symptoms, but her condition had worsened to the point where she was considered to be suffering from environmental illness.

Dr. Thomas' NAET testing determined that Marilyn was allergic to 40 different items. The list of substances producing an allergic reaction in her was formidable, including all egg and chicken products, calcium, milk protein, all fruits and vegetables containing vitamin C and B complex, all sugars, iron, vitamin A, fish, most minerals, salt, wheat gluten, and corn. In addition, Marilyn was allergic to most of the key brain chemicals known as neurotransmitters (SEE QUICK DEFINITION).

According to Dr. Thomas, Marilyn had major imbalances in her nervous, endocrine, and immune systems, such that her stress mechanism (her system's ability to tol-

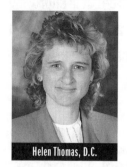

Helen Thomas, D.C.

According to Dr. Thomas, Marilyn had major imbalances in her nervous, endocrine, and immune systems, such that her stress mechanism (her system's ability to tolerate the stress of allergic reactions) was incapacitated. Dr. Thomas systematically cleared each of Marilyn's allergies with NAET. Progress was unmistakable and steady during this process.

erate the stress of allergic reactions) was incapacitated. Dr. Thomas systematically cleared each of Marilyn's allergies with NAET. Progress was unmistakable and steady during this process.

In about three weeks, her nausea began to recede; then within two months, her headaches lessened and her energy level started to pick up considerably. Five months after beginning the NAET treatments, Marilyn was able to wash every window in her house, clean all the rooms, and host a dinner party. In a subsequent letter to Dr. Thomas, Marilyn wrote: "I feel well and truly cared for, eased and comforted. Your treatments allowed my body to remember how well it could be."[2]

Nutritional Supplements

According to James Braly, M.D., who practices in Fort Lauderdale, Florida, if digestive disorders are compounding the allergies, which is usually the case, they will also need to be corrected before any significant improvement can occur.

"I find that many people with such complaints suffer from deficiencies in vitamin A, certain B vitamins, zinc, magnesium, and/or essential oils," Dr. Braly says. "Some people, especially as they get older or if their allergies are severe, also require digestive assistance in the form of pancreatic enzymes (SEE QUICK DEFINITION) and/or hydrochloric acid (HCl), so supplementing each meal with them can be helpful as well."

A **neurotransmitter** is a brain chemical with the specific function of enabling communications to happen between brain cells. Chief among the 100 identified to date are acetylcholine, gamma-aminobutyric acid (GABA), serotonin, dopamine, and norepinephrine. Acetylcholine is required for short-term memory and all muscle contractions. GABA works to stop excess nerve signals and thus keeps brain firings from getting out of control; serotonin does the same and helps produce sleep, regulate pain, and influence mood, although too much serotonin can produce depression. Norepinephrine is an excitatory neurotransmitter.

Vitamin C in high doses can have a dramatic effect in improving allergy symptoms due to its ability to counteract the inflammation responses that are part of the allergic condition.

To contact **James Braly, M.D.:** Immuno Laboratories, 1620 West Oakland Park, Fort Lauderdale, FL 33331; tel: 800-231-9197 or 954-486-4500; fax: 954-739-8583.

For more on **supplements**, see Chapter 10: Ending Nutritional Deficiencies with Supplements, pp. 260-291. For more on **probiotics**, see Chapter 5: Detoxifying the Body, pp. 132-163.

Both zinc and vitamin A play an important role in the production of secretory IgA (immunoglobulin A—SEE QUICK DEFINITION), a gastrointestinal antibody (SEE QUICK DEFINITION) secreted from the salivary glands in the mouth and from cells that line the digestive tract. "The IgA antibody latches on to what is perceived in the body as allergens or potential allergens in the foods that we eat," Dr. Braly explains.

"This action results in a protective coat of mucus being formed around these allergens and prevents them from being absorbed into the bloodstream. If you're zinc and vitamin-A deficient, you produce less secretory IgA, and therefore your susceptibility to food allergies increases." Zinc also plays a role in the production of the body's hydrochloric acid, which the body also needs for proper digestion to occur, says Dr. Braly.

Another group of nutrients that Dr. Braly employs to treat allergies is bioflavonoids (SEE QUICK DEFINITION). "Certain bioflavonoids are some of the most effective anti-allergy nutrients that I've come across," he says. "Many of my patients who are allergy prone, both to their diet and their environment, over a period of time stop having allergic reactions once these bioflavonoids start taking effect. Quercetin, my favorite bioflavonoid, taken orally along with bromelain, vitamin C, and glutamine, has produced wonderful results."

Quercetin is a natural bioflavonoid and nontoxic alternative to allergy and anti-inflammatory drugs. It works by stabilizing the mast cells, effectively preventing them from releasing histamine. Histamine produces the common symptoms of an allergic reaction.[3]

Finally, vitamin C in high doses can have a dramatic effect in improving allergy symptoms due to its ability to counteract the inflammation responses that are part of the allergic condition.

Probiotics—Since imbalances of intestinal flora are common among allergy sufferers, Dr. Chaitow stresses the need to restore bowel flora balance with a daily program of probiotics, or the use of friendly or beneficial bacteria that inhabit the intestines under healthy conditions. "*Lactobacillus acidophilus, Lactobacillus bulgaricus,* and the *bifidobacteria* are the key players in this process," Dr. Chaitow says. "But care must be taken to select the proper strains," he cautions. "To be effective, probiotic supplements should be freeze-dried, contain only the declared and desirable strains of the species, and have concentrations of the friendly bacteria of about one billion parts per gram. They should also be kept refrigerated."

Ayurvedic Medicine

In Ayurvedic medicine (SEE QUICK DEFINITION), allergies are viewed as a result of impaired digestion. "This is known as an *ama* condition," explains Virender Sodhi, M.D. (Ayurveda), N.D., of Bellevue, Washington. "In other words, the person with allergies is having trouble digesting proteins, carbohydrates, or fats, and this leads to a breakdown in the system that eventually creates the allergy."

Dr. Sodhi points out that the digestive system has a link to all allergies, not just those caused by food. "Proper digestion aids the body in clearing out toxins," he says. "When digestion becomes impaired, a greater threshold of toxins have to be dealt with and eventually the body becomes overwhelmed. This is what leads to the allergies. So, in Ayurvedic medicine we always start with the digestive system in order to treat allergies."

In the case of CFS, Dr. Sodhi's treatment focuses on eliminating toxins and allergies and improving digestion. He puts patients on diet modification and cleansing programs to get rid of the toxins and also works on psychosomatic elements to improve sleep patterns. Dr. Sodhi states, "If patients don't sleep well, growth hormones don't get triggered and the body cannot be repaired."

Some of the herbs used in Dr. Sodhi's

To contact **Virender Sodhi, M.D., N.D.:** 2115 112th Avenue NE, Bellevue, WA 98004; tel: 425-453-8022; fax: 425-451-2670.

treatment include *ashwaganda, amla, bala, triphala,* and lomatium, which are combined according to each patient's particular needs. *Acidophilus* is also part of the program. According to Dr. Sodhi, *vata* metabolic body types are more susceptible to CFS. Physically, *vata* people tend to be slender with prominent features, joints, and veins. Temperamentally, they are vivacious, energetic, and moody. Their energy characteristically fluctuates, with jagged peaks and valleys.

Maria, 45, had been experiencing progressively worsening fatigue for five years, to the point where she could not work at all. After being tested by hospitals and doctors, she was told nothing could be done for her and was given a prescription for antidepressants. Maria refused the medication and came to Dr. Sodhi. He placed her on his program, including a diet tailored to her specific medical history and body type. The diet consisted of vegetables, fruits, and fish, and no meat or dairy products. "Within three months of treatment, we were able to bring her test results down to normal. Now, she is working and functioning fine," reports Dr. Sodhi.

Environmental Illness and the Sick Building Syndrome

Left untreated, chronic fatigue syndrome can progress to environmental illness, in which the person becomes allergic to almost everything around them. Many sufferers of environmental illness are so reactive that they are forced to barricade themselves in a home cleared of all chemical products. Until fairly recently, no medical solutions were to be found for this perplexing disorder. Now, however, there are alternative medicine physicians who, in the course of treating the rising number of patients seeking their help after conventional medicine failed them, have developed effective protocols to reverse environmental illness.

The Meridian Center in Santa Monica, California, is the home of a team of doctors who have had great success in treating not only environmental illness, but chronic fatigue syndrome, fibromyalgia, digestive disorders, headaches, infertility, arthritis, and other chronic conditions that baffle conventional doctors. Specializing in reversing the negative health effects of toxic environments, both outside and inside the body, the Center itself was scrupulously designed and outfitted with environmentally friendly materials so it would not become yet another source of toxicity for clients.

Susan Lange, O.M.D., L.Ac., co-founder of the Meridian Center, knows from personal experience how important this is. She spent nearly twelve years figuring out how to recover from environmental illness herself and, in the process, traced its origins to her exposure to numerous toxins, some of which occurred in buildings where she had worked. Specialists in environmental medicine call it the "sick building syndrome." This is when the physical environment of a building—its construction materials, furnishings, paints, lighting, ventilation—directly contributes to the ill health of those living or working in it.

In Dr. Lange's case, her first exposure to a "sick building" was in England in the early 1980s. The clinic in which she worked had kerosene gas stoves and small cubicles with no ventilation. "This was a major source of petrochemical poisoning for me," she notes. In 1985, Dr. Lange did postgraduate acupuncture study in China in a hospital that was rife with mold and fungus. "You could actually see the mold running down the walls," she recalls.

Using Acupressure to Relieve an Allergy— A Self-Help Approach

Michael Reed Gach, Ph.D., director of the Acupressure Institute in Berkeley, California, has found that allergic reactions can often be relieved through acupressure, the use of fingertips in place of needles to stimulate acupoints. Dr. Gach explains, "As soon as you begin experiencing an allergic reaction, apply pressure on the point in the center of the webbing of your hand, between your thumb and index finger." (LI 4 on illustration below.)

"Gradually apply firm pressure onto the point, angling the pressure toward the bone that connects with the index finger," Dr. Gach instructs. He recommends keeping a constant pressure for at least two minutes while taking slow, deep breaths. Then repeat the process to the same point on your other hand. "This point works like an antihistamine," Dr. Gach further explains. "I have found that this simple technique can often quickly arrest an allergy attack, making it a useful self-help remedy that anyone can use."

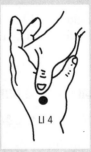

LI 4

Then, in a clinic in Los Angeles where Dr. Lange worked, the air-conditioning filters had not been cleaned or replaced for years, so the system was venting dirty air and microbial contamination. On reflection, Dr. Lange realized that she may have been carrying petrochemical residues in her system since birth. Dr. Lange's mother lived above a gas station and inhaled diesel fumes every day while she was pregnant with her. "She was throwing up all the time. It was a toxic womb—my cellular terrain [the biochemical condition and vitality of her cells] was damaged at an early age," she says.

Dr. Lange's system was further compromised in her early twenties when she picked up intestinal parasites (SEE QUICK DEFINITION) in India. According to one diagnosis at that time, she had amoebic hepatitis. Years of diarrhea, cramps, and pain ensued. Her doctors gave her a battery of tests, X rays, and conventional drugs such as Flagyl and cortisone, not understanding that what Dr. Lange most needed was a rebalancing of her intestinal flora with "friendly bacteria," or probiotics.

While the antibiotics were unsuccessful in killing the parasites, they did kill the beneficial microbes, allowing the "unfriendly," pathogenic bacteria to thrive. A friend introduced Dr. Lange to acupuncture and she started receiving treatments. "That helped me survive, but it didn't clear up everything," she comments. (However, it did lead to her studying acupuncture professionally.) Unfortunately, Dr. Lange found her system was too weak to handle the Chinese herbs prescribed for her parasites.

Allergic to Her Own House

The combination of environmental influences left Dr. Lange "incredibly ill" and her condition worsened over time. She had frequent heart palpitations and her ability to concentrate on her studies began to wane. She was allergic to about 70% of all foods and many other sub-

The "sick building syndrome" exists when the physical environment of a building—its construction materials, furnishings, paints, lighting, ventilation—directly contributes to the ill health of those living or working in it.

Electrodermal Screening

Electrodermal screening is a form of computerized information gathering, based on physics, not chemistry. A blunt, noninvasive electric probe is placed at specific points on the patient's hands, face, or feet, corresponding to acupuncture points at the beginning or end of energy meridians. Minute electrical discharges from these points serve as information signals about the condition of the body's organs and systems, useful for the physician in evaluation and developing a treatment plan.

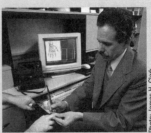

Photo: James H. Clark

stances—gas fumes and perfume nearly made her faint. "The term 'environmental illness' wasn't in use then," she recalls, "but when I walked into my own house, I felt like passing out."

Fortunately, Dr. Lange found that her system could handle homeopathy, so she used a series of homeopathic remedies to start detoxifying her system of all its poisons, starting with petrochemicals. According to electrodermal screening, these were the key toxins. She used Petrochem Antitox and Mercury Antitox, which are both complex homeopathic remedies; she also had the classical homeopathic remedy, *Sulphur*, in doses ranging from 6C to 200C, to help drain toxins and chemicals from her organs. (Dr. Lange cautions that these remedies were prescribed on an individual basis, and may not be appropriate for everyone.)

At the beginning, the most she could handle of the detoxification remedies was one drop daily in water (a normal dosage for Mercury Antitox and Petrochem Antitox is ten drops, three times a day). Any more than that and "my heart and head would pound." Gradually, Dr. Lange started feeling better and was able to increase the dosages to five drops a day. She also took a complex homeopathic remedy called *Ribes Nigrum*, which helps the kidneys to drain their toxins. For this, her dosage was two to three drops a day.

Electrodermal screening also indicated that she was seriously allergic to the mercury in her dental fillings. Complicating this was the fact that, when she was 16, major dental work had misaligned her bite. As she had grown up in Hong Kong and Malaysia, she had received numerous vaccinations for cholera, smallpox, and other tropical infections. These factors weakened her body's "terrain," leaving

Your Carpets Could Be the Culprit

Many people who are sensitive to chemicals, highly allergic, or laid low with chronic fatigue syndrome often tell their physicians that they suspected common household items, including carpets, were somehow poisoning them. Often doctors dismiss these associations as purely in the patient's head. Now there is substantial scientific data to support the claims of poisoning. Your carpet may be bad for your health and you may be better off with bare floors.

Rosalind Anderson, Ph.D., of Anderson Laboratories in Dedham, Massachusetts, analyzed the effect of gas emissions on laboratory mice, based on over 300 carpet samples obtained through retail stores, carpet mills, or from patients' homes. All carpets had been in use from one week to 12 years and none were older than 40 years. To get her disturbing results, Dr. Anderson performed over 500 different experiments. She found that carpet emissions decreased the breathing rate of mice immediately on contact, from a norm of 280 times per minute to a low of 235 after eight minutes of exposure. When the mice were removed from

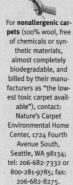

For **nonallergenic carpets** (100% wool, free of chemicals or synthetic materials, almost completely biodegradable, and billed by their manufacturers as "the lowest toxic carpet available"), contact: Nature's Carpet Environmental Home Center, 1724 Fourth Avenue South, Seattle, WA 98134; tel: 206-682-7332 or 800-281-9785; fax: 206-682-8275.

exposure to the carpet emissions, their respiration rates became normal again. Dr. Anderson next learned that one or more exposures of the mice to the carpet samples produced a range of alarming symptoms, including swollen faces, hemorrhaging beneath the skin surface, altered posture, loss of balance, hyperactivity, tremors, limb paralysis, convulsions, even death. Then she analyzed 125 carpet samples for signs of neurotoxicity, that is, emissions that harm brain cells or the nervous system. Dr. Anderson found that 90% produced at least one toxic effect and 60% produced three or more "severe neurotoxic effects" in at least 25% of the mice.

Over 200 different chemicals have been identified in the typical modern carpet, according to Dr. Anderson, and these can produce "diverse toxic effects" in humans, including flu-like symptoms, muscle pain, fatigue, tremors, headaches (lasting up to 16 weeks after exposure), memory loss, and concentration difficulties. When it comes to negative health effects from carpets, "this is not a psychological phenomenon," says Dr. Anderson.[4]

her vulnerable to illness. "Electrodermal screening enabled me to look back through my health history to see how my immune system had been damaged," she says. It also showed her the way to restore her health.

Eventually—it took three years to build up her system's vitality sufficiently to handle such a procedure—Dr. Lange had her mercury fillings removed and her dental bite corrected. To rebuild her immune system, she received two daily intravenous infusions of vitamin C (up to 10 g) combined with B complex (2 cc) and B12 (500 mg). She also took homeopathic Mercury Antitox to remove the mercury from her tissues. Within three weeks of removing the mercury fillings, her heart palpitations stopped and the chronic diarrhea began to lessen. "On a misery scale of one to ten, I had been a

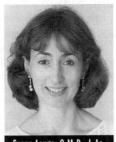

Susan Lange, O.M.D., L.Ac.

"The term 'environmental illness' wasn't in use then," Dr. Lange recalls, "but when I walked into my own house, I felt like passing out." Specialists in environmental medicine call it the "sick building syndrome."

ten, the highest. After this, I went down to a two. That's dramatic."

Next to go were the parasites. Dr. Lange discovered she still had the amoebae from her time in India, along with *Helicobacter pylori*, bacteria she had picked up in China and which is associated with stomach ulcers and chronic gastric pain. A combination of Chinese and other herbs (including artemisia, coptis, phellodendron, isitis, grapefruit seed extract, black walnut, and garlic) and an antibiotic eliminated the bacteria and, finally, the amoebae. After the parasites were gone, Dr. Lange steadily began to regain her health.

There was one more piece Dr. Lange had to address in order to fully heal and that was the psychological and emotional component of her illness. Looking back, Dr. Lange comments: "What kept me going was my commitment to getting well, but my biggest shift came when I faced and let go of the belief I was carrying that the world is dangerous and everything I put in my body is going to damage me."

An Environmentally Friendly Clinic

A personal, protracted experience with serious illness can be valuable training for a physician. Today, Dr. Lange's patients benefit from her long study of illness from the inside. Dr. Lange put her hard-won knowledge into practice in 1990 when she and her husband, Julian Lange, O.M.D., L.Ac., designed, outfitted, and launched the Meridian Center. She knew, and will never forget, that "sick patients require extra-special surroundings because they are so sensitized."

A doctor's office should not make patients feel sicker from spending time there, she says. "Being environmentally ill was a large motivation for me in putting the clinic together the way we did. Now that

Inside the Sick Building Syndrome

In the early 1980s, physicians began using the term "sick building syndrome" (SBS) to refer to a host of symptoms produced by low-grade toxic environmental conditions found in living, work, or office spaces. SBS symptoms are numerous: mucous membrane irritation of the eyes, nose, and throat, chest tightness, skin complaints (dryness, itching, abnormal redness), headaches, fatigue, lethargy, coughing, asthma, wheezing, chronic nasal stuffiness, temporary weight loss, infections, and emotional irritability. All of these depress the immune system, rendering the individual susceptible to long-term chronic illness and potentially to a cancer process.

"Indoor air pollution in residences, offices, schools, and other buildings is widely recognized as a serious environmental risk to human health," explains Michael Hodgson, M.D., M.P.H., of the School of Medicine, University of Connecticut Health Center in Farmington. Dr. Hodgson notes that most people in industrialized nations spend more than 90% of their time indoors, that indoor concentrations of pollutants (including toxic chemicals) are often "substantially" higher than found outdoors, and that small children, the elderly, and the infirm are likely to spend all their time indoors, leading to a permanent chronic exposure to low-grade toxic factors.

In most cases, problems with a building's engineering, construction, and ventilation system are the causes.

Studies suggest that symptoms occur 50% more frequently in buildings with mechanical ventilation systems. Among 2,000 office workers in Germany with work-related symptoms, there was a 50% higher than average rate of upper respiratory tract infections that were directly traceable to problems with mechanically ventilated buildings, reports Dr. Hodgson. A U.S. study found that 20% of office workers had job-related SBS symptoms, including a subjective sense of being less productive in their work.

Besides ventilation problems, other sources of indoor toxic pollution include volatile organic compounds released from particleboard desks, furniture, carpets, glues, paints, office machine toners, and perfumes. All contribute to "a complex mixture of very low levels of individual pollutants," states Dr. Hodgson. Bioaerosols are also indoor contaminants and originate as biological agents from mold spores, allergy-producing microbes, mites, or animal danders; then they are distributed through an indoor space by ventilation, heating, or air conditioning systems.

Of buildings classified as sources of SBS, one study showed that 70% have inadequate flow of fresh outside air. It also found that 50% to 70% of such buildings have poor distribution of air within the occupied space; 60% have poor filtration of outdoor pollutants; 60% have standing water that fosters biological growths; and 20% have malfunctioning humidifiers.[5]

I am well, I am acutely aware of the quality of energy in a building that is necessary for comfort and optimum health."

During her real life tutorial in illness and healing, Dr. Lange came across Bau-Biologie, the art and science of the "biological building."

Well-established in Germany, Bau-Biologie is about the impact of building environments on human health and how to use this knowledge to construct environmentally friendly interior spaces that support, not deteriorate, the health of those using them.

The Meridian Center, down to the finest detail, is a perfect demonstration of Bau-Biologie. Carpets are made of hypoallergenic nylon, free of formaldehyde, moth proofing, stain repellents, pesticides, and other toxic materials typically found in carpets. Formaldehyde, a highly toxic substance, is commonly found in many building materials and furnishings, from wood to upholstery fabrics.

Dr. Lange took great care to avoid using any products containing these or other injurious chemicals. Similarly, the Meridian Center was designed to minimize indoor air pollution, which in many cases can be worse—for its concentration of hazardous chemicals and toxic emissions from common household and workplace products—than outdoor smog and atmospheric pollution.

> A doctor's office should not make patients feel sicker from spending time there, Dr. Lange says. "Being environmentally ill was a large motivation for me in putting the clinic together the way we did. Now that I am well, I am acutely aware of the quality of energy in a building that is necessary for comfort and optimum health."

"All aspects of the clinic's interior—furniture, walls, paints, ceiling tiles, treatment tables, doors, fabrics, lighting, water, electrical installation, gowns, paper and cleaning products, even the plants—were selected for having the lowest environmental toxicity and for their ability to contribute to, not detract from, human health," says Dr. Lange. "Our facility and Bau-Biologie's principles demonstrate that it is possible to use materials that are environmentally safe and easily available."

Staff, patients, and visitors enjoy—relish—the clinic because "it's so free of the external disturbances experienced in ordinary living environments. The moment patients walk through the door, the healing process begins," she says. "To support the healing of the patient, we need facilities that are designed not to damage the envi-

To contact **Susan Lange, O.M.D., LAc.**: The Meridian Center for Personal and Environmental Health, 1411 5th Street, Suite 405, Santa Monica, CA 90401; tel: 310-395-9525; fax: 310-395-9235. For more information about **Bau-Biologie**, contact: Bau-Biologie and Ecology, Inc., P.O. Box 387, Clearwater, FL 34617; tel: 813-461-4371. For **Mercury Antitox** and **Petrochem Antitox,** contact: Apex Energetics, 1701 East Edinger Avenue, Suite A-4, Santa Ana, CA 92705; tel: 714-973-7733; fax: 714-973-2238.

ronment, but to bring positive regeneration to it—facilities that are not sick, but which are healing places for the body, mind, spirit, even the planet."

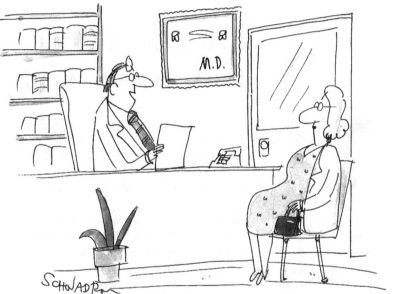

"I'M SENDING YOU TO A SPECIALIST WHO TREATS DRUG SIDE EFFECTS FROM DRUG SIDE EFFECTS."

CHAPTER 10

Ending Nutritional Deficiencies

WITH SUPPLEMENTS

THE CASE STORIES presented throughout this book show that nutritional deficiencies are often a feature of chronic fatigue syndrome. Yet, as with most of the factors involved in this disorder, it is difficult to tell which came first, the deficiencies or the immune breakdown of chronic fatigue syndrome (CFS).

The immune and other key physiological systems of the body need proper nutrients in order to maintain health. Without enough or the right kinds of nutrients, these systems cannot function at an optimum level. If the nutritional deficiency becomes chronic, breakdowns in function will occur. In addition, a body whose immune system is continually overactive, as it is in CFS, requires far more nutrients to keep it going than a healthy body does.

Unfortunately, a person with CFS is likely to be receiving *fewer* nutrients than someone who is healthy. This is because the various viruses, parasites, fungal overgrowths, and other infections characteristic of CFS are draining nutrients from the person suffering with CFS. In addition, with gastrointestinal disorders, many of the nutrients from food and even supplements are not being absorbed by the body.

Correcting the *underlying* problems that contribute to nutritional deficiencies is essential. Without that, nutritional supplementation may be wasted. There is no point in introducing into the body what it cannot absorb. Prescribing nutritional supplements without attending to the diet also lessens the likelihood of a successful outcome.

The nutritional testing detailed in Chapter 2 can pinpoint a patient's absorption problems and specific deficiencies in vitamins, minerals, amino acids, and essential fatty acids, among others. Test results can then be used as a guideline for designing a therapeutic program, monitoring its effectiveness, and modifying it as needed. Although every person with CFS is different and each program should be tailored to meet individual requirements, there are certain nutritional deficiencies that have been associated with CFS. In addition, there are specific nutrients that are useful for addressing symptoms and areas of dysfunction typical to CFS, such as weakened adrenal glands and an overworked immune system. As pointed out frequently in this book, restoring depleted immunity is a vital component in treating CFS.

Before we discuss dietary recommendations and useful supplements in detail, let's look at how two alternative medicine physicians employed nutritional supplements to reverse severe CFS.

CAUTION

Anyone currently under medical care, taking medications, or with a history of specific problems should always consult a physician (preferably one knowledgeable about diet and supplemental nutrients) before making any changes in diet or using supplements.

To contact **Guillermo Asis, M.D.:** The Marino Center for Progressive Health, 2500 Massachusetts Avenue, Cambridge, MA 02140; tel: 617-661-6225; fax: 617-492-2002; website: http://www.allhealth. com. For **Vitality Plus,** contact: Marino Health Store; tel: 800-456-LIFE or 617-661-6124.

Success Story: Back to Work in Three Months

When Elizabeth, 55, developed chronic fatigue syndrome, it became so severe she was disabled for eight months, unable to continue with her job. She sought help at the Marino Center for Progressive Health in Cambridge, Massachusetts. Guillermo Asis, M.D., ran tests to see if she had a *Candida albicans* yeast infection or an Epstein-Barr virus, cytomegalovirus, or Coxsackie virus infection, all of which are commonly associated with chronic fatigue syndrome. It turned out that Elizabeth's system registered a high level of Coxsackie; tests also showed that her system was deficient in DHEA (SEE QUICK DEFINITION), a key adrenal gland hormone.

Dr. Asis started Elizabeth on a daily oral supplement program including a multivitamin formula called Vitality Plus (four times), vitamin C (2,000 mg, twice), magnesium aspartate (400 mg, four times), the antioxidant glutathione (50 mg, twice), DHEA (20 mg on an empty stomach at bedtime), and melatonin (another key hormone which is made in the brain and regulates body cycles) taken at the dosage of 3 mg at bedtime.

Next, Dr. Asis began another more intensive supplement program for Elizabeth in which high doses of selected nutrients were delivered to her body by intravenous (IV) infusion. In this mixture Dr. Asis included vitamin C (35 g), magnesium (1.2 g), vitamin B5 (500 mg), sodium bicarbonate (615 mg) for a better pH balance (SEE QUICK DEFINITION), and vitamin B complex (1 cc).

The advantage of administering vitamin C through IV rather than taking it orally is that it will not produce diarrhea, even at high doses, says Dr. Asis. When vitamin C is ingested orally, the intestines have a set limit on how much of this substance they can absorb at a given time; when bowel tolerance is reached, temporary diarrhea results. Bowel tolerance for vitamin C varies among individuals, but it is probably in the area of 5,000-10,000 mg daily for a relatively healthy person.

Elizabeth received the IV mixture twice weekly while continuing the oral supplements. Within six weeks she was feeling better, Dr. Asis notes. In another six weeks, Elizabeth was able to return to work on a limited basis, gradually building up her strength and the length of her workday.[1]

Success Story: Supplement Prescription Reverses Chronic Fatigue

Marilyn, 47, endured ten years of recurrent colds, sore throats, sinusitis, bronchitis, and asthma. She attributed her chronic health problems to the dampness of her Northern California home. When she began experiencing fatigue and shortness of breath, Marilyn went to two different specialists. Both told her that she had an underfunctioning thyroid gland. Marilyn cut back her hours at work, but her symptoms returned whenever she attempted full-time employment.

Finally, Marilyn and her husband moved to Tucson, Arizona, in the hopes that the warm, dry climate might improve her condition. Although the Tucson climate helped with her asthma and bronchitis, Marilyn began experiencing problems with memory and concentration. In addition, her temperature, which was usually slightly below normal at 97.6° F, was elevated at a constant 99°-100° F. The blood tests Marilyn requested from her doctor showed that "nothing was wrong," even her thyroid was functioning "normally." Marilyn was unable to walk or do housework and had to rest after every minor physical exertion.

After learning about chronic fatigue syndrome in a health food store lecture, Marilyn sought out the help of John Dommisse, M.D., a Tucson-based physician who specializes in treating this debilitating illness. Although Marilyn's doctors in California and Arizona had already run general blood tests, Dr. Dommisse tested Marilyn specifically for nutrient and thyroid hormone imbalances. The additional testing revealed that Marilyn had severe deficiencies of vitamin B12 and the minerals chromium and manganese, and that her blood was carrying near-toxic levels of copper.

To get Marilyn's B12 levels back to normal, Dr. Dommisse administered injections of the vitamin (1,000 mcg) once a week for two months. After the initial injection treatment, Marilyn

> **Dr. Dommisse's testing revealed that Marilyn had severe deficiencies of vitamin B12 and the minerals chromium and manganese, and that her blood was carrying near-toxic levels of copper.**

was advised to supplement with B12 lozenges (2,500 mcg twice daily), to be taken under the tongue. Marilyn also took chromium (three tablets at 200 mcg each) and manganese (two tablets at 50 mg each) twice a day. To reduce the copper levels in Marilyn's body, Dr. Dommisse suggested that she only drink and cook with distilled or copper-filtered water.

After a few months on this program, Marilyn reported that her fatigue reduced by 50%, her temperature had returned to normal, and her chronic colds and sore throats had subsided. In addition, the correction of Marilyn's chromium and manganese deficiencies had contributed to an overall reduction in her appetite and increase in her metabolism. Marilyn dropped 50 pounds of excess weight as a result.

Dr. Dommisse then explored additional causes of Marilyn's fatigue, still only 50% improved. He tested her for candidiasis (an overgrowth of the yeast *Candida albicans*) and found Marilyn to have a minor case, but enough to be a problem. For the candidiasis, Dr. Dommisse prescribed 200 mg daily of Nizoral, a conventional antifungal medication. Dr. Dommisse also suggested that Marilyn treat her candidiasis with a no-sugar, no–white starch diet, which included

Improving the Mental Symptoms of CFS

Memory loss and mental confusion are common problems among CFS sufferers, but taking dietary supplements may help reverse these symptoms. Research now suggests that supplementing with the nutrients found in certain brain chemicals can support brain function and improve mental ability.

One of these brain chemicals is phosphatidyl-serine (PS), a large lipid molecule also found in trace amounts in lecithin derived from soybeans. PS, when given as a supplement, helps support both membrane functions in nerve cells and cell-to-cell communications. Since the 1970's, 34 clinical studies have demonstrated the effectiveness of PS supplements in improving mental abilities.

A Belgian study of 35 hospitalized patients, all of whom had mild to moderate loss of memory and mental ability, showed that taking PS at the rate of 300 mg per day for six weeks produced improvement in three different brain function rating scales. In Italy, a study involving 87 patients with moderate brain function loss linked PS to a strong improvement in attention, concentration, and short-term memory. Study participants also reported feeling less apathetic and withdrawn. In addition, the clinical studies found that PS has a remarkably good safety record, producing only minimal side effects in test subjects.

Lucas Meyer, Inc. has developed a means to produce the PS found in soy lecithin in commercially practical quantities. The PS-containing product—called LECIPS™—has been marketed as a dietary supplement geared toward improving brain function. The product's makers recommend an initial dose of 100-300 mg daily for one month, followed by a maintenance dose of 100-200 mg daily, noting that benefits in mental abilities will fade away if use of the substance is discontinued.[2]

supplements of *acidophilus* (1,000 mg, twice daily) and caprylic acid, an anti-*Candida* fatty acid (700-800 mg, twice daily).

Seven weeks after beginning this final stage of treatment, Marilyn's fatigue had disappeared entirely and it has not returned since. Marilyn no longer suffers from the nasal congestion that caused her to leave northern California, and her insomnia and shortness of breath have ceased. Even better, Marilyn now has enough energy to exercise daily and has returned to full-time work. "Of all the doctors that treated me in the past six years, all meticulously recorded my symptoms of chronic fatigue," Marilyn says, "but despite the batteries of blood tests and MRI scans, they never tested me for the factors that eventually led to my cure."[3]

Diet and Nutrition in Chronic Fatigue

The leading nutritional problem in the United States today is "over-consumptive undernutrition," or the eating of too many empty-calorie junk foods, says Jeffrey Bland, Ph.D., a biochemist and nutrition expert based in Gig Harbor, Washington. Although people in the United States consume plenty of food, it is not the right kind of food. Almost two-thirds of an average American's diet is made up of fats and refined sugars having low to no nutrient density.

Consequently, the remaining one-third of the average diet is counted on for the essential nutrients needed to maintain health, which may or may not be from high-nutrient-density food. Insufficient nutrient intake weakens overall physiological and mental performance, robs the body of its natural resistance to disease, and leads to premature aging. Chronic nutritional deficiencies can obviously contribute to the domino effect of disorders which characterizes CFS.

Without a healthy diet, nutritional supplementation is like sprinkling a few drops of water on parched earth. Michael Murray, N.D., naturopathic educator and author of *Encyclopedia of Nutritional Supplements*, says that attention to diet is crucial in reversing CFS.[4] "Your energy level is directly related to the quality of the foods you routinely ingest."[5] In his estimation, a healthy diet avoids "empty" foods low in nutrients and high in sugar and fat. Instead, it concentrates on high-nutrient, high-protein, complex-carbohydrate foods—vegetables, grains, beans, fish, and poultry (care should be taken to avoid mercury toxins in fish and antibiotics in poultry). He advises eliminating caffeine and alcohol. There are many reasons to do so, but perhaps foremost is to avoid further stress on the adrenal glands and the liver.

Dr. Murray also cautions that, as food allergies may be undermining your nutrient intake, it is important to identify them and take measures to avoid the problem foods. To prevent the development of allergies, don't always eat the same foods, but rather include a variety

> **Michael Murray, N.D., naturopathic educator and author of *Encyclopedia of Nutritional Supplements*, says that attention to diet is crucial in reversing CFS. "Your energy level is directly related to the quality of the foods you routinely ingest."**

For more on **food allergies and CFS**, see Chapter 9: Addressing the Allergy Connection, pp. 232-258.

Deficiencies in vitamin B12, folic acid, pantothenic acid, vitamin C, iron, potassium, zinc, and phosphorus have been implicated in fatigue. Supplementation with these nutrients has had beneficial effects on people with chronic fatigue.

and rotate what you eat.[6] In addition, Dr. Murray and most alternative medicine physicians recommend drinking eight to ten glasses of pure water daily.

Nutritional Deficiencies and Chronic Fatigue Syndrome

Medical science has long held that healthy adults do not need supplementation if they consume a healthful, varied diet, but the U.S. Department of Agriculture (USDA) has found that a significant percentage of the American population receives well under 70% of the U.S. Recommended Daily Allowance (RDA) for vitamin A, vitamin C, B-complex vitamins, and the essential minerals calcium, magnesium, and iron.[7]

A separate study found that most typical diets contained less than 80% of the RDA for calcium, magnesium, iron, zinc, copper, and manganese, and that the people most at risk were young children and women, adolescent to elderly.[8] It is sobering to consider that the situation is even worse than these numbers indicate, because the RDA in itself is judged by many nutritionists to be below the amount most individuals actually need of a given nutrient.

This is especially true in the face of the numerous factors in modern life which drain us of nutrients and thus raise the levels we require. Even when we eat a healthy diet (which, as stated above, most people in the U.S. don't), the food we are getting is not as nutrient-rich as it once was. Most of the soil in which food is grown in the United States has been depleted by poor farming practices and the use of pesticides. Even organic farming, unless the land was always farmed organically, has to contend with the poor soil produced by decades of conventional farming. Additionally, environmental pollution (both chemical and electromagnetic), stress and other lifestyle patterns, and certain medications create even greater nutrient requirements.

Historically, if patients had no overt symptoms or disease, doctors regarded them as healthy and adequately nourished. Today, doctors and scientists are beginning to recognize mild and moderate nutritional deficiencies, the symptoms of which may often be subtle, overlapping, and varied, according to D. Lindsey Berkson, M.A., D.C., of Santa Fe, New Mexico. For example, the first signs of B-vitamin deficiency may include subtle changes in behavior: an inability to concentrate, insomnia, and mood swings.

Other symptoms of nutritional deficiencies can include fatigue, muscle weakness, nervousness, mental exhaustion, confusion, and anemia. It has been reported that marginal deficiencies of vitamins A, C, E, and B6 may also reduce immuno-competence, impairing the body's ability to ward off disease and repair tissues.[9] Do these symptoms sound familiar? All are characteristic of CFS.

When nutritional deficiencies are combined with the other elements of CFS, once again, the balance can tip toward developing the disorder. Research has clearly linked CFS with deficiencies in magnesium, essential fatty acids, and the amino acids carnitine and methionine. Further, deficiencies in vitamin B12, folic acid, pantothenic acid, vitamin C, iron, potassium, zinc, and phosphorus have been implicated in fatigue. Supplementation with these nutrients has had beneficial effects on people with chronic fatigue.[10] Deficiencies associated with other symptoms of CFS, such as muscle weakness and depression, are discussed in the following section under the relevant nutrient.

Nutritional Supplements for Fibromyalgia Relief

Many of the supplements discussed in this chapter are beneficial for treating fibromyalgia, but Chanchal Cabrera, M.N.I.M.H., a clinical herbalist practicing in Vancouver, British Columbia, has found the following to be especially useful:

Niacinamide—A form of niacin (vitamin B3), high doses (900-4,000 mg daily in divided doses) of niacinamide are effective in reducing musculoskeletal imflammations, but should only be taken under a physician's supervision.

Lipotropic factors (substances that remove and prevent fatty deposits)—A combination of the lipotropic factors phosphatidyl choline (lecithin, a neurotransmitter precursor), inositol (component of vitamin B complex), and methionine (an amino acid) can aid in liver function, helping to detoxify the system and correct any excessive fat deposits which reduce blood circulation and can lead to painful blood clots. Methionine is integral to cartilage so it can improve the strength of joint tissues. The dosage is one

To contact **Chanchal Cabrera, M.N.I.M.H.:** Gaia Garden Herbal Dispensary, 2672 West Broadway, Vancouver, BC, Canada V6K 2G3; tel: 604-734-4372; fax: 604-734-4376. The initials M.N.I.M.H. stand for Member of the National Institute of Medical Herbalists, a British designation used in Canada to indicate professional status as an herbalist.

gram of each per day, taken in combination.

Vitamin E—This antioxidant's effective anti-inflammatory action suppresses the breakdown of cartilage while stimulating cartilage growth. A dose of 400-1,200 IU a day is recommended.

Vitamin C—This antioxidant nutrient is vital for tissue repair and, when taken in combination with vitamin E, will contribute to the stability of cartilage. The recommended dosage is to bowel tolerance (the point just prior to diarrhea).

Eicosapentaenoic acid (EPA)—An essential fatty acid found in most fish oils, EPA is an anti-inflammatory. An effective dosage is 1.8 grams daily.

Selenium—This antioxidant mineral works in combination with vitamin E and inhibits inflammation. Selenium blood levels tend to be low in fibromyalgia sufferers. The recommended dosage is 200 mcg per day.

Zinc—This antioxidant mineral is necessary for tissue repair and may be deficient in people with fibromyalgia. An effective dosage is 25-50 mg daily.

Magnesium malate—A lack of magnesium can result in aluminum buildup in the brain which can, in turn, produce fibromyalgia symptoms. Magnesium (1,000-1,500 mg daily) taken in a combination formula with malic acid is an effective supplement.

Lifestyle Changes and Supplements Can Aid Chronic Fatigue

Julian Whitaker, M.D., author of *Dr. Whitaker's Guide to Natural Healing* (Rocklin, CA: Prima Publishing, 1995), uses a nutritional supplement and lifestyle adjustment program to successfully treat chronic fatigue syndrome. The program "is based on a simple truism of nondrug health care: a multifactorial problem is best addressed with a multifactorial solution," explains Dr. Whitaker. "The Whitaker Wellness Program, on its own, will often lead to complete recovery from chronic fatigue. The major factors that determine your energy levels and the status of your immune system are diet and lifestyle. Once you improve these factors, the rest is easier."

For a subscription to *Dr. Julian Whitaker's Health & Healing*, a monthly newsletter, contact: Health & Healing, 7811 Montrose Road, Potomac, MD 20854; tel: 301-424-3700. To contact Julian Whitaker, M.D.: Whitaker Wellness Institute, 4321 Birch Street, Newport Beach, CA 92660; tel: 714-851-1550; fax: 714-851-9970.

■ Start practicing the Whitaker Wellness Program. Adopt a healthy lifestyle, which means paying attention to nutrition and getting plenty of exercise. Definitely quit using tobacco, alcohol, and recreational drugs. Take a megavitamin/mineral supplement daily so that your intake is well above the Recommended Daily Allowance (RDA).

Add to this a strong antioxidant program including vitamins C (3,000-8,000 mg daily) and E (1,200 IU daily). Then fortify everything with extra amounts of magnesium (1,000 mg daily), potassium (about 400 mg daily), and essential fatty acids from evening primrose, flaxseed, black currant seed, borage, and fish oils. Finally, eat a diet high in complex carbohydrates and low in fats.

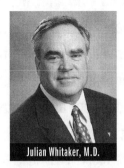

Julian Whitaker, M.D.

"The Whitaker Wellness Program, on its own, will often lead to complete recovery from chronic fatigue," says Dr. Whitaker. "The major factors that determine your energy levels and the status of your immune system are diet and lifestyle. Once you improve these factors, the rest is easier."

■ Strengthen your immune system vitality by taking calf thymus extracts (two tablets of ThymuPlex brand, each containing 375 mg of active calf thymus components, twice daily with your meals). The wonder herb echinacea is also a powerful ally here, in dosages of 2-4 ml (one to two teaspoons) of tincture three times daily.

■ Strengthen your adrenal glands. Most CFS sufferers have adrenal malfunction due to chronic stress and inadequate nutrition. Useful are oral bovine adrenal extracts (dosage depends on your individual constitution and condition) and Siberian ginseng extract (100 mg three times a day).

Dietary Guidelines: Why You Need Fats in Your Diet

Nutritional biochemist **Patricia Kane, Ph.D.**, offers the following observations about the importance of having the proper amount of fat in the diet and the dangers of having the wrong kinds:

In the interest of staying slim—this is especially true of women—butter and cream are rejected in favor of margarine and hydrogenated (semi-solid) fats. This is terribly unfortunate because saturated, hydrogenated fats, typified by margarine—a category called trans-fatty acids (SEE QUICK DEFINITION)—create havoc in a person's neurochemistry, negatively affecting every system of the body.

At the same time, these inappropriate food choices lead to nutrient depletion because the body is not given the kind of fat it *needs* from

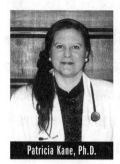

Patricia Kane, Ph.D.

When your diet no longer supplies the necessary raw materials—many of them derived from fats—for running the body efficiently, lots of things go wrong and the body—and brain—starts to shut down, says Dr. Patricia Kane.

EDITOR'S NOTE

Patricia C. Kane, Ph.D., is a nutritional biochemist specializing in traumatic brain injury, seizure disorders, autism, and developmental delay. Dr. Kane is the author of *Food Makes the Difference* (1985) and *The Neurochemistry and Neurophysics of Autism* (1996), director of nutritional biochemistry at the Kaplan Institute in Orangevale, California, and director of medical research for Carbon Based Corporation in Incline Village, Nevada. To contact Dr. Kane: Carbon Based East, Five Osprey, Millville, NJ 08332; tel: 609-825-2200 or 609-825-8333; fax: 609-825-2143.

the diet for proper body function. The fats we need are called essential fatty acids. The foods many people choose in their diet, increasingly, are not nutrient-dense, such as a white flour bagel, a salad with non-fat dressing, or pasta, and thereby fail to provide essential ingredients for body processes.

When your diet no longer supplies the necessary raw materials—many of them derived from fats—for running the body efficiently, lots of things go wrong and the body—and brain—starts to shut down. Prozac is only a few more wrong meals away. In the contrast between *trans*-fatty acids and *essential* fatty acids, you have the cause and cure of depression.

Trans-fats, or hydrogenated manmade fats, were synthesized originally to extend shelf life of commercial products. But the production of trans-fatty acids for human consumption is the most devastating nutritional mistake ever made. In the effort to make foods last longer in the supermarket, all traces of essential fatty acids (such as omega-3s) are obliterated from processed foods, and trans-fats or partially hydrogenated oils take their place.

The absence of omega-3 (SEE QUICK DEFINITION) essential fatty acids in Western diets has contributed to an alarming increase in a number of diseases that appeared only infrequently 100 years ago. A lack of the essential fatty acids and cofactors (such as minerals and vitamins) to handle fat, along with the consumption of trans-fats, is more often the cause of obesity and cardiovascular disease than is eating cholesterol-rich foods. After all, the body *needs* some cholesterol. That's because cholesterol is needed to produce a cascade of crucial hormones including pregnenolone, testosterone, progesterone, estradiol, estrone, and cortisol, among others.

It's not just cholesterol that is needed in the diet. You need fats, too. Like proteins, fats (lipids) are building blocks of the body's essential structures. The membrane of every cell and organelle is a thin envelope of fat that encases and protects the internal biochemical components; within this fatty envelope are thousands of proteins that facilitate communication and transport—acting like gates—across the cell membrane.

Fatty acids strongly influence the *fluidity* of cell membranes, which means the ability of the cell wall to change shape to allow red blood cells through with life-sustaining nutrients. These biomembranes literally control and signal all activities inside and outside the cell; the brain, it's important to know, is 60% lipids. Perhaps you can begin to sense the kind of trouble likely to result when there is a disturbance in or deficiency of the right kind of fats in the body.

Disturbances in fatty acid metabolism (its energy changes and chemical conversions) are reflected through every system of the body, including many physical and mental disorders.

Let me express the problem with trans-fatty acids with an image. The more unsaturated the fat, the more it vibrates, and the longer the chemical "tail," the faster the vibration. An unsaturated fat has a "tail" that is extremely vibratory in nature, and this vibration is good. But a saturated fat or trans-fatty acid is rigid and has little movement.

A trans-fatty acid sits like cement inside you, shutting everything down such as hormone production, and replacing the good, necessary fats (omega-3s and -6s) with something harmful to health. You can't do anything with a trans-fatty acid except burn it for calories; basically, its activity is to poison your system and generate an abnormal, undesirable biochemistry.

The use of trans-fatty acids shuts down the fatty acid metabolism within the immune, endocrine, and central nervous systems. High quality fatty acids obtained through the diet are essential for the synthesis of hormones called prostaglandins which control all interactions among cells. Further, your body needs specific fatty acids to maintain the integrity of

QUICK DEFINITION

A **trans-fatty acid** is a chemically and structurally altered hydrogenated vegetable oil (such as maragrine), in which the double bonds linking hydrogen atoms is changed from a "cis" (atoms bonded on the same side of a chain) to a "trans" form (atoms bonded on opposite sides of a chain), considered more stable. Trans-fatty acid (TFA) composition of commercially prepared hydrogenated fats varies from 8-70% and comprise about 60% of the fat found in processed foods. It is estimated that Americans consume over 600 million pounds annually of TFAs in the form of frying fats. TFAs can increase the risk of heart disease by 27% when consumed as at least 12% of the total fat intake. TFAs also reduce production of prostaglandin (hormones that act locally to control all cell to cell interactions) and interfere with fatty acid metabolism.

Omega-3 and **omega-6 oils** are the two principal types of essential fatty acids, which are unsaturated fats required in the diet. The digits "3" and "6" refer to differences in the oil's chemical structure with respect to its chain of carbon atoms and where they are bonded. A balance of these oils in the diet is required for good health. The primary omega-3 oil is called alpha-linolenic acid (ALA) and is found in flaxseed (58%), canola, pumpkin and walnut, and soybeans. Fish oils, such as salmon, cod, and mackerel, contain the other important omega-3 oils, DHA (docosahexaenoic acid) and EPA (eicosapentaenoic acid). Omega-3 oils help reduce the risk of heart disease. Linoleic acid or cis-linoleic acid is the main omega-6 oil and is found in most plant and vegetable oils, including safflower (73%), corn, peanut, and sesame. The most therapeutic form of omega-6 oil is gamma-linolenic acid (GLA), found in evening primrose, black currant, and borage oils. Once in the body, omega-3 and omega-6 are converted to prostaglandins, hormone-like substances that regulate many metabolic functions, particularly inflammatory processes.

the gastrointestinal tract lining, cell walls (to ensure smooth traffic of nutrients and signals across cellular membranes), and to produce hormones and immune system cofactors. Trans-fatty acids must be *completely avoided* to protect your immune, endocrine, and central nervous systems. ■

An A to Z of Nutritional Supplements for CFS

The following is a guide to supplements which address the deficiencies often found in CFS as well as the specific disorders characteristic of the illness. Dietary sources of nutrients are listed where appropriate as an additional means of remedying a deficiency.

Vitamins

The key function of vitamins is to support the activity of the enzymes and coenzymes in the body, but all essential processes are impaired by vitamin deficiency. Vitamins and enzymes work together in the body to maintain all chemical reactions, including energy production.

Vitamin A–As one of the primary antioxidants (SEE QUICK DEFINITION), vitamin A protects the body from free-radical (SEE QUICK DEFINITION) damage. It also helps the body ward off disease by: 1) strengthening the immune system through the stimulation of T-cell activity; 2) contributing to the health of the thymus, which is integral to immune health since one of this gland's functions is to activate T cells; and 3) maintaining the health of the skin and mucous linings of the digestive tract, sinuses, lungs, bladder, and other organs which are the first line of defense in keeping disease-causing microorganisms from entering the body. Chronic infection, as in CFS, depletes the body of vitamin A, and a vitamin A deficiency leaves the body more vulnerable to infection, so the cycle of deficiency deepens.

Research indicates that, in addition to increasing immune response, controlled high-dosage supplementation with vitamin A may significantly reduce fatigue.[11] This may be due in part to vitamin A's role in the production of red blood cells, a shortage of which is the condition known as anemia, characterized by fatigue. A person's red blood cell level may not have dropped to the range defined as anemia, but may be in short enough supply to produce fatigue. A compromised immune system obviously contributes to fatigue as well.

Dietary sources particularly high in vitamin A include liver, chili peppers, carrots, dried apricots, sweet potatoes, and leafy greens.[12] Supplemental dosages of vitamin A for CFS vary, but should not be above 20,000 IU daily without physician supervision, according to Susan Lark, M.D., of Los Altos, California.[13]

Beta carotene—Beta carotene, classified as a carotenoid, is the pigment that accounts for much of the color in the plant world and is the dominant pigment in most fruits and vegetables. As an antioxidant and precursor to vitamin A, converted by the body as needed, beta carotene performs the functions of vitamin A. It also has antioxidant and immune-enhancing properties not found in vitamin A.[14]

These include increasing the numbers of key immune cells—T, B, and natural killer (NK) cells—as well as macrophage (SEE QUICK DEFINITION) activity. As a decrease in the numbers and function of NK

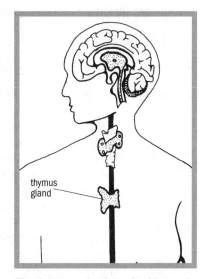

thymus gland

The thymus, a ductless gland located beneath the sternum, is part of the body's lymphatic system and one of the seven endocrine glands. The thymus activates bone marrow or stem cells to respond to foreign or abnormal cells (bacteria, toxins, tumor cells, or transplanted tissue). After being activated, these cells develop into T lymphocytes (the "T" stands for thymus-derived), the "workers" of the cell-mediated immune system that will respond to antigens (foreign substances) but not to the body's own tissues. Specifically, thymic proteins activate the T4 helper cells to locate foreign or abnormal cells (viruses, bacteria, parasites, or tumor cells). Once the invading pathogen is found, the T4 cells secrete immune proteins (particularly, interleukin 2) which activate T8 killer cells, which then seek out and destroy the specific invader. The thymus reaches its maximum size at puberty, then its function and size gradually decline throughout life. T cells already in circulation will continue to function, but are less able to proliferate and are less cytotoxic (able to destroy invading organisms).

In chronic fatigue, the mitochondria (the energy factories of cells) are damaged by several or all of the factors associated with the disorder—viruses, bacterial infection, *Candida* overgrowth, allergies, and chemical sensitivities.

cells (SEE QUICK DEFINITION) is characteristic of CFS,[15] beta carotene supplementation is highly useful for this in addition to its other immune-supporting abilities. Dr. Murray's dosage for immune enhancement is 25,000-300,000 IU daily.[16] As with vitamin A, carrots and sweet potatoes are high in beta carotene.

Vitamin C (ascorbic acid)—There is now solid evidence that vitamin C, another of the primary antioxidants, is essential for optimal functioning of the immune system.[17] It is vital to the health of white blood cells and their production of antibodies (SEE QUICK DEFINITION), as well as the manufacture of interferon which acts as an antiviral. NK cells are only active if they contain relatively large amounts of vitamin C.[18] Vitamin C also reduces pain and inflammation. Further, it is vital to the adrenal glands (located above the kidneys) in which the concentration of vitamin C is the highest in the body.[19] Thus, vitamin C supplementation offers both immune and adrenal support—two critical components in any program to reverse CFS.

Low levels of vitamin C have been linked to fatigue.[20] In a study of 411 dentists and their wives, vitamin C intake and fatigue were inversely related. The low vitamin C users had double the mean number of fatigue symptoms compared to the relatively high vitamin C users.[21] Robert F. Cathcart, M.D., of Los Altos, California, uses massive doses of vitamin C to treat CFS patients because he terms CFS a "free-radical disease involving damaged mitochondria."

In CFS, the mitochondria (the energy factories of cells) are damaged by several or all of the factors associated with the disorder—viruses, bacterial infection, *Candida* overgrowth, allergies, and chemical sensitivities. "The damaged mitochondria become the major source of free radicals," Dr. Cathcart explains. Further, mitochondria normally refuel vitamin C in its scavenging of free radicals, replacing the electrons vitamin C gives up in the process.

Damaged mitochondria are unable to perform this function and the vitamin C is used up after one bout with a free radical. Once again, the vicious cycle of CFS is in operation here. Massive doses of vitamin C are useful, then, to both bolster the immune system and to provide an ongoing supply for free radical destruction in the face of the mitochondria's inability to refuel the vitamin.[22]

In treating CFS, Murray Susser, M.D., of Santa Monica, California, uses intravenous infusions of vitamin C, along with other vitamins and minerals. As an oral supplement for CFS patients, Michael Murray, N.D., recommends 500-9,000 mg a day of vitamin C in divided doses.[23] The foods highest in vitamin C are not citrus fruits, as generally thought, although they do have significant amounts. Red chili peppers have over seven times the vitamin C as oranges, the leafy greens kale and collard have over three times more, and broccoli contains over twice as much.[24]

An **antibody** is a protein molecule containing about 20,000 atoms, made from amino acids by B lymphocyte cells in the lymph tissue and set in motion by the immune system against a specific foreign protein, or antigen. An antibody is also referred to as an immunoglobulin and may be found in the blood, lymph, colostrum, saliva, and the gastrointestinal and urinary tracts, usually within three days after the first encounter with an antigen. The antibody binds tightly with the antigen as a preliminary for removing it from the system or destroying it.

Ester C or esterified vitamin C is a combination of several forms of vitamin C. It has all of the same healthful properties and benefits, but is more quickly absorbed by the body and less seems to be eliminated in the urine as compared to standard vitamin C. Non-acidic, it is also less likely to cause gastrointestinal distress.[25]

Vitamin E (alpha tocopherol)—The third in the triumvirate of antioxidants formed by vitamins A, C, and E, vitamin E is among the major nutrients required for strong immune response to infection. It is also one of the body's primary agents for protecting cell membranes, including protection against the effects of environmental pollutants.

Since chemical toxicity is often a factor in CFS, this is a further reason to include vitamin E in a supplement protocol for the disorder. In addition, vitamin E has antihistamine effects and can stop inflammation.[26] It also improves circulation which can be of benefit for the muscle pain and weakness associated with CFS and fibromyalgia. For CFS patients, Dr. Murray recommends a dosage of 200-400 IU daily.[27] Dietary sources include polyunsaturated vegetable oils, leafy green vegetables, avocados, nuts, seeds, and whole grains.

Vitamin B Complex—The B vitamins act as a team to help speed up chemical reactions and support overall energy metabolism. Each assists in the utilization of the others. Since they are essential for red

Case Study: Vitamins and Exercise Help Reverse Fibromyalgia

Ellen, 54, suffered from chronic low back pain, muscle soreness, general achiness, fatigue, and depression. She endured years of clinical testing and various drug treatments without getting a diagnosis or relief of her symptoms. Frustrated by her lack of progress with conventional doctors, Ellen sought help from Mary Olsen, D.C., a chiropractor based in Huntington, New York.

Dr. Olsen identified Ellen's condition as fibromyalgia by testing the 18 trigger points associated with that disorder. Eleven of these points must be sore to the touch to qualify as fibromyalgia, according to the conventional medical definition. In Ellen's case, 16 of the sites were tender.

Dr. Olsen prescribed a three-part treatment program for Ellen. First, she used acupressure on Ellen's trigger points, applying pressure in eight-second intervals and repeating the treatment three times at each site. The trigger points in fibromyalgia are actually muscles in spasm and those near the spine often pull it out of alignment. Dr. Olsen administers acupressure to massage the trigger point, chiropractic to realign the spine, and applied kinesiology to prevent the trigger point from injuring the spine again. Ellen saw Dr. Olsen three times a week until her spine began to respond to treatment, and monthly thereafter.

Second, Dr. Olsen prescribed vitamin supplements specifically tailored to fibromyalgia. From her clinical experience, Dr. Olsen has found that fibromyalgia sufferers tend to have low levels of B vitamins and malic acid. The supplement formula she typically uses for this deficiency includes vitamin B1 (25 mg), vitamin B6 (75 mg), manganese (2.5 mg), and malic acid (300 mg). "In most cases, I notice a dramatic improvement within 48 hours of beginning the vitamin therapy," Dr. Olsen says. Ellen took this formula two to eight times daily, as needed.

Third, Ellen began a moderate exercise program, performing a 10- to 15-minute stretching routine five days a week and walking for 20 minutes three times weekly. The exercise would help raise her serotonin levels which, in turn, would reduce her fatigue. Dr. Olsen emphasizes

QUICK DEFINITION

Acupressure is an ancient Chinese massage technique based on acupuncture, but employing gentle pressure of the fingers instead of needles on the meridian points to clear these energy pathways and stimulate the organs. Many acupressure techniques can be self-administered. Finger pressure should be steady and firm and may be applied to a point for 10 seconds or less to one minute, depending on the individual.

Applied kinesiology, first developed by George Goodheart, D.C., of Detroit, Michigan, is the study of the relationship between muscle dysfunction (weak muscles) and related organ or gland dysfunction. Applied kinesiology employs a simple strength resistance test on a specific indicator muscle that is related to the organ or part of the body that is being tested. If the muscle tests strong, maintaining its resistance, it indicates health. If it tests weak, it can mean infection or dysfunction. For example, the deltoid muscle in the shoulder shares a relationship to the lungs and therefore is a good indicator of any problems there.

that her patients never exercise to the point of pain and this aspect of treatment needs to vary according to the individual. Many people with fibromyalgia are too tired to exercise at all, she says. Dr. Olsen usually waits until the person's condition has improved through vitamin therapy before beginning the exercise program. In Ellen's case, she was able to start exercising relatively quickly.

After one year of treatment, Ellen reported that her low back pain was gone, her muscle aches had subsided, and her energy level had increased considerably. As her condition improved, Ellen began exercising more, which further boosted her energy level. Her increased energy (and relief from pain) also elevated her mood and Ellen no longer suffers from depression.

To contact **Mary Olsen**
D.C.: 42 High Street, Huntington, NY 11743; tel: 516-421-1248.

blood cell formation, B-complex deficiency produces anemia (reduced red blood cells), the main symptom of which is fatigue. Fatigue and depression have both been linked to B-vitamin deficiency. Deficiencies of any one or more of the B vitamins also interfere with the immune system's ability to fight disease.

Vitamin B1 (thiamin) and vitamin B2 (riboflavin) primarily serve in the maintenance of mucous membranes, formation of red blood cells, and metabolism of carbohydrates, the body's most efficient energy source. Brewer's yeast is an excellent source of both of these vitamins.

Vitamin B3 (niacin) is vital for oxygen transport in the blood, and fatty acid and nucleic acid formation. As the primary component of two coenzymes, it is vital to the actions of more than 150 enzymes. Without these enzymatic reactions, our body's energy production would shut down in the blink of an eye. Brewer's yeast is also a good source of B3, as are whole grains, particularly rice.

Vitamin B5 (pantothenic acid) is vital for synthesis of hormones and support of the adrenal glands. Pantothenic acid deficiency is cited as a source of fatigue.[28] It is also associated with insomnia and depression. Dietary sources of B5 are brewer's yeast, liver, and soybeans.

Vitamin B6 (pyroxidine) strongly influences the immune and nervous systems. It aids in fat and protein metabolism, DNA/RNA synthesis, hemoglobin function, and tryptophan metabolism (which in turn affects mood and level of alertness).[29] B6 is essential in the production of prostaglandin E1, which is necessary for normal thymus

B vitamins should be taken in a B-complex form because of their close interrelationship in metabolic processes.

"In my experience, when their other problems are also treated, many people respond dramatically to B12 injections," says Dr. Teitelbaum.

function and regulation of T cells. Prostaglandin deficiency affects mood and can increase fatigue.[30] Brewer's yeast, whole grains, and sunflower seeds are good dietary sources of this B vitamin.

Vitamin B12 (cobalamin) is virtually absent in vegetable food sources which means vegetarians are frequently low in this vitamin. It is essential for normal formation of red blood cells and the maintenance of the nervous system and mucous membrane linings (important to prevent pathogens from entering the body). A New Zealand study found that injection of vitamin B12 in CFS patients helped normalize imbalances in their red blood cells.[31] Other research has demonstrated that B12 supplementation appears to improve CFS symptoms.[32]

According to conventional medicine, a person's B12 level is considered normal when it is above 208 picograms per deciliter. However, even when blood tests reveal normal B12 levels, supplementation may be warranted. In a study of 28 people who suffered from fatigue but whose B12 levels tested normal, all 28 felt significantly better after receiving injections of B12 twice a day for two weeks.[33] Vitamin B12 deficiencies have resulted in severe nerve and brain damage when the patients' levels were as high as 300 picograms per deciliter.[34]

The renowned Framingham Heart Study (the health of 5,209 people monitored since 1948) reveals evidence of deficiencies of B12 at levels over 500.[35] According to Jacob Teitelbaum, M.D., author of *From Fatigued to Fantastic: A Manual for Moving Beyond Chronic Fatigue and Fibromyalgia*, the standard for B12 was originally established at the level that prevents anemia, but this amount of B12 does not meet the requirements of the brain and nervous system.

Despite the tendency of conventional medicine to scoff at the efficacy of B12 injections, Dr. Teitelbaum uses them in treating CFS. "In my experience, when their other problems are also treated, many people respond dramatically to B12 injections," he says. "I have found that treating patients with B12, even if their levels are technically normal, often results in marked improvement."[36]

Folic Acid (folate, folacin)—Part of the B vitamin family, folic acid is essential for blood formation, especially red and white blood cells, and RNA/DNA synthesis. Folic acid deficiency has been linked to fatigue.[37] In a study of 38 patients, researchers found that supplementing with folic acid (10 mg daily) produced a regression of fatigue, lassitude, and depression in two to three months.[38] Leafy green vegetables have high concentrations of folic acid; not surprising when you consider that its name derives from the same root as the word *foliage*. As with the other B-complex vitamins, brewer's yeast is an excellent source of folic acid.

Biotin–Another member of the B vitamin group, biotin is equally essential to food metabolism and the release of energy. A deficiency of biotin produces fatigue, lack of appetite, depression, and muscle pains. Biotin assists in the synthesis of nucleic, amino, and fatty acids. Good food sources for biotin include brewer's yeast, liver, and soybeans.

Minerals

Some would argue that monitoring mineral deficiencies is even more important than vitamin deficiencies as the body doesn't manufacture minerals and they are difficult to liberate from food sources. Like vitamins, minerals are a basic part of all cells. They play an essential role in the body's regulatory functions. The actions of minerals are highly interrelated, to each other and to vitamins, hormones, and enzymes. No mineral can function in the body without affecting others.

Dosages are not included here for most of the minerals because supplementation is a more delicate process than in the case of antioxidant vitamins, for example. Balancing the minerals with each other is vital and needs to be precisely tailored to meet the individual's imbalances and deficiencies.

Calcium–Necessary for strong bones and teeth, calcium also serves as an essential cofactor in cellular energy production and nerve and heart function. Magnesium is involved in the body's uptake of calcium. As magnesium is one of the most common deficiencies implicated in CFS, calcium is likely to be lacking as well. Low levels of calcium can result in muscle cramps and emotional irritability, two symptoms of CFS and fibromyalgia.

In addition to relaxing blood vessels and calming muscle tension, calcium supplementation can ease stress and anxiety. Given the particularly dependent interaction of the two minerals, calcium and magnesium supplements should be taken in ratio, although calcium is best absorbed at bedtime and magnesium in the morning.

Dietary sources of calcium include dairy products, tofu, kelp, leafy green vegetables, and brewer's yeast.

Chromium–Many people with CFS suffer from hypoglycemia (low blood sugar). Chromium is beneficial because it stabilizes insulin production, thereby regulating the body's ability to convert and process glucose for energy and thus blood sugar levels. Anything that helps better control blood sugar levels can substantially improve immune function. The United States appears to be a chromium-deficient nation, probably due to our overindulgence in refined grain products.[39] Chromium is contained in the outer bran portion of grains, so much of it is lost in the production of white flour. In addition, a high intake of white sugar tends to deplete the body of chromium since our chromium needs increase in proportion to blood sugar levels.[40]

In addition to whole grains, brewer's yeast and meat are good sources of chromium. As a supplement, chromium picolinate is the preferred form for those with food sensitivities because it is yeast free. It is also more easily absorbed by the body.

Germanium–Among other functions, this element enhances the availability of oxygen to cells, which promotes cell health. Between 20% and 50% of CFS patients given germanium experienced substantial to marked relief of their symptoms.[41] Germanium may accomplish this by stimulating the production of interferon (proteins released by white blood cells) which blocks the spread of viruses and stimulates other immune "workers" in turn.[42] Germanium is not available in food and can only be obtained via a supplement.

Iodine–Iodine is part of the structure of the thyroid hormones T3 and T4, which regulate our body's energy usage as well as numerous body functions. Iodine's effects are far reaching, since the metabolism of all the body's cells—except for brain cells—is influenced by thyroid hormones. Iodine deficiency most typically results in hypothyroidism (SEE QUICK DEFINITION) which is characterized by many of the symptoms of CFS, including fatigue, general weakness, depression, headaches, and memory lapses. Dietary sources of iodine are cod liver oil, certain fish, shrimp, kelp, chard, turnip greens, cantaloupe, sunflower seeds, and sea salt.

Iron–Iron is essential to red blood cell synthesis, oxygen transport, and energy production through food metabolism. Low iron levels in the blood are commonly paired with anemia and have been linked to fatigue.[43] Once again, testing as normal for iron doesn't necessarily mean that supplementation won't have an effect. In a study of chronically fatigued, but not anemic, women, 66% experienced improvement after iron supplementation.[44]

Iron-rich foods include kelp, blackstrap molasses, lecithin, certain nuts and seeds, millet, and parsley.

Magnesium—Magnesium is required for ATP (SEE QUICK DEFINITION) synthesis in the body. As you may recall, ATP is our source of energy. Magnesium is a cofactor in more than 300 enzymatic reactions involving energy metabolism and nerve function. Magnesium also aids in the uptake of calcium and in transporting potassium into cells. The daily intake of magnesium in the United States has decreased from 450-485 mg daily in the early 1900s to 185-235 mg per day currently, probably as a result of magnesium-depleted farming soil and a diet high in processed foods. The RDA is at least 350 mg daily and, as discussed earlier, RDAs are often lower than the optimum level for the body. Obviously, a lot of Americans are walking around with magnesium deficiency.

ATP stands for adenosine triphosphate, a substance found in all cells, particularly muscle, and responsible for energy. When enzymes split ATP, energy is released (12,000 calories/mole of ATP) from the high-energy phosphate bonds. This bond can be instantly split on demand whenever energy is required to run cellular functions. Then ATP becomes ADP. When energy is returned, it becomes ATP again. ATP is often called the cell's *energy currency* because it can be continually spent and remade again in a matter of minutes.

Magnesium deficiency results in impaired energy production and has been clearly linked with CFS. Its symptoms resemble the CFS laundry list: tiredness, weakness, muscle pain, nausea, anorexia, learning disability, and personality change. In a study at the University of Southampton in England, 20 CFS patients had lower red blood cell magnesium levels than healthy volunteers. In a companion study, 32 CFS patients had a once-weekly injection of either magnesium or a placebo for six weeks. Of those receiving the magnesium, 80% had reduced symptoms and improved energy while less than 20% of those on placebo injections reported improvement. The red blood cell magnesium levels returned to normal in those who had the magnesium injections.[45]

Research has shown that combining magnesium with malic acid, a fruit acid found in apples which is also crucial to the formation of ATP, is useful in the treatment of chronic fatigue syndrome as well as fibromyalgia. In the case of fibromyalgia, low magnesium is what keeps muscles

For more on **thyroid hormones and chronic fatigue**, see Chapter 6: Reversing Hidden Thyroid Problems, pp. 164-189.

What It Takes to Absorb Some Calcium: Nutrients That Aid and Hinder Its Absorption

The mere fact that you take a calcium supplement or eat a calcium-rich food doesn't mean that your body actually absorbs this essential nutrient. According to Melvyn R. Werbach, M.D., assistant clinical professor at the U.C.L.A. School of Medicine, specific interactions among nutrients can either hinder or aid the absorption of calcium, and of any targeted nutrient.

Knowledge of nutritional interactions should be regarded "as an essential component of good medical practice," Dr. Werbach urges in his new book, *Foundations of Nutritional Medicine*, and not as "an 'alternative' or 'complement' to conventional medicine." Based on his review of a great number of clinical studies, which he summarizes in his book, Dr. Werbach offers the following observations about calcium.

■ **Bioavailability.** This term indicates the body's ability to process, absorb, retain, and use a nutrient from a dietary or supplemental source. If you are taking a calcium

supplement, the most efficient absorption typically occurs in individual doses of 500 mg or less, says Dr. Werbach.

You are also likely to absorb more calcium if you take vitamin D concurrently; you may absorb five times more calcium from milk than spinach; and some individuals can glean more usable calcium from dairy products than from supplements. If you take a calcium supplement with foods, this increases your absorption by 10%. Late evening intake is the most effective time and calcium in a whole-bone extract tends to be better absorbed than simple calcium salts. Of calcium salts, calcium citrate appears to be among the most bioavailable, but be careful here, because calcium citrate can increase your absorption of dietary aluminum.

■ **Aiding absorption.** On the positive side, particular nutrients can enhance the absorption or retention of calcium. These include iron, lactose (milk protein), the amino acid lysine (in amounts up to 800

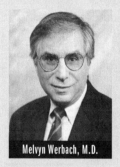

Melvyn Werbach, M.D.

> You are also likely to absorb more calcium if you take vitamin D concurrently; you may absorb five times more calcium from milk than spinach; and some individuals can glean more usable calcium from dairy products than from supplements, explains Dr. Werbach.

mg, if taken at the same time as a calcium source), potassium, sodium bicarbonate, vitamin D, vitamin B6, and vitamin A. Glucose (simple sugar) can increase calcium absorption by 20% if taken at the same time as a calcium source.

■ **Hindering absorption.** Other nutrients can decrease the amount of calcium absorbed by the intestines. These include fatty acids, fiber, phytates (found in the bran layer of cereal grains), and uronic acid (found in the fiber content of fruits and vegetables). Oxalates, concentrated in certain leafy green vegetables such as spinach, can block the absorption of calcium if these foods are consumed alone, but not if they are eaten with other calcium-containing foods. A high daily level of zinc supplementation (140 mg) can reduce calcium absorption if, at the same time, a person has an especially low level (200 mg or less) of calcium intake from the diet.

■ **Increasing calcium loss.** Certain substances can increase the amount of calcium excreted in the urine, thereby decreasing overall calcium levels in the body. These include caffeine, protein, sugar (offsetting its ability to increase absorption), refined carbohydrates, sodium, and foods high in phosphorous (meat, grains, soft drinks) if consumed in large amounts.

■ **Drug interactions.** Certain categories of drugs and specific drugs can also interfere with calcium absorption, reports Dr. Werbach. For example, glucocorticoids (cortisol and cortisone) can reduce the

Melvyn R. Werbach, M.D., is the author of *Foundations of Nutritional Medicine: A Sourcebook of Clinical Research* (1997). Available from: Third Line Press, Inc., 4751 Viviana Drive, Tarzana, CA 91356; tel: 818-996-0076 or 800-916-0076; fax: 818-774-1575; e-mail: tip@third-line.com.

amount of calcium in the blood. With prolonged use, tetracyclines (a class of antibiotics) can begin to deplete calcium stores in the body.

Digoxin (a heart drug) and ethacrynic acid (used to induce urination) increase the amount of calcium excreted in the urine; and isoniazid (an antibiotic for tuberculosis) curtails the production of vitamin D which is necessary for absorbing calcium. If used for a long time, methotrexate (a chemotherapy agent), phenytoin (an anticonvulsant for epilepsy), and phenobarbital (a sedative) can block calcium absorption and lead to calcium depletion.

■ **General cautions.** Keep your calcium to phosphorous intake at a ratio of less than 2:1 to avoid an excess of calcium which can cause reduced bone strength. Consuming calcium in excess of 2 g daily can make your parathyroid gland (located in the throat and concerned with calcium metabolism) overactive. Calcium needs to be maintained in ratio to magnesium.

If you are a woman taking estrogen and have a low magnesium intake, calcium supplementation may increase your risk of thrombosis (blood clotting that can lead to a heart attack). Calcium carbonate, such as from ground oyster shells, can produce constipation. Calcium supplements, especially from natural materials (such as limestone rock) may contain toxic metals, such as lead. In one study of 70 different brands, 25% exceeded lead safety levels, while a second study of one brand of dolomite revealed higher than desirable levels of aluminum, arsenic, cadmium, and lead.

Daniel Peterson, M.D., one of the doctors treating patients in the original outbreak of CFS in Incline Village, Nevada, has found that 40% of CFS patients benefit from taking magnesium and malic acid.

CAUTION

Most physicians recommend that the malic acid/magnesium supplement be taken on an empty stomach, but some people have reported intestinal problems. If this occurs, the supplement should be taken with food or the dosage reduced.

in a state of spasm, so supplementation can aid in relieving this painful symptom. Jay Goldstein, M.D., uses the magnesium/malic acid combination in treating both CFS and fibromyalgia. "Fibromyalgia pain may respond within 48 hours while fatigue may take about two weeks," he states.[46] Daniel Peterson, M.D., one of the doctors treating patients in the original outbreak of CFS in Incline Village, Nevada, has found that 40% of CFS patients benefit from taking magnesium and malic acid.[47]

A study by Guy D. Abraham, M.D., and Jorge D. Flechas, M.D., showed positive results for the reversal of fibromyalgia with magnesium and malic acid supplementation. Fifteen patients with fibromyalgia who took magnesium (300-600 mg daily) and malic acid (1,200-2,400 mg daily) experienced subjective improvement in their symptoms within the first 48 hours. Over an eight-week period of supplementation, their degree of muscle tenderness and pain dropped from 19.6 to 6.5, according to medical scores.[48]

Dietary sources of magnesium include tofu, kelp, leafy green vegetables, whole grains, nuts, seeds, raisins, dried figs, and blackstrap molasses.

Manganese—Manganese is an important catalyst and cofactor in many enzymatic processes and reactions, including energy metabolism, regulation of blood sugar, and thyroid hormone functions.[49] It is part of the main antioxidant enzyme, superoxide dismutase (SOD), and there is some evidence that it may help to counteract the immune-suppressive effects of stress hormones (corticosteroids) which have been shown to be elevated in people with CFS. Manganese may also increase the binding ability and other activities of white blood cells.[50] Manganese can be found in whole grains, leafy green vegetables, dried fruit, and nuts.

Phosphorus—A member of the nitrogen family, this element occurs in combined form in phosphate which plays a major role in energy production and activation of B vitamins. Phosphorus is also a component of RNA/DNA, bones, and teeth. Research has shown that phosphorus deficiency can produce fatigue.[51] High-protein foods like milk, cheese, meat, and fish are also high in phosphorus.

Potassium—Potassium is a primary electrolyte (SEE QUICK DEFINITION), important in controlling pH (acid/base) and water balance. It plays a role in nerve function and helps maintain cell integrity by regulating the transfer of nutrients into the cells. Potassium supports the adrenal glands, which is important for CFS sufferers as these glands are often severely impaired from a protracted period of functioning in a continual state of stress response.

Fatigue and muscular weakness are the most common symptoms of potassium deficiency.[52] A review of studies involving a total of nearly 3,000 patients found that 75% to 91% of those treated with potassium and magnesium aspartates (1 g of each salt daily) experienced "pronounced relief of fatigue," usually after four to five days.[53]

Potassium is found in fruits, vegetables, whole grains, nuts, and seeds. According to Dr. Susser, it is important to balance potassium intake with salt intake and the ratio should be greater than five (potassium) to one (sodium).[54]

Selenium—This element is an important constituent of the antioxidant enzyme system (glutathione peroxidase) which protects tissues against free radical damage. Selenium works synergistically with vitamin E, meaning that the two nutrients mutually reinforce the body's immune defenses. A deficiency in selenium can depress immune function.[55] Studies have shown that supplementation with selenium enhances immune function by increasing the ability of lymphocytes and NK cells to rid the body of harmful microorganisms.[56] Dietary sources of selenium are wheat germ, Brazil nuts, bran, and red Swiss chard.

Zinc—This mineral is a cofactor in numerous enzymatic processes and reactions crucial for healthy body function. Like selenium, zinc supports many aspects of the immune system. It is necessary for the free radical–quenching activity of the enzyme SOD (superoxide dismutase). A deficiency of zinc can lead to depressed activity of NK and other immune cells.[57] B cells use up zinc when they make antibodies, so someone who has been fighting infection for a prolonged period, as

QUICK DEFINITION

Electrolytes are substances in the blood, tissue fluids, intracellular fluids, or urine which conduct an electrical charge, either plus or minus. Examples include acids, bases, and salts, such as potassium, magnesium, phosphate, sulfate, bicarbonate, sodium, chloride, and calcium. Electrolytes provide inorganic chemicals for cellular reactions and control mechanisms, such as the conduction of electrochemical impulses to nerves and muscles. Electrolytes are also needed for key enzymatic reactions involved in metabolism, or the release of energy from food.

in CFS, is likely to be deficient in zinc.

Declining levels of zinc are implicated in the shrinkage of the thymus gland (an endocrine gland located behind the sternum) which occurs with age. Zinc supplementation can help restore the thymus and thus bolster the immune system. Research links zinc deficiency with fatigue[58] and indicates that supplementing with zinc improves muscle strength and reduces muscle fatigue.[59] Oysters contain high concentrations of zinc. Whole grain wheat, wheat germ, and pumpkin seeds are also good food sources.

Additional Supplements

The following nutritional supplements are also helpful in the treatment of CFS:

Amino Acids—Amino acids are the building blocks of protein. Since amino acids work as a team and in ratio to each other, it is important to identify specific deficiencies and design a precise supplement program based on the results. Amino acid deficiencies and imbalances are common in CFS. Carnitine[60] and methionine[61] seem to be the ones most implicated.

Carnitine is vital to mitochondial energy production. Low carnitine levels have been found in CFS patients.[62] In addition, a more severe deficiency correlates with a greater degree of fatigue.[63] Carnitine deficiency may also account for the muscle pain and weakness and the post-exercise exhaustion typical of CFS.[64]

Among its other functions, methionine helps the liver to detoxify. Given the probable overload on the liver due to an elevated level of chemical toxins in a person with CFS, supplementation with methionine can assist the liver in its detoxification function. Methionine also aids in reducing the body's uptake of mercury, thereby freeing immune cells to focus on the viruses and other opportunistic infections involved in CFS. Mercury dental fillings can deplete methionine through the continual need they present for detoxification.

This is also true of glutathione, another amino acid that aids in detoxification. Glutathione reduces free-radical damage to cells, prevents depletion of other antioxidants, and activates certain immune cells. "The ability of cells to maintain an adequate glutathione status is critical to our health," states Jay Lombard, M.D., author of *The Brain Wellness Plan: Breakthrough Medical, Nutritional, and Immune-Boosting Therapies*. To raise glutathione levels, Dr. Lombard recommends a combination of N-acetyl cysteine or NAC (an amino acid precursor of glutathione; 1 g daily on an empty stomach), lipoic acid

A Guide to Taking Supplements

Jeffrey Bland, Ph.D. and Lindsey Berkson, D.C., offer these recommendations and advisories to follow when taking nutritional supplements:

■ Nutritional supplements should be taken with meals to promote increased absorption. Fat-soluble vitamins (such as vitamin A, beta carotene, vitamin E, and the essential fatty acids linoleic and alpha linolenic acid) should be taken during the day with the meal which contains the most fat.

■ Amino acid supplements should be taken on an empty stomach at least an hour before or after a meal, and taken with fruit juice to help promote absorption. When taking an increased dosage of an isolated amino acid, be sure to supplement with an amino acid blend.

■ If you become nauseated when you take tablet supplements, consider taking a liquid form, diluted in a beverage.

■ If you become nauseated or ill within an hour after taking nutritional supplements, consider the need for a bowel cleanse or rejuvenation program prior to beginning a course of nutritional supplementation.

■ If you are taking high doses, do not take the supplements all at one time, but divide them into smaller doses taken throughout the day.

■ Take digestive enzymes with meals to assist digestion. If you are taking pancreatic enzymes for other therapeutic reasons, be sure to take them on an empty stomach between meals.

■ Take mineral supplements away from the highest fiber meals of the day as fiber can decrease mineral absorption.

■ When taking an increased dosage of an isolated B vitamin, be sure to supplement with a B complex.

■ When taking nutrients, be sure to take adequate amounts of liquid to mix with digestive juices and prevent side effects.

(a vitamin-like substance necessary for ATP production; 200 mg daily with food), and selenium (no more than 200 mcg daily with food).[65]

For more on **glutathione**, see Chapter 4: Restoring Immune Vitality, pp. 127-129.

Shari Lieberman, Ph.D, C.N.S., a clinical nutritionist based in New York City, considers glutathione a must for people with environmental sensitivities whose detoxification organs and systems have been overloaded and are in need of support. "Glutathione is a powerful antioxidant that works inside our cells. It is also used in many of the body's detoxification mechanisms," Dr. Lieberman says.

Chlorella–Chlorella (*Chlorella pyrenoidosa*, a freshwater single-celled green algae) has numerous benefits for CFS sufferers. One, it is a first-string detoxifying agent, capable of removing alcohol from the liver and heavy metals (such as cadmium and mercury), certain pesticides,

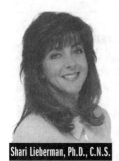

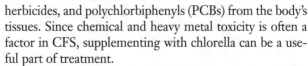
Dr. Lieberman has found that EFA supplementation (three to six capsules daily of high-potency fish oil) is particularly useful for people with fibromyalgia. "It works like a natural cortisone to decrease inflammation," she reports.

Shari Lieberman, Ph.D., C.N.S.

For more information on **chlorella**, contact: Nature's Balance, Inc., 10705 North Main Street, Suite 307, Archdale, NC 27263; tel: 800-858-5198 or 910-434-4102; fax: 910-434-3119. Sun Wellness, Inc., 4025 Spencer Street, Unit 104, Torrance, CA 90503; tel: 800-829-2828 or 310-371-5515; fax: 310-371-0094.

For more on **chlorella** in mercury detoxification, see Chapter 7: Eliminating Heavy Metal Toxicity, p. 203, 205.

herbicides, and polychlorbiphenyls (PCBs) from the body's tissues. Since chemical and heavy metal toxicity is often a factor in CFS, supplementing with chlorella can be a useful part of treatment.

Two, chlorella contains 60% protein, including all the essential amino acids, as well as high levels of beta carotene and chlorophyll. This has clear benefits for the nutrient-depleted state of most people with CFS. Three, chlorella can absorb toxins from the intestines, help relieve chronic constipation, favorably alter the bacterial flora content of the bowel, and eliminate intestinal gas.

Chlorella can assist in reversing the digestive disorders common to CFS. Finally, both scientific documentation and reliable anecdotal reports indicate that chlorella is effective in helping to reduce the symptoms of viral and bacterial infections, low blood sugar, and anemia, among other disorders. With multiple infections the symptomatic centerpiece of CFS and the other two conditions frequently present as well, chlorella has obvious application in these areas.

Chlorella's far-reaching effects may be due to its ability to increase albumin levels in the body. Albumin, continually secreted by the liver, is the most abundant protein found in the blood. It acts as a major natural antioxidant, contributing an estimated 80% of all neutralizing activity against free radicals in the blood that would otherwise damage cells and tissues. Strengthening the immune system is an important feature in any CFS treatment program.

Coenzyme Q10—Coenzyme Q10 (coQ10), also known as ubiquinone, is vital to the mitochondria and thus to energy production. A powerful antioxidant, it also improves oxygenation and helps to prevent toxicity. In the event of a coQ10 deficiency, common among CFS sufferers,

ATP production is seriously impaired. CoQ10 is found in every plant and animal cell.

The fact that vegetarians tend to have almost double the blood levels of coQ10 as compared to meat eaters seems to indicate that plants have a higher percentage, but food sources don't deliver high amounts of coQ10 and supplementation is therefore the best way to derive therapeutic benefits.[66] Supplementing with coQ10 has been shown to improve symptoms of CFS.[67] A general dosage for CFS is 25-50 mg three to four times daily; for fibromyalgia, 30-200 mg per day.[68]

Essential Fatty Acids—Essential fatty acids (EFAs—SEE QUICK DEFINITION) are vitamin-like compounds that cannot be made in the body and must be ingested through the foods you eat. Without EFAs, your organs cannot manufacture prostaglandins, substances that are key regulators of immune, digestive, cardiovascular, and reproductive functions. Furthermore, cell membranes consist mainly of lipids (fats) which are highly susceptible to free-radical damage. EFAs help to protect against this damage. EFAs also aid in reducing the release of serotonin; elevated brain serotonin levels may be a factor in CFS and help to explain the severe fatigue. Research has found that too much serotonin is as detrimental as too little.

Research suggests a link between CFS and low levels of essential fatty acids.[69] A study of 63 patients with post-viral fatigue syndrome who also had low EFA levels found that three months of supplementation with a combination of evening primrose oil and fish oil resulted in normal EFA levels and highly significant improvement in all the individual symptoms, including fatigue, aches and pains, and depression.[70] Evening primrose oil contains GLA (gamma-linoleic acid), a particularly powerful EFA. For CFS patients, Dr. Murray suggests flaxseed oil, one tablespoon per day.[71]

Dr. Lieberman has found that EFA supplementation (three to six capsules daily of high-potency fish oil) is particularly useful for people with fibromyalgia. "It works like a natural cortisone to decrease inflammation," she reports. Sometimes she adds GLA (one or two 240-300 mg capsules

QUICK DEFINITION

Essential fatty acids (EFAs) are unsaturated fats required in the diet. Omega-3 and omega-6 oils are the two principal types. The primary omega-3 oil is called alpha-linolenic acid (ALA) and is found in flaxseed (58%), canola, pumpkin and walnut, and soybeans. Fish oils, such as salmon, cod, and mackerel, contain the other important omega-3 oils, DHA (docosahexaenoic acid) and EPA (eicosapentaenoic acid). Linoleic acid or cis-linoleic acid is the main omega-6 oil and is found in most plants and vegetable oils, including safflower (73%), corn, peanut, and sesame. The most therapeutic form of omega-6 oil is gamma-linolenic acid (GLA), found in evening primrose, black currant, and borage oils. Once in the body, omega-3 and omega-6 are converted to prostaglandins, hormone-like substances that regulate many metabolic functions, particularly inflammatory processes.

CAUTION

Alternative practitioners sometimes recommend dosages higher than those currently considered safe by conventional medicine. The scientific literature and numerous clinical trials generally support these elevated dosages for short periods of time but should be taken with medical supervision.

daily), but not in the form of evening primrose oil because, according to her, the latter also contains an acid which is pro-inflammatory.

Quercetin—A bioflavonoid (SEE QUICK DEFINITION) found in fruits and vegetables, quercetin is known as a vitamin C "helper," which means it enhances the beneficial activities of vitamin C by increasing its absorption. As an antioxidant, quercetin provides the body with protection against environmental stresses that can result in allergies. It also inhibits the release of histamine, the substance that produces the symptoms of an allergic reaction. Further, quercetin is an effective antiviral. All of these functions are beneficial for CFS. Commercially, quercetin can be found in blue-green algae.

How Nutrients Work Together

Vitamins and minerals help regulate the conversion of food to energy in the body and can be separated into two general categories: energy nutrients, which are principally involved in the conversion of food to energy; and protector nutrients, which help defend against damaging toxins derived from drugs, alcohol, radiation, environmental pollutants, or the body's own enzyme processes.

"The B-complex vitamins and magnesium are examples of energy nutrients," says nutritionist Jeffrey Bland, Ph.D., "for they activate specific metabolic facilitators called enzymes, which control digestion and the absorption and use of proteins, fats, and carbohydrates. These nutrients often work as a team, their mutual presence enhancing the other's function."

In the process of converting food to energy, free radicals are produced which can damage the body and set the stage for degenerative diseases. Protector nutrients, such as vitamin E, beta carotene, vitamin C, and the minerals zinc, copper, manganese, and selenium, play a critical role in preventing or delaying these degenerative processes. Vitamins A, C, and E work together as a team, protecting against breakdown and helping each other maintain adequate tissue levels.

Lindsey Berkson, D.C., of Santa Fe, New Mexico, notes that vitamins and minerals are what make the chemical and electrical circuitry of the body work, and that the body's functioning is therefore profoundly affected by how nutrients either work together or against each other. Nutrients can help each other or inhibit each other when taken simultaneously. For example, iron is best absorbed when taken separately from pancreatic enzymes and should also not be taken with vitamin E, says Dr. Berkson. There are also certain nutrients that can help "potentiate" the other nutrients. For example, vitamin C taken with iron provides the maximum absorption of the iron.

CHAPTER 11

Healing Psychological and Emotional Factors

AT THE START of this book, Jesse Stoff, M.D., spoke of learning the "lessons of the disease." Why did *this* person get *this* illness *now*? Illness is more than a matter of imbalanced physiology. There are *always* psychological and emotional aspects to every health problem and unless these are thoroughly addressed no cure, from no matter how holistic or alternative a source, will ever be complete and lasting. This chapter focuses on the *person* who has the chronic fatigue and how their lifestyle—their ways of thinking, acting, and being—contributes to, or seeds, the problem, and keeps it in place.

Illness is more than a matter of imbalanced physiology. There are always psychological and emotional aspects to every health problem and unless these are thoroughly addressed no cure, from no matter how holistic or alternative a source, will ever be complete and lasting.

Lifestyle choices can contribute to chronic fatigue. For example, the style of high-paced overachievement—some call it workaholism—that characterizes the lives of many CFS sufferers prior to becoming sick. Sometimes in a curious way, getting laid out with unremitting fatigue is the only way some people will ever take the time to focus on their *internal* world. Alternative medicine competently addresses the psychological and emotional side of all illnesses, including chronic fatigue, recognizing the uniquely *individual* factors in each patient. In other words, all chronic fatigue patients do not have the same psychology, but all chronic fatigue patients have psychological issues that participate in their illness. These mental and emotional factors constantly interact with—sometimes directing, other times following—the person's physiological condition.

Let's begin by looking at a case which brings together a number of the components discussed throughout the book. Enzyme, hormonal, and nutrient deficiencies as well as allergies all contributed to Michelle's fibromyalgia, but psychological and emotional factors were as significant as the physical imbalances in creating her illness. **Norman Levin, M.D.**, of Aldie, Virginia, who is board certified in internal medicine, rheumatology, and chelation therapy, explains how mental-emotional factors must be addressed to successfully reverse a chronic condition such as fibromyalgia and how this involves asking the right questions of your disease:

Success Story: Michelle Stops Carrying the Weight of the World

Before seeing me, Michelle, 39, had suffered from severe muscle pain for about two months. On the surface, it seemed ironic that a woman as physically active as Michelle should develop the classic symptoms of fibromyalgia. Michelle taught a full-time schedule of aerobics classes, and ran around constantly to keep up with her two young children. She was the kind of person who tried to do and be everything for everybody. As we discovered, this attitude was at the core of her muscle aches.

When a person has problems with muscle spasms or muscle irritability, often there is an absolute or relative deficiency of magnesium in the body. Almost as a general rule, I will give the Meyer's cocktail (SEE QUICK DEFINITION) to patients with fibromyalgia or muscle spasms to get sufficient magnesium into their systems. Often, a standard blood test for magnesium levels does not reveal the true magnesium status. First, a regular blood test does not necessarily tell you the amount of magnesium available in the

QUICK DEFINITION

The **Meyer's Cocktail** is an intravenous vitamin and mineral protocol developed in the 1970s by John Meyers, M.D., a physician at Johns Hopkins University in Baltimore, Maryland. It contains magnesium chloride hexahydrate (5 cc given), calcium gluconate (2.5 cc), vitamin B2 (1,000 mcg/cc; 1 cc given), vitamin B5 (100 mg/cc; 1 cc given), vitamin B6 (250 mg/cc; 1 cc given) the entire vitamin B-complex (100 mg/cc; 1 cc given), and vitamin C (222 mg/cc; 6 cc given). The solution is slowly injected over a 5-15 minute period. The "Cocktail" is indicated for patients with chronic fatigue, depression, muscle spasm, asthma, hives, allergic rhinitis, congestive heart failure, angina, ischemic vascular disease, acute infections, and senile dementia.

"Michelle was the kind of person who tried to do and be everything for everybody. As we discovered, this attitude was at the core of her fibromyalgia," says Norman Levin, M.D.

For more about **magnesium deficiency**, see Chapter 10: Ending Nutritional Deficiencies With Supplements, pp. 260-291. For more about **allergies**, see Chapter 9: Addressing the Allergy Connection, pp. 232-258. For more about the **Comprehensive Digestive Stool Analysis**, see Chapter 2: Testing, pp. 42-47. For more about **enzymes**, see Chapter 8: Replenishing Enzyme Deficiencies, pp. 212-231.

Enzymes are specialized living proteins fundamental to all living processes in the body, necessary for every chemical reaction and the normal activity of our organs, tissues, fluids, and cells. There are hundreds of thousands of these "Nature's workers." Enzymes enable the body to digest and assimilate food. There are special enzymes for digesting proteins, carbohydrates, fats, and plant fibers. Specifically, protease digests proteins, amylase digests carbohydrates, lipase digests fats, cellulase digests fiber, and disaccharidase digests sugars.

body because most of it is stored inside the cells. Second, even ascertaining how much magnesium exists in the cells (intracellularly) is not the final answer because the reading could be normal yet the patient may respond favorably to extra doses of magnesium (as was the case with Michelle).

In addition to considering magnesium supplementation, it is often advisable to run a delayed allergy hypersensitivity test on a person with fibromyalgia symptoms. Frequently, there are hidden food or substance allergies that can aggravate the symptoms, although the reaction may not take place until hours—12 hours is not uncommon—after eating the food, thereby displacing our attention from the allergen itself. For example, you could eat wheat and have a migraine headache the next day, or have some corn and experience an arthritis flare-up 24 hours later. In addition, you may think you're on a healthy diet but, in fact, you may be allergic to one of the "healthy" foods you're eating. For instance, drinking organic carrot juice may contribute to your physical symptoms if you're allergic to carrots.

Michelle's allergy test indicated she was reactive to most dairy products (Romano cheese, yogurt, and whole butter, in particular), tuna fish, raspberries, cherries, coffee, food additives and preservatives (MSG, saccharine, sodium benzoate), and environmental chemicals such as cleaning products, benzene, and trichloroethylene. As a first measure, Michelle began avoiding these substances.

Next, we used a laboratory test called the Comprehensive Digestive Stool Analysis to see how her digestion and intestines were working. The results indicated large amounts of residual fats and vegetable fibers, which told us that Michelle had a nutrient malabsorption problem. I put her on a digestive enzyme formula called Digestin that contains the primary enzymes (SEE QUICK DEFINITION) for each food group (fats, proteins, carbohydrates, and fibers), hydrochloric acid (the stomach's principle digestive juice), and ox bile (to aid the small intestine in its digestive processes).

Concurrently, I put Michelle on several other nutrients and formulations. She took esterified vitamin C to bowel tolerance (the point just before diarrhea); the ester form is better absorbed. She took Fibroplex to provide nutrients for muscle energy. Specifically, this formula contains magnesium, malic acid, manganese, and vitamins B1 and B6. Providing magnesium and malic acid in adequate amounts often produces favorable benefits for fibromyalgia, possibly by removing aluminum from the body.

In addition, Michelle took a supergreens concentrate called Greens Plus twice daily as a powder added to water or juice. The purpose here was to provide a full natural nutrient array in organic form that could be easily assimilated by the body. The product contains a large amount of chlorophyll, which is a natural, easily absorbed source of magnesium. Michelle also took vitamin B12 as a capsule that dissolves and is absorbed under the tongue. She responded better to B12 when it could enter her body without having to pass through her digestive tract.

After checking Michelle's DHEA (SEE QUICK DEFINITION) levels, which tested low, I started her on 5 mg daily of this hormone. I had her slowly increase her DHEA intake until she achieved the maximum benefit and before she started experiencing adverse side effects (in her case, 25 mg daily). Most people tolerate DHEA well but, because it is a precursor hormone, it can turn into other hormones, such as estrogen or testosterone, in the bodies of some women. This can lead to side effects of abnormal bleeding, breast tenderness or swelling, acne, or unusual hair growth.

I also had Michelle take 5 mg of the hormone melatonin (widely used to rebalance disturbed sleep/wake cycles) at bedtime to aid her sleeping, which was a major problem for her. Finally, Michelle consulted a chiropractor who used a deep-muscle massage technique called myotherapy (SEE QUICK DEFINITION) to release "trigger points" in her musculature. These are specific points on the body known to carry and concentrate stress; releasing them through massage is an effective contribution to overall pain reduction.

After about four weeks of following this program (including the once-weekly Meyer's cocktail), Michelle

QUICK DEFINITION

DHEA (dehydroepiandrosterone) is naturally produced by the human adrenal glands and gonads with optimal levels occurring around age 20 for women and age 25 for men. After those ages, DHEA levels gradually decline so that a person 80 years old produces only a fraction of the DHEA they did when they were 20. As an antioxidant, hormone regulator, and the building block from which estrogen and testosterone are produced, DHEA is vital to health. Low DHEA levels have been associated with cancer, diabetes, multiple sclerosis, hypertension, obesity, AIDS, heart disease, Alzheimer's, and immune dysfunction illnesses. Test subjects using supplemental DHEA reported improved sleeping patterns, better memory, an improved ability to cope with stress, decreased joint pain, increases in lean muscle, and decreases in body fat. No serious side effects have been reported to date, although acne, oily skin, facial hair growth on women, deepening of the voice, irritability, insomnia, and fatigue have been reported with high DHEA doses.

For more information about **esterified vitamin C (Ester C)**, see Chapter 10: Ending Nutritional Deficiencies With Supplements, pp. 274-275.

reported considerable gains. Her digestion was improved, she was coping better with stress, and she felt more at peace with herself and in greater control of her life. She told me, "I feel like I have more energy. I feel less shaky, the muscle spasms aren't as bad, and I'm starting to get a little perspective on my condition."

The perspective Michelle was gaining had to do with insight into why she had fibromyalgia. She was highly motivated to get well, willing to do the hard psychological inner work and to make the life changes such insight required. In a sense, she had to, because she had reached the point where the pain was so severe she could no longer function. Pain had forced her to cut back on her aerobics classes and teach only the much less demanding water aerobics. Then she had to give that up as well.

When I urged her to ask herself about the message of her condition, Michelle began to see that she always strove to be the super mom, super wife, super teacher, and the super performer in every situation or relationship. Her striving wasn't egotistical, but came out of her caring and industriousness. Michelle saw how everybody leaned on her and how, because she felt this was her role, she could never say no—and it was too much. Michelle understood how she had developed severe, almost total body pain that forced her to stop in her tracks. She saw what she had been doing and appreciated that she could no longer do it nor did she want to. Finally, Michelle realized that it was okay to say no and to ask for help.

Not everyone with fibromyalgia will fit this pattern, but there is a certain general trend to the psychological factors involved in chronic muscle pain of this type. A person feels burdened and overwhelmed, as if everybody is leaning on their body, as if they are carrying the world's weight on their shoulders. So the "weight" goes to the muscles which eventually complain, using the body language of aches and spasms.

As the nutrients, dietary restrictions, and psychological work took effect over the next several months, Michelle recovered almost completely. Now she has returned to her active schedule and to teaching aerobics full-time; in fact, she is an instructor for other people with fibromyalgia.

The successful reversal of chronic pain, such as fibromyalgia, may certainly require the use of multiple nutrients, enzymes, hormones, and dietary changes, but you must also examine the patient's state of mind and life conditions. Rather than a patient asking why did this illness happen to me, which is the common complaint, the better question might be why is this illness happening at all. Often when patients probe their

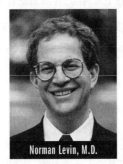

Norman Levin, M.D.

"Not everyone with fibromyalgia will fit the same pattern, but there is a certain general trend to the psychological factors involved in chronic muscle pain. A person feels burdened and overwhelmed, as if they are carrying the world's weight on their shoulders," states Dr. Norman Levin.

own life circumstances—to see how they feel about what is happening—the why behind the illness becomes clear and the condition usually clears up more quickly and thoroughly than expected. ∎

Lifestyle Choices and Personality Characteristics in CFS

If the psychological side of fibromyalgia is the sense of carrying the weight of the world on your shoulders, the state of mind underlying chronic fatigue syndrome might be expressed something like this: you're only okay if you're producing. This is a generalization of the psychological state underlying a complex health condition and of course each patient has their own *particular* cluster of emotional issues which may be contributing to their illness. Yet numerous practitioners experienced in treating CFS have noted that people who develop the syndrome tend to be overachievers.

"Every single person I have seen with CFS was an overachiever," states Shari Lieberman, Ph.D., C.N.S., a nutritional specialist in New York City. "These were people who, when they got flu or another sickness, refused to give in to it, didn't rest enough, and quickly went back to a full schedule of work and exercise. These people are go-getters. The common thread is that their CFS was precipitated by an illness in which they didn't take care of themselves enough."

If fibromyalgia is carrying the weight of the world on your shoulders, chronic fatigue syndrome is you're only okay if you're producing. "Every single person I have seen with CFS was an overachiever," says Shari Lieberman, Ph.D., C.N.S.

John Diamond, M.D., director of the Triad Medical Center in Reno, Nevada, also observes that all of his patients with chronic fatigue syndrome are overachievers. His discipline, which includes homeopathy, a medical science that emphasizes the psychological side of illness, has schooled him in looking for these factors. The self-image of these chronic fatigue patients is "locked into or associated with their personal productivity," he says. Driven by the pressure to succeed, their bodies eventually break down. "As a physician, I have to go backwards into my patients' histories to trace the whole issue," says Dr. Diamond. "Invariably, I find that my chronic fatigue syndrome patients have terrible life skills and poor habits. That kind of insulting treatment of their system adds up and the body finally says, 'no more.'"

Jacob Teitelbaum, M.D., concurs that CFS sufferers tend to be type-A personalities. These are people who are accomplishment-oriented, driven, operating on deadlines, usually anxious—a term often used to describe people prone to heart attacks. Such people often live in what Dr. Teitelbaum calls "role entrapment" before they become ill. "Role-entrapped people were taught that they have to be the *perfect* spouse or the *perfect* parent or the *perfect* employee. The 'superwoman' complex is a good example. CFIDS can be your body's way of getting out of the roles in which you are trapped," he explains.[1] In addition to the psychic discomfort of attempting to fulfill someone else's idea of what you should be, trying to live up to these roles creates a tremendous amount of stress in people's lives. A high stress level is a common feature in those who get CFS.

An important question to ask is this: what is stress? Dr. Stoff, for one, defines stress as "the internal state that results when the capacity to adapt to what is has been exceeded."[2] When this condition persists, the immune system is weakened and the body becomes vulnerable to breakdown. "Excessive stress is like putting the welcome mat out for the first 'evil' germ (be it EBV, cytomegalovirus, or Coxsackie virus) that feels like setting up camp," says Dr. Stoff.[3]

Operating at an ongoing high stress level also overloads the adrenal glands which then leads to fatigue, as the adrenals are integral to energy production. You may recall from an earlier discussion that CFS patients tend to have high levels of cortisol (one of the adrenal hormones), indicating that the adrenal glands are overworking. Clearly, taking steps to reduce the stress in your life is an important part of reversing the patterns that contributed to your CFS. Maoshing Ni, D.O.M., Ph.D., L.Ac., a practitioner of traditional Chinese medicine who has treated many people with CFS sums up the process involved: "I describe my patients as people who, before treatment, were *gulping* coffee. After treatment, they learn how to *sip* tea."

Your illness may have forced you out of your previously stressful mode of living, but it is important when you begin to recover through the various methods covered in this book that you do not resume your old habits. A first step might be to find out what *you* want to do in your life, how you *want* to spend your time. It is vital to the healing process that patients begin to get to know themselves better, says Dr. Stoff. "Self-awareness will reveal many harmful patterns and make them healthier. It is not merely an intellectual exercise," he states.

This is what Dr. Stoff means by learning the lessons of your disease. It's also what Dr. Teitelbaum has in mind when he says: "Although you likely view your illness as an enemy, you should let it become your ally."[4] Making it an ally by doing the hard internal work of sorting through the emotional and psychological components of your illness will, when combined with the treatments for the physical factors involved, result in lasting recovery.

> "Role-entrapped people were taught that they have to be the *perfect* spouse or the *perfect* parent or the *perfect* employee. The 'superwoman' complex is a good example. Chronic fatigue can be your body's way of getting out of the roles in which you are trapped," Dr. Teitelbaum explains.

For more information about **CFS and the meaning dimension**, see Chapter 6: Reversing Hidden Thyroid Problems, pp. 164-189.

Homeopathy Can Provoke Emotional Healing

Homeopathic treatment of CFS and other chronic illnesses begins by eliminating the immediate symptoms, then progresses to the older,

Stressed Out—A Pervasive Western Problem

Although the concept of stress—being "stressed out" or "under constant stress"—may be commonly discussed today, its role as a contributing factor in many diseases is underappreciated. Estimates suggest that as much as 70% to 80% of all visits to physicians' offices are for stress-related problems. Chronic stress directly affects the immune system and, if not effectively dealt with, can seriously compromise health.

Stress is a pervasive problem among Americans, according to a 1996 poll of corporate executives. For example, 44% of employees polled said their work load is excessive compared to 37% in 1988; 43% are bothered by excessive job pressure; and 55% worry considerably about their company's future; 25% of both men and women feel stressed out at work every day, another 12% feel it almost every day, and another 38% feel it once to several days a week.[5]

Research in psychoneuro-immunology, or PNI, has shown that the immune and nervous systems are linked by extensive networks of nerve endings in the spleen, bone marrow, lymph nodes, and thymus gland (a primary source of T cells). At the same time, receptors for a variety of chemical messengers—catecholamines, prostaglandins, thyroid hormone, growth hormone, sex hormones, serotonin, and endorphins—have been found on the surfaces of white blood cells. Such connections serve to integrate the activities of the immune, hormonal, and nervous systems, enabling the mind and emotional states to influence the body's resistance to disease.[6]

Stress can be defined as a reaction to any stimulus or interference that upsets normal functioning and disturbs mental or physical health. It can be brought on by internal conditions, such as illness, pain, emotional conflict, or psychological problems, or by external circumstances, such as bereavement, financial problems, loss of job or spouse, or relocation. Stress, when it becomes chronic, is often unrecognized by the person whose body is experiencing it; one begins to accept it as a fact of life, without being aware of how it is actually compromising all bodily function and preparing the foundation for illness.

More specifically, research confirms that high levels of emotional stress increase one's susceptibility to illness. Unrelieved, chronic stress begins taxing and eventually weakening, even suppressing, the immune system. Stress can also lead to hormonal imbalances which, in turn, interfere with immune function. Of all the body's systems, stress damages immune function the most. It does so by overly activating the sympathetic part of the autonomic nervous system, the part that controls the "fight-or-flight" response and initiates adrenaline and cortisol release.

underlying "layers" of the condition. One of these layers may be unresolved emotions the patient has been suppressing, often for many years. An emotional imbalance of this kind has as strong an impact as a physical malady on the overall health of the body. Homeopathic remedies help the patient release the stored emotions. If all the layers of an illness are not addressed, healing is incomplete and, as mentioned above, relapse or the development of a different disease or disorder is likely.

In the following section, **John Diamond, M.D.**, a physician specializing in homeopathy (SEE QUICK DEFINITION) and other alternative modalities, describes a multi-layered case of CFS and the homeopathic treatment of each layer, including the emotional component of the illness:

Success Story: Reversing a 14-Year Episode of Chronic Fatigue

When Rebecca, 38, first came to me, she had already seen eight conventional physicians for her multifaceted condition. She had chronic fatigue, depression, joint, muscle, and low back pain, migraine headaches, and severe pelvic and anal pains. Often her knees hurt and her legs would feel heavy. According to standard laboratory tests, Rebecca had a low white blood cell count, indicating her immune system was seriously weakened; it also showed she had a high level of Epstein-Barr virus (SEE QUICK DEFINITION), which is often the case in CFS patients.

Rebecca had used three different antidepressants but none had lifted her depression. Earlier, a physician had put her on Synthroid, a standard drug for inflammation of the thyroid gland (thyroiditis). Rebecca also felt claustrophobic, had frequent panic attacks, was afraid of new medications, was chronically constipated, and had, in her own words, "no energy." Rebecca had been on antibiotics since she was 20 for pelvic inflammatory disease, but they failed to resolve this problem. She told me she had pain in her pelvis "all the time."

Here is how Rebecca described her state: "When I get a bad pain attack in my back or pelvis, it comes over me in waves and I need to go and hide away in my bedroom and just get under the covers and rest. Sometimes it's for days. The energy just ebbs out of me. When I have no energy, my pelvis aches and throbs. I have to sit down to stop the pain. It feels like my uterus will just about drop out of me."

Homeopathy was founded in the early 1800s by German physician Samuel Hahnemann. Today, an estimated 500 million people worldwide receive homeopathic treatment; in Britain, homeopathy enjoys royal patronage. Homeopathy is now practiced according to two differing concepts. In classical homeopathy, only one single-component remedy is prescribed at a time in a potency specifically adjusted to the patient; the physician waits to see the results before prescribing anything further. In complex homeopathy, typified by *Hepar compositum*, a prescription involves multiple substances given at the same time, usually in low potencies.

Epstein-Barr virus (EBV) is a herpes-like virus thought to be the cause of infectious mononucleosis and Burkitt's lymphoma. It is contracted through the cells in the lining of the mouth and throat, and can therefore be spread by sharing utensils, kissing, and unsanitary habits. EBV symptoms, frequently duplicated in other conditions, include debilitating fatigue, fever, swollen glands, arthritic symptoms, multiple allergies, and difficulties in concentrating. People with chronic fatigue syndrome often have a high level of EBV antibodies in their blood, but EBV is no longer regarded (as it was in the 1980s) as the sole or even necessarily a contributing cause for chronic fatigue.

Controlled Exercise Can Help Chronic Fatigue

Postexercise exhaustion is on the CDC's list of chronic fatigue syndrome symptoms. Many people with CFS experience a worsening of their symptoms after exercise. However, according to a study published in the *British Medical Journal*, graded (or gradually increasing) exercise can actually produce lasting benefit for some CFS patients. The study of 66 people with CFS consisted of three groups: 1) participants in a graded exercise program; 2) a control group of flexibility training and relaxation therapy instead; and 3) 22 control subjects who "crossed over" into the exercise program after the first 12 weeks of the study.

The graded exercise consisted mainly of walking, but some cycling or swimming if desired, and the sessions initially lasted between five and 15 minutes, increasing at the rate of one or two minutes per week to a maximum of 30 minutes. If patients experienced increased fatigue, they were advised to continue at the same level of exercise for an extra week. This allowed their bodies to adjust to the increase in aerobic activity.

Of the 29 patients in the exercise group, 16 (55%) considered themselves "much" or "very much" better than at the start of the trial, compared to 8 out of 30 (29%) in the control group. In the crossover group, 12 out of 22 (55%) rated themselves as better following the exercise phase. Follow-up interviews revealed that the benefits of graded exercise appeared to continue even after the program had ended, with 68% reporting they still felt better three months after the study ended.

Researcher Peter D. White, M.D., speculates that graded exercise—not simple exercise by itself—may work by functioning as a type of behavior therapy. "Graded exercise can reduce the anxiety and apprehension understandably felt by many CFS patients, who have learned that unstructured exercise tends to cause relapses of their condition," Dr. White says. "By making the exercise graded and agreed upon by the patient, he or she is able to feel more in control."[7]

Further, she had memory and concentration problems, craved salty foods, was usually hot and sweaty while she slept, and woke frequently at night only to stare emptily at the bedroom wall just as she had done as a child. She told me that all aspects of her problem worsened at the age of 24, which I later learned was when she got married to a man who already had three young children.

I asked her about her childhood. "It was terrible," she said. Both parents had been alcoholics and addicted to drugs. Her two older brothers were heavy drinkers and had sexually abused her. Rebecca said her mother hated her because she was competing for her husband's affections. Rebecca's mother repeatedly told her she was a "worthless child," that she was "a nothing, less than a dog."

Beginning at age six, Rebecca became a surrogate mother for the household since her mother was chronically drunk. Rebecca did all the chores around the house. Meanwhile, her father was drunk most of the time and often violent. Her parents argued and fought frequently and, when they did, Rebecca would retreat to her bedroom and stare at the wall. In sum, she was extremely passive, quiet, and depressed as a child.

At 18, she had an abortion, about which she felt exceedingly guilty, and moved out of the family house. She began drinking steadily, and drifted around until she married at the age of 24. She moved to another town with her husband and his children. Consider what she did here: Rebecca duplicated the situation she had lived with as a child. She became the surrogate mother again which was, truly, the last thing she wanted to do. Eventually her biology decided this arrangement was not what she needed and shut her down with a mass of symptoms.

What Electrodermal Screening Showed—

As part of my medical practice, I regularly use electrodermal screening (EDS—SEE QUICK DEFINITION) to identify hidden energy blockages in the body. It is also an effective way to get beyond times when a patient prefers not to admit a fact from their history or perhaps literally does not remember it; at such times, these hidden facts may be the key to a case. My electrodermal evaluation of Rebecca showed highly inflammatory conditions in her tonsils and pharynx.

A "normal" EDS reading is about 50, but for Rebecca the needle hovered between 70 and 80. It also indicated trouble in her spleen, liver, kidneys, intestines, and uterus. In some instances there was a sudden change in the readings, from a high to a low value; in the elec-

---

Massage Therapy Can Reduce the Pain of Fibromyalgia

Twenty-one of 26 fibromyalgia patients experienced reduced pain and general improvement after receiving massage therapy. The study discovered a relationship between a fibromyalgia patient's degree of pain and an increase in blood levels of myoglobin (the oxygen-carrying protein of the muscle tissue). The pain may be the outcome of myoglobin leaking from the muscles. Along with the pain reduction after massage, there was a gradual decline in the high levels of myoglobin in the patients' blood.[8]

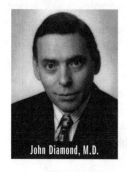

John Diamond, M.D.

The first time you see a patient, you need to give remedies that will get the physiological system working properly again, removing from the body all the obstacles to healing, says Dr. Diamond. Then you can give a single remedy and the body will respond.

QUICK DEFINITION

Electrodermal screening is a form of computerized information gathering, based on physics, not chemistry. A blunt, noninvasive electric probe is placed at specific points on the patient's hands, face, or feet, corresponding to acupuncture points at the beginning or end of energy meridians. Minute electrical discharges from these points serve as information signals about the condition of the body's organs and systems, useful for the physician in evaluation and developing a treatment plan.

A **homeopathic nosode** is a super-diluted remedy made as an energy imprint from a disease product, such as bacteria, tuberculosis, measles, bowel infection, influenza, and about 200 other substances. The nosode, which contains no physical trace of the disease, stimulates the body to remove all "taints" or residues it holds of a particular disease, whether it was inherited or contracted. Only qualified homeopaths may administer a nosode.

trodermal screening world, we call this an "indicator drop" and it is a bad sign. It suggests that the organ is leaking energy and may be undergoing severe degeneration, starting at an energy level and moving into a more tangible deterioration.

On the basis of all the evidence I collected about her symptom picture, it seemed clear to me that there was a strong link between her history of childhood sexual abuse and her chronic pelvic problems. In my approach to homeopathy, the first time you see a patient, you need to give remedies that will get the physiological system working properly again. This means removing from the body all the obstacles to healing. Then, according to classical homeopathy, you can give a single remedy and the body will respond by healing completely.

Removing the Obstacles to Healing—I prepared a remedy program for Rebecca consisting of six components. My prescribing philosophy in this case was to give her the strongest remedies possible. Her immune system needed major stimulation after 14 years of not working correctly. First, I gave her a homeopathic nosode (SEE QUICK DEFINITION) of Epstein-Barr virus (EBV) at a strength of 200C which she would take once weekly for a month. This would help her body start to eliminate the high levels of EBV in her tonsils, liver, and kidneys. Second, I gave Rebecca a nosode called Viricin to be taken once daily. This broad-based formula contains all the main viruses including EBV but at a low potency. I wanted to be sure to catch all the virus problems.

Third, Rebecca took *Rehmannia 6*, a remedy composed

of Chinese herbs, to address the energy imbalance in her kidneys as evidenced by her night sweats. She took three tablets, three times daily. Fourth, I prescribed a homeopathic formula for detoxification. This was a combination of three low-dose "drainage" remedies (SEE QUICK DEFINITION), called Liquiessences, for the lymph, kidneys, and liver in potencies of 1X and 2X (one and two successive dilutions and successions or vigorous shaking). Rebecca took these drops three times daily.

Drainage remedies comprise low potency homeopathic substances and tinctures (alcohol extractions) of both Chinese and Western herbs. The concept of drainage derives from French homeopaths who were interested in applying homeopathy at a grosser, physiological level rather than at the level of "mentals" (psychological, emotional, and spiritual factors). Drainage remedies encourage the lymphatic system, liver, kidneys, blood, tissues, intercellular spaces, fat, and skin to eliminate, or "drain," their toxins, thus keeping them from circulating in the body or being deposited in other tissue. The best known drainage remedies are *Solidago* and *Berberis* for the kidney; *Taraxacum, Silymarin* and *Carduus* for the liver; *Hydrastis* as a general drainage; and *Myosotis* for the lymphatic system.

Fifth, I selected a single homeopathic remedy called *Sepia* 12C according to classical homeopathic prescribing. Rebecca took *Sepia* once daily. This remedy comes from squid ink and its oceanic origins (and other psychological and physiological factors) perfectly matched Rebecca's condition—even her choice of words, such as "waves" and energy "ebbs." In fact, her expression that her uterus felt as if it might "fall out" is typical of the type of images that consistently are presented by patients needing *Sepia*. The sense of her uterus falling out, the sexual abuse, the abortion, and the subsequent guilt are all connected. It was as if, on a psychological or metaphorical level, Rebecca wanted to get rid of her uterus, to push it out so the experience would be gone from her life along with the organ that bore its memory.

Sixth, I addressed her chronic constipation and years of excessive antibiotic intake by giving her Multiflora, a "friendly bacteria" or probiotics product. This blend contains *acidophilus* and *bifidus* cultures and fructo-oligosaccharides (which are helpful "fast food" for the beneficial bacteria). She took two capsules, three times daily to start restoring the normal population levels and balance of intestinal microflora previously destroyed by all the antibiotics.

The day after she took the *Staphysagria*, Rebecca's anger welled up so strongly that she was mad at everyone in her life— husband, children, and parents, says Dr. Diamond. She took an angle iron and smashed up her garage door until all her anger was discharged. From that moment, the remaining pelvic pain disappeared and has not returned.

To contact **John Diamond, M.D.**: Triad Medical Center, 4600 Kietzke Lane, M-242, Reno, NV 89502, tel: 702-829-2277; fax: 702-829-2365. Dr. Diamond is coauthor with William Lee Cowden, M.D., of *An Alternative Medicine Definitive Guide to Cancer* (Tiburon, CA: Future Medicine Publishing, 1997). To order, call 800-333-HEAL.
For more information about **Multiflora ABF** (available only to licensed health-care practitioners), contact: UAS Laboratories, 5610 Rowland Road, Suite 110, Minnetonka, MN 55343; tel: 800-422-3371 or 612-935-1707; fax: 612-935-1650. For **Viracin**, contact: Natural Botanicals, P.O. Box 1596, Ferndale, WA 98248; tel: 360-384-5656 or 800-232-4005; fax: 360-384-1140. For **Liquiessences**, contact: Professional Health Formulas, P.O. Box 80085, Portland, OR 97280; tel: 503-245-2720 or 800-952-2219; fax: 503-452-1239. For ***Rehmannia 6***, contact: ProBotannix, 9250 Geronimo Road, Irvine, CA 92718; tel: 800-909-4372; fax: 714-457-6039.

EDITOR'S NOTE

Some readers may find this expression of sudden anger to be unusual or perhaps strange, even alarming. In homeopathy, such a release of suppressed emotional energy is considered a hallmark of the healing process. The modern science of psychoneuroimmunology (PNI) has demonstrated convincingly that emotions "talk" to human biochemistry, affecting immune response, and either support or hinder healing, and that this system runs in a continuous feedback loop. Your body *listens* to your thoughts and your thoughts *follow* the trend of your physiology. Chinese medicine has always correlated body organs with emotions, such as liver/anger, lungs/grief.

Confronting Her Past—Rebecca left my office with these six remedies and instructions to take them all concurrently. I didn't hear from her for a month. When she called, her report was highly encouraging. Her pelvic pain had worsened the first several days on the remedies and was followed by a copious vaginal discharge of, in her words, a "smelly yellow liquid." This went on for three days, but when it stopped, she felt "so much better."

A temporary worsening of symptoms followed by an often powerful discharge then rapid improvement is typical of how homeopathic remedies work. I interpreted the discharge as her body's way of getting rid of what was ailing in her pelvis. In a sense, her body materialized all the emotional toxins (from parental abandonment, sexual abuse, and other traumatic factors from her personal history) and forcibly expelled them from her body.

It was understandable, therefore, that during the period of her vaginal discharge Rebecca was exhausted. As soon as it was finished, her energy began increasing daily until she estimated her energy level was 80% improved. After a week, she was sleeping better and her constipation gave way to normal, daily bowel motions. She stopped feeling cold and stopped craving salt; her panic attacks disappeared and she was no longer fearful about taking new medicines. (Initially, Rebecca had been highly resistant to the remedies and I had to persuade her that it was in her best interest to take them.)

She reported that emotionally she felt remarkably better and that the pain had receded from her anus and pelvis and was localized over the bladder and uterus. Overall, the pain had decreased by 50% but, for me, this wasn't good enough. I was left with a woman whose physical symptom picture had markedly improved yet she still had 50% pain in her pelvis. Using electrodermal screening, I found that there was no longer any evidence of Epstein-Barr virus anywhere in her system and the only organ carrying any imbalance was her uterus.

To address this underlying imbalance, I gave her a

single homeopathic remedy called *Staphysagria* (larkspur seeds) at a medium strength of 200C. This remedy often helps break open a condition of internalized anger. Rebecca came to my office a month later with good and surprising news. The day after she took the *Staphysagria*, her anger welled up so strongly that she was mad at everyone in her life—husband, children, and parents. She telephoned the latter and directly confronted them with their neglect and abuse of her as a child. She had avoided them for years before this moment. Then she took an angle iron and smashed up her garage door until all her anger was discharged. From that moment, the remaining pelvic pain disappeared and has not returned. ■

Success Story:
Resolving the Emotional Core of Chronic Fatigue

Deeply suppressed grief can be as debilitating as the unexpressed anger which was the central emotion contributing to Rebecca's illness. The following case illustrates the role of both grief and anger in long-standing CFS and, again, how homeopathy can assist in releasing the stored emotions.

Homeopath Judith A. Lewis, R.N, N.D., of Mill Valley, California, consulted with Rhonda, 43, who worked part-time as an editor. She had suffered from chronic fatigue syndrome, genital herpes, and chronic allergies for nearly 15 years, and from an underactive thyroid (hypothyroidism— SEE QUICK DEFINITION) for eight years. Rhonda had previously consulted nearly two dozen practitioners of alternative medicine and had been put on various herbal treatments, intestinal cleansers, and allergy elimination diets. She had received multiple remedy homeopathic medicines and undergone extensive psychotherapy, and was currently taking a conventional drug for her thyroid imbalance.

> The result [of these experiences] was deeply suppressed grief and anger. To release and clarify these strong emotions, Dr. Lewis gave Rhonda *Naturum Muriaticum* 30C and during the next month, Rhonda's buried emotions began to surface and be released, and her overall mental state improved.

As a younger person, Rhonda had been athletic and excelled in her studies; as an adult, she was a perfectionist and hard worker, but prone to depression, with a defeatist attitude. She was impatient and

"This case shows clearly how a powerful but unaddressed emotional experience can set in motion a complicated and chronic illness pattern," observes Dr. Lewis. "When you release the triggering emotion, then the body is able to start eliminating the secondary physical symptoms."

overly self-critical, reports Dr. Lewis. Her 25 physical symptoms included sleeping a great deal, allergies, bloating, constipation, a feeling of body-wide toxicity, frequent headaches, a diminished libido, sluggish digestion, and recurrent bouts of genital herpes about every six weeks.

To start the treatment, Dr. Lewis recommended Rhonda take *Nux Vomica* 12X (homeopathic poison nut), two daily for 10 days. This remedy would clear away the confusing energy picture in Rhonda's system produced by having received so many different herbs and homeopathic mixes over the years. *Nux Vomica* would also help to drain toxins from Rhonda's liver. Dr. Lewis also suggested that Rhonda start a supplement program including kelp herbal extract (one teaspoon, three times daily), vitamin A (10,000 IU daily), vitamin C (6-10 g daily), vitamin E (400 IU daily), and a balanced vitamin B complex pill daily. In addition, every day Rhonda was to drink an herbal tea made of dandelion, burdock, ginger, and red clover.

One month after beginning this program, Dr. Lewis gave Rhonda a single dose of *Carcinosin* 200C. This is a nosode made from homeopathically potentized cancer cells. The purpose here, Dr. Lewis explains, is to remove the energy residue (called "miasm"—SEE QUICK DEFINITION) of a strong family history of cancer; it would otherwise remain in her system as a subtle but persistent interference in her complete healing.

During Dr. Lewis' lengthy initial interview with her, Rhonda revealed that she had experienced three deaths in close succession shortly before she became sick. Two close family members and a family pet had died suddenly; in addition, Rhonda had had a shocking near-death experience. The result was deeply suppressed grief and anger, observes Dr.

Lewis. To release and clarify these strong emotions, Dr. Lewis gave Rhonda *Naturum Muriaticum* 30C (homeopathic common salt). During the next month, Rhonda's buried emotions began to surface and be released, and her overall mental state improved.

Her digestive problems had worsened, however. In a subsequent follow-up interview, Rhonda revealed that she had contracted severe dysentery while traveling abroad. Dr. Lewis believed that this microbial contamination was still upsetting Rhonda's digestion, so she prescribed one dose of *Bacillus* No. 7 (a homeopathic bowel nosode) to remove all energy taints of this infection. At this point, Rhonda had considerable emotional upheaval; some symptoms had improved but many had relapsed, which is typical of the healing process in homeopathy, says Dr. Lewis.

During the fifth month of treatment, Dr. Lewis gave Rhonda a single stronger dose of *Naturum Muriaticum*, and during the sixth month, she further increased the strength of the single dose. During this period, Rhonda experienced several outbursts of grief and anger. "This was a sign of progress because emotions lie deeper than the physical symptoms," says Dr. Lewis. At the end of this period, Rhonda's thyroid was back to normal and she discontinued her thyroid medication after having been dependent on it for six years. In addition, she was no longer experiencing herpes outbreaks.

Rhonda reported herself to be 85% improved and "liberated from chronic fatigue after 15 years." Her energy levels felt normal again and she was able to work almost full-time. Rhonda initiated new social contacts and began a new relationship, also for the first time in 15 years. All her digestive and allergy problems had disappeared; her sleeping patterns were normal again; and as far as her mental state and bodily functions were concerned, Rhonda's chronic fatigue was entirely an experience of the past. "This case shows clearly how a powerful but unaddressed emotional experience can set in motion a complicated and chronic illness pattern," observes Dr. Lewis. "When you release the triggering emotion, then the body is able to start eliminating the secondary physical symptoms.

QUICK DEFINITION

A **homeopathic miasm**, as originally described by Samuel Hahnemann, the 19th-century German founder of homeopathy, is a subtle taint or energy residue of previous illness, which recurs over generations. As an inherited predisposition for chronic disease that is far more subtle than anything genetic, miasms are broad-focused, predisposing individuals and families to specific illnesses, such as tuberculosis or cancer. According to Hahnemann, three miasms underlie all chronic illness and parallel broad stages in the history of human experience with primary disease states. They are the *Psoric* miasm (from *psora,* meaning "itch"), the *Syphilitic* miasm (deriving from syphilis), and the *Sycotic* miasm (arising as a residue of gonorrhea). Some homeopaths add a fourth *Cancer* miasm, and a fifth *Petroleum* miasm.

To contact **Judith Lewis, R.N., N.D.:** tel: 415-381-4727.

Releasing the Trapped Emotions Underlying Fibromyalgia

Alternative medicine practitioner Christiane Northrup, M.D., author of *Health Wisdom for Women*, believes that fibromyalgia has a strong emotional element. Negative feelings of despair and resentment, from job stress, family problems, or even childhood memories, get "trapped" in the muscles and constrict them. To release trapped emotions, Dr. Northrup recommends the following steps which she says can often produce good results in three to six weeks:[9]

For information on **Alpha Sun** and **Omega Sun blue-green algae**, contact: Grain & Salt Society, P.O. Box DD, Magalia, CA 95954; tel: 800-867-7258; or contact Cell-Tech at 800-927-2527. For **malic acid**, contact: Emerson Ecologics, 18 Lomar Drive, Pepperell, MA 01463; tel: 800-654-4432; fax: 800-718-7238.

■ Exercise: Even though it seems you can't move your muscles, you must keep moving every day; your pain will actually diminish as you build a consistent exercise program.

■ Rest and Relax: Sleep 8-10 hours nightly, go to bed before 10 p.m. and get up at the same time every morning.

■ Meditate: Even 15 minutes a day will help balance your brain chemicals, or neurotransmitters.

■ Balance the Prostaglandins: Keep your prostaglandin hormone levels in balance by eating no more than 500 calories per meal; keep your diet low in refined carbohydrates and fats, and moderate in protein.

■ Increase Your Serotonin: Use blue-green algae in a progressive, four-week supplementation program to enhance levels of this important neurotransmitter. First week: Take two Cell-Tech digestive enzymes with Alpha Sun or Omega Sun blue-green algae capsules before breakfast and lunch. Also take two capsules of *acidophilus* with algae, 30 minutes before breakfast. Second week: Add to this one capsule of Alpha Sun and Omega Sun before breakfast. Third week: Continue this while increasing the algae intake to 2-4 capsules three times daily with meals. Fourth week: Continue with this regime, increasing the algae if necessary. This will increase your serotonin levels and have an antidepressant effect.

■ Use Supplements: Take magnesium (300-600 mg daily); malic acid (1,200 mg daily, divided into three doses, building to 2,400 mg if pain persists after two weeks); all the B vitamins (100 mg each, daily); and manganese (10-20 mg).

Lifting the Depression Associated with Chronic Fatigue

Most people with CFS, fibromyalgia, and environmental illness suffer from depression. The impact of these debilitating disorders on one's life is enough in itself to induce depression, but there are numerous biochemical factors which may be causing the persistently low feelings. These include hormonal imbalances, nutritional deficiencies, hypoglycemia (low blood sugar), allergies and sensitivities, chemical or heavy metal toxicity, and viral or fungal infections.[10] Note that all of these factors have been discussed earlier in this book as agents that help cause chronic fatigue.

For **antidepressant herbs**, see Chapter 12: Correcting Chronic Fatigue With Herbs, pp. 318-338.

Observe the continuous cycle of illness. The factors that create CFS produce depression as well, and this, in turn, suppresses immune function. Then, the more compromised the immunity becomes, the worse the deficiencies and imbalances; this then leads to a deepening of the depression and the cycle continues.

Evidence indicates that depression is an outcome rather than a precipitating factor in CFS, but some in the conventional medical establishment still view CFS as a psychogenic or psychosomatic ailment (having mental as opposed to physical origins) and believe the depression associated with it is a sign of these origins. However, even the U.S. Centers for Disease Control now acknowledges that most CFS patients report their depression and anxiety as starting *after* the onset of the illness. On this basis, the CDC is willing to grant these symptoms as being "secondary reactions to CFS."[11]

The fact that people with CFS led very active lives before getting sick supports this conclusion since depression is characterized by low energy and a sense of immobilization. In addition, the depression of CFS tends to lift as the person begins to feel better. "A reactive depression to the extreme fatigue of CFS should not be surprising," says Leon Chaitow, N.D., D.O. "Those with CFS have often been suffering debilitating symptoms for a number of years, barely acknowledged by the medical establishment, and have been offered little appropriate treatment other than a 'chin up' attitude and handfuls of antidepressants."

However, just as unresolved emotions may be contributing to CFS, they may be a factor in the depression experienced in the illness as well. The following section demonstrates how deep depression and the associated CFS can be reversed with traditional Chinese medicine (TCM—SEE QUICK DEFINITION). **Marie Hoshimi-Wilkes, Ph.D., N.D., O.M.D.,** of Las Cruces, New Mexico, describes how emotional and psychological factors are often a source of physical imbalances and how she uses TCM to address these elements:

To contact **Marie Hoshimi-Wilkes, N.D., Ph.D., O.M.D.:** Oriental Medicine Plus, 120 West Chestnut, Las Cruces, NM 88005; tel: 505-647-8077.

Lift Depression Without Prozac

An estimated 12 million people worldwide (six million Americans) take Prozac for depression, resulting in annual sales of $2 billion for Eli Lilly and Company, Prozac's maker. Why further enrich this drug company when safer, inexpensive alternatives exist to successfully elevate your mood? According to naturopathic physician and educator Michael T. Murray, N.D., lifestyle, dietary, and psychological therapies can serve as natural antidepressants and keep you Prozac free.

■ Lifestyle—First, make sure your depression does not have an organic, physiological cause, such as diabetes, cancer, or heavy metal toxicity, or is not due to a food allergy or overuse of prescription drugs. Then know that it is highly beneficial to create a mental attitude that is positive and optimistic, says Dr. Murray. Set achievement goals, practice affirmation. Quit smoking, reduce or eliminate your intake of caffeine and alcohol, exercise regularly, practice a relaxation and stress reduction exercise every day for at least ten minutes, and laugh more.

■ Dietary—Nutrient imbalances or deficiencies can contribute to chronic depression, says Dr. Murray. "Correcting an underlying nutritional deficiency can restore normal mental function and relieve depression," he adds. Among Dr. Murray's recommendations: reduce your fat intake; eat at least five daily servings of fresh fruits and vegetables; minimize your consumption of refined sugars and salt; eat much more fiber and complex carbohydrates (whole grains); and keep your protein intake moderate.

■ Supplements—Start correcting the nutritional foundation of your health with a daily high-potency multiple vitamin and mineral formula, says Dr. Murray. In addition, he suggests taking daily folic acid (800 mcg), vitamin B12 (800 mcg), vitamin B6 (50-100 mg), and flaxseed oil.

■ Herbs—As an additional antidepressant support, Dr. Murray recommends using *Ginkgo biloba*. For people over 50, take 80 mg, three times daily, with addition folic acid (1,200 mcg). For people under 50, take St. John's Wort extract, 300 mg, three times daily.

■ Amino Acids—Deficiencies or imbalances in the body's levels of amino acids, which are essential protein building blocks, can also contribute to depression. Dr. Murray suggests 2,000 mg of D- or L-phenylalanine, or 1,000 mg of L-tyrosine, taken once daily, before breakfast.

■ Insomnia—Depression often brings a disruption of normal sleeping rhythms. Helpful here are melatonin (3 mg) before bedtime; valerian herbal extract (150-300 mg) taken 30 minutes before bedtime; or GABA (gamma aminobutyric acid, an amino acid derivative), taken at 200-400 mg, 30 minutes before bedtime.

"Adopting these guidelines is all that the majority or people with depression will need to do to elevate their mood," says Dr. Murray.[12]

Success Story:
Freeing Chronic Fatigue's Depression

The statement from Chinese medicine that over 90% of all diseases have a psychological and emotional origin continually influences my work. I believe you cannot possibly heal somebody through Chinese medicine without working through a great deal of their psychological and emotional issues. As soon as you start getting the body well, these deeper causes of the physical symptoms will begin to surface.

You have to work on them, because otherwise they will come back up into the body again and produce more symptoms. I use acupuncture, moxibustion (SEE QUICK DEFINITION), herbs, counseling, even flower essences and color therapy, to give the patient enough strength to start looking at the deeper problems with clarity. Chronic fatigue syndrome, from my perspective, is about deep-seated emotions, deeply repressed feelings of anger, even self-hatred, that have finally affected the immune and digestive systems, producing a host of symptoms, as the case of Elaine illustrates.

Elaine, 45, came to me with deep depression and extreme exhaustion. She had low energy, no concentration, bad memory, fevers, sweat, chills, poor sleep, dizzyness, cold extremities, high blood pressure, respiratory problems, irregular periods, and back, neck, and muscle pain. She was defensive and ready to cry, even at innocuous remarks. She had been previously treated for a chronic bladder and kidney obstruction, and was still sporadically unable to urinate. Elaine had suffered these chronic symptoms for four years.

In Chinese medicine terms, she had kidney yang deficiency, which means she didn't have enough yang, or active, fiery energy in her kidneys, leaving her sluggish, passive, inactive, fearful, tired, holding water, and with no willpower. During her first 90-minute session, I inserted needles on all the organ points on her back, especially her kidney points, and then followed it with moxibustion to strengthen her vital energy—to bring up her *qi*, or vital body energy. I also made suggestions as the needles remained in place: "Elaine, I'm working on your kidneys now, so let's release fear and anxiety. It's safe to release fear." This had immediate effects.

Elaine knew she had deeply buried emotions, but didn't know how to process them. All the time I was treating her physically, I was also working with the emotional and psychological energies

QUICK DEFINITION

Traditional Chinese medicine (TCM), originating in China over 5,000 years ago, is a comprehensive system of medical practice that heals the body according to the principles of nature and balance. A Chinese medicine physician considers the flow of vital energy (*qi*) in a patient through close examination of the patient's pulses, tongue, body odor, voice tone and strength, and general demeanor, among other elements. Underlying imbalances and disharmony in the body are described in terminology analogous to the natural world (heat, cold, dryness, or dampness). The concept of balance, or the interrelationship of organs, is central to TCM. In TCM, imbalances are corrected through the use of acupuncture, moxibustion, herbal medicine, dietary therapy, massage, and therapeutic exercise

In **moxibustion**, a dried herb called moxa (usually mugwort) is burned over the skin at a specific acupuncture point. The moxa may be attached to a special acupuncture needle or in a freestanding cone set on a slice of ginger; its slow burning provides a penetrating heat. The purpose is to warm the blood and *qi* (basic life force energy flowing through energy pathways), particularly when a patient's energy picture is cold or damp.

Nutritional Deficiencies Associated with Depression

Nutritional biochemist Patricia Kane, Ph.D., of Millville, New Jersey, has observed distinct nutritional deficiencies among patients diagnosed with depression. Dr. Kane cites the case of Sylvia, 29, who had suffered a prolonged depression lasting for three years. Initially, she had complained of chronic fatigue and mood swings; later, she reported digestive difficulties and food allergies, and although she had avoided conventional drugs, she was on the verge of taking Prozac.

A comprehensive blood test revealed the nutritional, or biochemical, side of Sylvia's depression. It showed she was either deficient or in excess of 31 substances, indicating "a deeply imbalanced biochemistry," says Dr. Kane. "Most generally stated, Sylvia's blood status was an 80% match with the known 'disease pattern' for depression. Further, Sylvia's blood nutrient status deviated by 31% from the healthy norm." For the most part, Sylvia was 10% deficient in many key nutrients. Basically,

To contact **Patricia C. Kane, Ph.D.**: Carbon Based East, Five Osprey, Millville, NJ 08332; tel: 609-825-2200 or 609-825-8333; fax: 609-825-2143.

owing to her dietary choices (low in natural fat, high in synthetic fats, or trans-fatty acids), Sylvia didn't have enough of the essential raw materials for her body to produce the hormones, proteins, and other substances necessary for a healthy physiology, Dr. Kane explains.

"Most often, a depressed person will have lower than average amounts of five substances, namely, blood urea nitrogen, chloride, cholesterol, potassium, and uric acid." Sylvia's pattern matched four out of five of these criteria: her blood urea nitrogen (nitrogen in urea form in the urine) was 33% low; cholesterol 80%; potassium 33%; and uric acid (a crystalline acid from nitrogen metabolism) 64%; her chloride was high at 57% above the norm. Usually, high chlorides are correlated with epilepsy or high anxiety, while low chlorides are often found with depression. Three other markers consistently associated with depression were also low in Sylvia's blood chemistry, specifically, iron, creatinine, and albumin, says Dr. Kane.

associated with the physical symptoms. Her back went into spasms and ripples as she started coming in contact with these old painful feelings made available through the needles, such as sexual abuse by her uncle, grief over the death of a malformed infant, deep guilt taken on from her dead mother, profound sadness over the fact she had never known her father. She was also now in a marriage that had been abusive for years; before seeing me, she had resigned herself to living with it.

After the first session, Elaine's spirits lifted and she was able to have a sense of humor and objectivity about her condition. I gave her five flower essences (SEE QUICK DEFINITION) to take hourly to help further lift her mood; they were Self Heal, California pitcher plant, St. John's Wort, Scotch broom, and fuchsia. After her second session, I prescribed a mixture of Chinese herbs to improve her energy, to help the bladder and kidney problem, and tone her digestion. These included *Foti*, to nourish and detoxify the blood; *fructus Lycii*, to help liver and kidney energy; *fu-shen*, for calming the spirit; *dong quai*, to build up the blood; aconite, to bring up yang energy; astragalus, for the night sweats; plus cinnamon, licorice, and diascoria. She took these twice a day, in liquid form, for about three months; I modified the mix according to her symptoms.

> **Elaine knew she had deeply buried emotions, but didn't know how to process them. Her back went into spasms and ripples as she started coming in contact with these old painful feelings made available through the needles, says Dr. Hoshimi-Wilkes.**

I also employed color therapy each session, using a German-made Vegalux color generator to project different colors (through little flashlights at the tips of fiber optic tubes) onto her skin. Color therapy is a soothing, energy-building adjunct to acupuncture. For example, I used orange on her lower abdomen for endocrine insufficiency, and blue and yellow on her feet to release stress and prenatal feelings. I left the colors in place for 40 minutes a session.

Doing the Deep Work—As the needles, moxibustion, flowers, color, and herbs built up her energy, Elaine began to have a lot of emotional releases and psychological insights, which surprised and encouraged her. She is a good patient, willing to do the hard work of healing.

During her second session, Elaine said it was as if an animal were trying to eat her up from the inside, devouring all her energy. Another time she said she felt she had a "hole" in her body (or what I might call an energy field) out of which energy kept leaking. All this time she had been

QUICK DEFINITION

Flower remedies comprise subtle liquid preparations made from the fresh blossoms of flowers, plants, bushes, even trees, to address emotional, psychological, and spiritual issues underlying physical and medical problems. The approach was pioneered by British physician Edward Bach in the 1930s, when he introduced the 38 Bach Flower Remedies, based on English plants. Today, an estimated 20 different brands of flower remedies, based on plants native to many landscapes, from Australia to India to Alaska, offer about 1,500 different blends for a diverse range of psychological conditions.

It all comes down to what we say in alternative medicine: you have to treat the whole person of body, mind, and spirit. You cannot just treat the body or the spirit alone, because they're part of the same system, says Dr. Hoshimi-Wilkes.

making drawings of volcanoes that could only blow steam and lava out their sides, not their tops. In a later session, we focused on her so-called victimhood. I said to her: "Why don't you make your own heart affirmation while I'm treating you. Give me words that tell me who you truly are, not the victimized person you think you are."

After six treatments, Elaine had enough energy to resume doing things she couldn't do for years and to confront the fact that her marriage was not satisfactory. This is what her healing was about: having the energy to face her life issues and bad marriage and to make the necessary changes. It means now, after only eight sessions spread over three months, she's strong enough to move courageously to take control of her life again.

Elaine is about 70% cured and I'm confident the treatment is working, as her energy is steadily improving. Elaine's illness was probably brewing for seven years before she came to me, and for about three years before all the symptoms started. Her newborn child's death seven years earlier might have triggered it all, producing a deep sadness and feeling of futility. The body follows these emotional clues and begins to weaken. Then as the person starts to get physically well, these old, buried issues start to come up again and must be dealt with as part of the healing process.

It all comes down to what we say in alternative medicine: you have to treat the whole person of body, mind, and spirit. You cannot just treat the body or the spirit alone, because they're part of the same system. ■

How Homeopathy Can Help Fibromyalgia

In a double-blind trial, 24 patients with fibromyalgia experienced "statistically significant" improvement after taking one of three homeopathic remedies indicated for their particular condition and individual make-up: *Arnica* (mountain daisy), for muscle fatigue, characterized by aches, pains and exhaustion; *Bryonia* (wild hops), typically used in cases of arthritis and rheumatism; and *Rhus tox* (poison ivy), often the first remedy administered when there is stiffness and pain.[13] Another study confirmed these results.[14]

Lifestyle choices can contribute to
chronic fatigue. For example, the style of high-
paced overachievement—some call it
workaholism—that characterizes the lives of many
CFS sufferers prior to becoming sick.
Sometimes in a curious way, getting laid out with
unremitting fatigue is the only
way some people will ever take
the time to focus on their internal world.
Alternative medicine competently addresses
the psychological and emotional side of all illnesses,
including chronic fatigue,
recognizing the uniquely individual
factors in each patient.

12

Correcting Chronic Fatigue With Herbs

HERBAL MEDICINE can be of great assistance in the treatment of chronic fatigue syndrome. Herbs can help strengthen weakened body systems and relieve symptoms, ranging from uncomfortable to debilitating, produced by this weakness. Herbs are a practical and desirable therapy because they provide their benefits without the side effects so frequently experienced with conventional drugs. Each herb has one or more specific healing property, an advantage enabling the skilled herbalist to design a treatment program targeting specific ailments or imbalances. For example, ginseng is useful in chronic fatigue because it is both an adaptogenic herb, meaning it increases resistance to stress by support-

> **Using herbal medicines as the primary therapeutic modality, Dr. van Benschoten sees a response in 85% to 90% of his patients. "The time necessary to completely resolve the situation can vary from as short as four to six weeks to as long as 12 to 18 months."**

ing the adrenal glands, and a tonic, meaning it builds overall vital energy by nurturing and enlivening the entire system.

Although there are no universal remedies, particularly for a complex condition such as chronic fatigue, there are a number of herbs which have proven useful for the syndrome. Many alternative medicine physicians have developed herbal protocols that have been effective for their CFS patients. For example, Susan M. Lark, M.D., author of *The Chronic Fatigue Self Help Book*, recommends ginkgo,

Siberian ginseng, oatstraw, ginger, licorice, and dandelion root to improve energy levels and combat depression in CFS sufferers. Those who have the accompanying symptoms of anxiety and insomnia should look into passionflower, chamomile, hops, and valerian root, she says. To support a faltering immune system, always a factor in chronic fatigue sufferers, Dr. Lark relies on garlic, echinacea, and goldenseal.[1] However, before starting any program you should consult a qualified herbalist to ensure that the herbs you take meet your individual needs.

As another example, Matt van Benschoten, O.M.D., M.A., C.A., of Reseda, California, uses herbal medicine to treat the viral infections and immune suppression found in CFS patients. "The initial therapy has to be focused on antiviral measures," he says. "Once that's accomplished and the virus is well eliminated, you can begin to address some of the secondary factors that cause the weakness in the immune system, such as stress-induced weakness, problems in the intestinal tract, heavy metal poisoning (such as dental mercury), and low-level pesticide poisoning." Prescriptions are individualized for each patient, he says.

Using herbal medicines as the primary therapeutic modality, Dr. van Benschoten sees a response in 85% to 90% of his patients. "The time necessary to completely resolve the situation can vary from as short as four to six weeks to as long as 12 to 18 months," says Dr. van Benschoten, "depending upon the duration of the illness and other accompanying health problems." Many of the herbs Dr. van Benschoten employs in treating CFS and its attendant conditions are found in the herbal glossary beginning on page 321.

Herbs That Can Help Chronic Fatigue

- Immune-building—astragalus, echinacea, garlic, ginger, ginkgo, ginseng, goldenseal, nettle
- Adrenal Support—ginseng, licorice
- Antimicrobial—astragalus, echinacea, garlic, ginger, goldenseal, licorice, St. John's Wort
- Fatigue—ginseng, oatstraw
- Brain function—ginkgo, ginseng
- Sleep Disorders—chamomile, hops, passionflower, St. John's Wort, valerian
- Joint and Muscle Pain—cayenne, chamomile, nettle, peppermint, valerian
- Allergies—chamomile, ephedra, milk thistle
- Digestive Disorders—astragalus, cayenne, chamomile, dandelion, ginger, goldenseal, licorice, peppermint
- Anxiety—chamomile, hops, kava-kava, passionflower, valerian
- Depression—oatstraw, St. John's Wort

Success Story: Cayenne Contributes to Fibromyalgia Relief

The following case highlights how herbs (in this case, cayenne) can occupy a central role in the treatment program for fibromyalgia.

Henrietta, 42, had consulted seven doctors over a two-year period before receiving the correct diagnosis of post-traumatic fibromyalgia and successful treatment by chiropractor Dennis Zinner, D.C., of San Francisco, California. The stress of those two years "amplified her syndrome," comments Dr. Zinner. In addition to constant pain and lack of proper sleep, that time was made more difficult by "the missed diagnosis, the stress of facing a work lay-off, and the worry that other people think your symptoms are all mind-derived."

In Dr. Zinner's assessment, Henrietta's post-traumatic fibromyalgia resulted from a work-related injury to her left shoulder at age 40, with subsequent lower back pain. When she was 15, Henrietta sustained two bone fractures in her lower back from a car accident; at age 34, her family physician diagnosed osteoarthritis in her lower back; at 41, she sprained her wrist, and at 42, she had surgery for breast cancer.

At the time she began treatment with Dr. Zinner, Henrietta complained of left shoulder pain, neck pain leading to severe headaches, constant severe pain in her lower back, hips, and feet, ankle swelling, and general physical impairment affecting sitting, walking, and job performance. In addition, she had generalized fatigue, morning stiffness, depressive episodes, irritable bowel syndrome, and nonrestful sleep. Henrietta had discomfort in all 18 of the tender point sites common to fibromyalgia, and her conditions worsened under stress. "With new studies, we are discovering that fibromyalgia is a neuromuscular problem in which, for reasons we do not yet know, the muscles stay in contraction and do not relax," explains Dr. Zinner.

To contact **Dennis Zinner, D.C.**: 2920 Post Street, Suite 202, San Francisco, CA 94115; tel: 415-885-5563; fax: 415-921-2281. For a source of **capsaicin cream**, contact: En Garde Health Products (Chirozone), 7702-10 Balboa Boulevard., Van Nuys, CA 91406; tel: 800-955-4MED (4633).

The first step in Dr. Zinner's treatment plan for Henrietta was to apply a microcurrent probe at each of the 18 tender point sites on her body, three times weekly. Second, he applied deep heat (for 15 minutes) to Henrietta's two most painful sites to decrease muscle spasm. At home, Henrietta repeated the procedure using a moist heating pad. Third, Dr. Zinner instructed Henrietta to massage capsaicin cream into her sore points four times daily. Capsaicin is a pungent alkaloid of cayenne pepper that has a warming effect on the body.

Fourth, for her sleeping disorders, Dr. Zinner prescribed the hormone melatonin (6 mg, taken 30 minutes before bedtime). He also made chiropractic adjustments, as needed, to areas related to the location of the 18 tender spots. Dr. Zinner further advised Henrietta to do regular aerobic exercise followed by heat treatment such as a whirlpool.

Dr. Zinner notes that the use of capsaicin has two benefits. First, it dissolves the sensation of pain. Second, capsaicin usefully depletes bodily reserves of substance P, believed to be overabundant in patients with fibromyalgia. Substance P intensifies and perhaps prolongs muscle inflammation and pain. In other words, too much Substance P may be a factor that prevents fibromyalgia from going away. Research has shown that capsaicin can be effective in the treatment of fibromyalgia. The Medical College of Wisconsin in Milwaukee treated 45 people suffering from primary fibromyalgia with capsaicin (0.025%) cream for four weeks. The patients reported less tenderness in the spots treated and a significant increase in their grip strength.[2]

After six months of regular therapy, Henrietta reported a change in her pain from "constant severe" to "constant slight to moderate" with only occasional severe episodes. Her improvement continued under Dr. Zinner's fourfold program. "Henrietta's outcome was good. She is back to living her life," says Dr. Zinner. "She has returned to school full time to get a degree on child development and she works part-time at the school. She sees me every three months for a treatment but she is managing her infrequent episodes of pain."[3]

Substance P is a polypeptide (several amino acids bonded together) made naturally in the body and normally present in minute amounts in the nervous system and intestines. It stimulates the expansion and contraction of the smooth muscles in the intestines and elsewhere. Substance P is also involved in the secretion of saliva and the functioning of the peripheral and central nervous system, notably the pain response. Substance P is released in response to physical injuries to tissues and muscles and is overabundant in patients with fibromyalgia (chronic muscle pain). In turn, this stimulates the release of histamine, causing tissue swelling and inflammation, smooth muscle contraction, and pain transmission. Substance P also suppresses serotonin, another neurotransmitter (a brain chemical that conducts nerve "messages"); under healthy conditions, serotonin inhibits the overabundance of Substance P. It is regarded as one of the most potent compounds affecting smooth muscle contraction and inflammation.

A Glossary of Herbs to Help Chronic Fatigue Syndrome

The following are some of the many herbs that can help alleviate the numerous symptoms of chronic fatigue, such as extreme debilitating fatigue, joint and muscle pain, memory problems and poor concentration, depression, anxiety, allergies, gastrointestinal complaints, and sleep disorders. Antimicrobial herbs (antivirals, antifungals, and antibiotics) and herbs that strengthen the immune system, provide adrenal support, or aid the liver in its toxin-filtering function are also designated in what follows.

Astragalus *(Astragalus membranaceus)*

A medicinal staple in Chinese medicine, astragalus is an energy tonic known for its healing abilities in chronic conditions in which weakness is a major factor. It exerts a potent influence on the immune system, increasing the production of white blood cells (important immune "workers"). It also aids the immune system by acting as an antiviral and antibacterial agent.[4] In addition, it facilitates digestion. Its system-wide strengthening abilities have lead many alternative medicine physicians to include astragalus in their herbal protocol for CFS.

Cayenne *(Capsicum annuum)*

Cayenne or red pepper is an effective systemic stimulant, meaning it invigorates the physiological activities of the body. It is especially helpful for the circulatory and digestive systems, stimulating blood flow and strengthening the heartbeat and metabolic rate.[5] It is used to treat insufficient peripheral circulation, characterized by cold hands and feet, frequently a symptom of CFS. It also helps ward off colds.[6] Externally, it is used for muscle and joint pain.[7]

Chamomile (German or wild, *Matricaria recutita*; Roman, *Anthemis nobilis)*

The flower of the chamomile plant produces a calming effect, easing anxiety and reducing tension.[8] It can thus be helpful with overall anxiety, sleep disorders, and muscle tension. Its calming property has a beneficial effect on the gastrointestinal system as well. In addition, it stimulates digestive secretions, so it can improve digestive function.

In Europe, chamomile is recognized as a digestive aid, a mild sedative, and an anti-inflammatory, notably in antibacterial oral hygiene

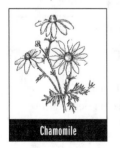

Chamomile

and skin preparations.[9] Its anti-inflammatory properties also reduce allergic response. In Germany, chamomile is licensed as an over-the-counter drug for internal use against gastrointestinal spasms and inflammatory diseases of the gastrointestinal tract.

Dandelion *(Taraxacum officinale)*

As both a liver and digestive tonic, as well as a blood cleanser and diuretic (urine-increasing agent), dandelion can aid in detoxification of the body.[10] The liver is a filter for toxins and, as such, serves as one of the body's main detoxification mechanisms. As testimony to dandelion's powerful influence on the liver, severe hepatitis has been reversed by dandelion tea along with dietary restrictions in as short a period as a week.[11]

Given the chemical or heavy metal toxicity frequently involved in chronic fatigue syndrome, dandelion can help cleanse the body of these toxins and support the liver in its toxin-eliminating function. As a digestive tonic, dandelion may also help clear up the gastrointestinal complaints associated with CFS.

Echinacea *(Echinacea angustifolia)*

Due to its widely demonstrated immune-enhancing qualities, echinacea is a standard ingredient in many doctor's herbal regimens for CFS. Combining equal parts of tinctures of echinacea, goldenseal, and myrrh results in an even more powerful immune booster.

Often called purple cone-flower, echinacea refers to several species of plants that are generally found in the Great Plains region of North America, where it was the most widely used medicinal plant of the Native Americans in that area. They used echinacea for its external wound-healing and anti-inflammatory properties. Echinacea is widely used in Europe and becoming more well known in the United States for its immune-stimulating properties; most popularly, for its ability to help relieve flus and the common cold.

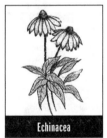

Echinacea

Over 180 over-the-counter echinacea products are marketed in Germany alone, including extracts and fresh-squeezed juices from both the roots and leaves of echinacea.[12] The German government has approved oral dosage of echinacea for use in recurrent infections of the respiratory and urinary tracts, progressive systemic disorders such as tuberculosis, leukosis (abnormal growth of white blood cells), connective tissue disease, multiple sclerosis, and, when applied topically, for surface wounds with a poor tendency to heal. Liquid echinacea preparations have been shown to have immune-stimulating activity when administered both orally and parenterally (denoting any medication route other than the intestine, e.g., intravenously).

Specifically, echinacea increases the number of leukocytes (white blood cells) and splenocytes (white blood cells of the spleen) and enhances the activity of granulocytes (granular white blood cells) and phagocytes (cells that have the ability to ingest and destroy substances, such as bacteria, protozoa, and cell debris).[13]

Due to its widely demonstrated immune-enhancing qualities, echinacea is a standard ingredient in many doctor's herbal regimens for CFS. Combining equal parts of tinctures of echinacea, goldenseal, and myrrh results in an even more powerful immune booster. The recommended dosage is one teaspoonful of this blend three times a day.

Ephedra or *Ma-huang (Ephedra sinica)*

Ephedra is a medicinal plant that has been cultivated for over 5,000 years in China, where it was used for asthma and hay fever-like conditions. Also known as *ma-huang*, the stems contain two primary alkaloids, ephedrine and pseudoephedrine, which are primary ingredients

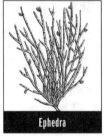

Ephedra

in conventional over-the-counter decongestant and bronchial drugs. Ephedrine has a marked peripheral vasoconstricting (causing constriction of the blood vessels) action. Pseudoephedrine is a bronchodilator (able to dilate the windpipe), approved for use in asthma and certain allergy medicines.

Ma-huang and its extracts are found in a number of herbal formulas that are designed to increase energy and reduce appetite. Both ephedrine and pseudoephedrine have properties that stimulate the central nervous system (CNS), ephedrine being more active. The CNS activity of these alkaloids has been characterized as being stronger than caffeine and weaker than methamphetamine (a central nervous system stimulant). Ephedra can be useful in the treatment of CFS both for its anti-allergy and energy-stimulating abilities.

CAUTION

CFS sufferers should consult a qualified practitioner before taking this herb and it should be used with caution or avoided by those with high blood pressure, diabetes, glaucoma, and related conditions where hypertensives are contraindicated.

Garlic *(Allium sativum)*

Garlic is probably the most well-recognized medicinal herb. It is used by traditional medicines all over the world and its applications are as varied as its geographical distribution. The chemistry and pharmacology of garlic is well studied; over 1,000 research papers have been published in the past 25 years.

Garlic and its preparations are known for their antibiotic, antifungal, and antiviral activity; for use in clearing congested lungs and for coughs, bronchitis, and sinus congestion; as a preventive measure for flus and the common cold; and for intestinal worms, dysentery, certain ulcers, gout, and rheumatism.[14] Garlic has shown an ability to aid certain immune functions, particularly increasing natural killer cell (SEE QUICK DEFINITION) activity.[15] Studies indicate general benefits from almost any type of garlic, be it raw garlic, dried garlic, garlic oil, or a prepared commercial product.[16]

Natural killer cells are a type of nonspecific, free-ranging immune cell produced in the bone marrow and matured in the thymus gland. NK cells can recognize and quickly destroy virus and cancer cells on first contact. "Armed" with an estimated 100 different biochemical poisons for killing foreign proteins, they can kill target cells without having encountered them previously. As with antibodies, their role is surveillance, to rid the body of aberrant or foreign cells before they can grow and produce cancer or infection.

Ginger *(Zingiber officinalis)*

In addition to its popular food-flavoring qualities, ginger is widely used as a medicinal herb in traditional Chinese and Ayurvedic medicines, often added to herbal formulas to increase digestion and the activity of other herbs. Ginger helps combat respiratory infections, improves circulation, aids the body in releasing toxins by promoting sweating, and eases intestinal complaints. All of these functions are useful in the treatment of CFS.

Ginkgo *(Ginkgo biloba)*

Ginkgos are the oldest living trees on earth. Their leaves contain compounds called ginkgolides which are the biochemical substances responsible for ginkgo extract's healing properties. Ginkgo is an antioxidant and also improves blood circulation, particularly to the brain.[17] Increasing capillary circulation and thus facilitating greater oxygen flow to brain cells, ginkgo is known for its ability to improve cognitive function. In Germany, it is licensed for the treatment of cerebral dysfunction including the following symptoms: difficulty in memory, dizziness, tinnitus, headaches, and emotional instability coupled with anxiety.

At least three volumes of technical papers on the chemistry, phar-

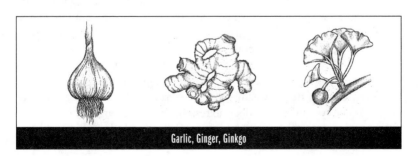

Garlic, Ginger, Ginkgo

Ginkgo is an antioxidant and also improves blood circulation, particularly to the brain. Increasing capillary circulation and thus facilitating greater oxygen flow to brain cells, ginkgo is known for its ability to improve cognitive function.

macology, and clinical studies of *Ginkgo biloba* extract have been published.[18] In a 1995 study, Alzheimer's patients received either 80 mg of ginkgo extract or a placebo three times daily. Among the patients taking ginkgo, significant improvement was noticed in cognitive function. Memory and attention span increased in the first month of supplementation. Another study of ginkgo, involving people over the age of 50, showed that 40 mg taken three times daily for 12 weeks significantly improved overall cognitive function in individuals with mild to moderate memory impairment.[19]

Ginseng

Ginseng has an ancient history and as such has accumulated much folklore about its actions and uses. Common varieties are Oriental ginseng (*Panax ginseng*) and American ginseng (*Panax quinquefolius*). The genus name *Panax* is derived from the Latin word panacea meaning "cure all." Many of the claims that surround ginseng are exaggerated but it is clearly an important remedy, receiving attention from researchers around the world.[20]

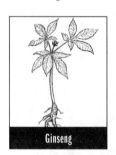
Ginseng

Ginseng has many healing properties that are useful in the treatment of CFS. One of the oldest general tonics from traditional Chinese medicine, ginseng sharpens mental abilities, concentration, and alertness, improves stamina, and delays the onset of fatigue after physical exercise.[21] It is a powerful adaptogen (SEE QUICK DEFINITION),[22] aiding the body to cope with stress, primarily through effects upon the functioning of the adrenal glands.[23] Ginseng has antioxidant,[24] antihepatotoxic (liver-protecting),[25] and hypoglycemic[26] effects.

The main application is with weak, debilitated, stressed, or elderly people, where these properties can be especially helpful.[27] In addition, ginseng may lower blood cholesterol[28] and stimulate a range of immune system[29] and endocrine responses.[30] If ginseng is abused, however, serious side effects can occur, including headaches, skin problems, and other reactions. For this reason, the proper dosage for the individual should be determined and respected.

Another variety of ginseng, Siberian ginseng or eleuthero (*Eleutherococcus senticosus*), has a very low toxicity. Copious clinical and laboratory research has been con-

Initial findings from controlled experiments indicate that Siberian ginseng produces a dramatic reduction of total disease occurrence, especially in diseases related to environmental stress.

ducted on Siberian ginseng in the former Soviet Union. Initial findings from controlled experiments indicate that Siberian ginseng produces a dramatic reduction of total disease occurrence, especially in diseases related to environmental stress.[31] There is a long list of illnesses that improve with the use of this herb, including chronic fatigue, chronic gastritis, diabetes, and atherosclerosis (hardening of the arteries).

Goldenseal *(Hydrastis canadensis)*

One of the most widely used American herbs, goldenseal is considered to be a tonic remedy that stimulates immune response and is directly antimicrobial itself. In addition, because of its bitter effects, goldenseal can help in many digestive problems, from peptic ulcers to colitis.[32] Its bitter stimulation helps in loss of appetite, and the alkaloids it contains promote production and secretion of digestive juices.

Goldenseal's antimicrobial properties are due to berberine.[33] This alkaloid, found in a number of other herbs as well, has marked antimicrobial activity. Its inhibiting effects have been demonstrated against bacteria, protozoa, and fungi, including *Staphylococcus*, *Streptococcus*, *Candida albicans*, and *Giardia lamblia*,[34] which are often implicated in CFS. Berberine has also been shown to activate macrophages (cells that digest cell debris and other waste matter in the blood).[35]

Hops *(Humulus lupulus)*

Hops has been used as a bittering and preservative agent in brewing for centuries. In Germany, hops is licensed for use in states of unrest and anxiety as well as sleep disorders, due to its calming and

QUICK DEFINITION

Adaptogens are substances that provide a non-specific effect on the entire body by increasing resistance to stress and toxins (physical, chemical, or biological) and promoting a balancing or normalizing condition. The key function of adaptogens is support for the adrenal glands, which are located near the kidneys and activated in response to stress. Chronic stress can overwhelm the adrenals, leading to symptoms including fatigue, reduced immune function, and poor blood sugar metabolism. Adaptogens help reinvigorate and support the adrenals, enabling the body to deal more effectively with stress. In addition to adrenal support, adaptogens enhance central nervous system activity, provide protection for the liver, act as antioxidants, and increase stamina. Herbs that are considered adaptogenic include Asian and Siberian ginseng, *Ashwagandha*, *Astragalus*, *Codonopsis* ("*Dangshen*"), and *Schizandra*.

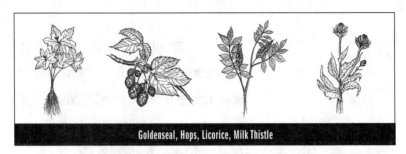

Goldenseal, Hops, Licorice, Milk Thistle

sleep-inducing properties. European medicinal plant researchers have approved the use of hops for such conditions as nervous tension, excitability, restlessness, and sleep disturbances, and as an aid to stimulate appetite. Unlike other types of sedatives, there are neither dependence nor withdrawal symptoms reported with the use of hops, nor are there any reports of adverse side effects.[36]

Kava-Kava *(Piper methysticum)*

An extract of the kava-kava plant (a slow-growing bushy perennial) acts as a natural tranquilizer. According to E. Lehmann, M.D., and colleagues, when 29 patients with diagnosed anxiety (including panic disorder and general tension) took kava-kava at the rate of 100 mg three times daily for four weeks, and were then evaluated using three standard psychological profiles of anxiety, all measures were significantly lower. No side effects or adverse reactions occurred, and benefits were noted as early as the first and second weeks.[37]

In another study of 101 people, 100 mg of kava-kava extract taken three times daily produced significant improvement in anxiety and tension of nonpsychotic origin. The effects were noted from the eighth week of supplementation. Specifically, 20% of those taking kava-kava were rated "very much improved" according to a standard anxiety scale, while only 10.5% of the placebo group received a similar rating. After 24 weeks of taking the herbal extract, the percentages were 53.1% of the kava group and 30.2% of those taking a placebo.[38]

Licorice *(Glycyrrhiza glabra)*

Licorice is another traditional herbal remedy with an ancient history. Modern research has shown it to have beneficial effects on the endocrine system, adrenal glands, and liver. It is also a systemic anti-inflammatory.[39] Constituents of this herb, called triterpenes, are metabolized in the body into molecules that have a similar structure to the adrenal cortex hormones, which is possibly the basis for licorice's anti-inflammatory action and its effectiveness in cases of adrenal insufficiency.[40]

As overworked adrenal glands are characteristic of CFS, licorice has obvious application. In addition, glycyrrhizin, one of the triterpenes, inhibits liver cell injury from chemicals, another benefit for CFS sufferers.[41] Glycyrrhizin prevents the growth of several viruses, inactivating herpes simplex virus particles irreversibly.[42] Licorice is used as a treatment for digestive problems such as gastritis, peptic ulceration, and abdominal colic. It is also effective for bronchitis, coughs, and other bronchial problems.

The *Quarterly Review of Natural Medicine* cited a case report of successfully treating chronic fatigue syndrome with licorice dissolved in milk (2.5 gm per 500 ml daily). The logic behind using licorice for CFS is sound, according to the article. Glucocorticoid levels are often low in CFS patients and licorice can reverse this deficiency. The authors of the article recommend following up initial licorice treatment with Oriental ginseng and eleuthero as long-term adrenal support.[43]

In a study of 101 people, 100 mg of kava-kava extract taken three times daily produced significant improvement in anxiety and tension. The effects were noted from the eighth week of supplementation.

Milk Thistle *(Silybum marianum)*

Historically this herb has been used in Europe as a liver tonic. In addition, it is an antihistamine and an anti-inflammatory, and therefore inhibits allergic response. A wealth of laboratory and clinical research on this herb is revealing exciting data about reversal of toxic liver damage as well as protection from potential hepatotoxic agents, such as chemicals.[44] These properties are of use in the case of CFS for improvement of liver function to help the body deal with toxic overload and easing of the allergies which usually accompany the syndrome.

Nettle *(Urtica dioica)*

Nettle is one of the most widely used herbs in the Western world. Throughout Europe, it is employed as a general tonic and detoxifying remedy. It is both a circulatory and immune stimulant. A lectin (plant protein) found in the plant's leaf promotes lymphocyte production.[45] Traditional use of nettle in the treatment of allergic rhinitis (hayfever)

There is a small possibility of affecting electrolyte balance with extended use of large doses of licorice. It can cause retention of sodium, thus raising blood pressure. The whole herb has constituents that counter this, but it is best to avoid licorice in cases of hypertension or kidney disease, or during pregnancy. It is important to clarify here that the kind of licorice effective in CFS patients is licorice root, which contains glycyrrhizic and glycyrrhetinic acids, not the deglycyrrhizinated form of licorice from which these acids have been removed.

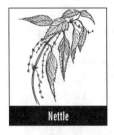
Nettle

is gaining research support.[46] Fresh nettle has been used as a safe diuretic (urine-increasing agent), and thus is helpful in assisting the body in flushing toxins.[47] Again, all of these healing abilities have application to CFS.

Noni: A Tahitian Plant with Many Healing Qualities

Among the lay healers of Tahiti, the reputation of the noni fruit (*Morinda citrifolia*) as a medicinal food ranks high. The plant itself is found throughout French Polynesia and can grow as high as 20 feet, bearing noni fruits the size of potatoes. In Malaysia, it is known as Mengkudu and is used for urinary problems, coughs, and painful menstruation, while in the Caribbean, people know it as the Pain Killer Tree. People throughout the region have long used the noni fruit as a dietary staple.

Anecdotal reports suggest that juice from this fruit can be significantly helpful in numerous health conditions, such as chronic fatigue syndrome, hypertension, wounds and infections, ulcers, skin rashes, digestive disorders, PMS, colds, influenza, arthritis, and cancer. Mitchell Tate, director of the Center for Lifestyle Disease in St. George, Utah, reports using noni to prevent sore throats and bacterial infections after his family was exposed to strep infection. Tate further reports that while researching noni at the University of Honolulu in Hawaii (noni also grows in Hawaii), he found that "a significant amount of research had been done on the plant and that most of it substantiated claims by the Tahitians."

One laboratory study showed that noni was effective as an antiseptic against nine types of infectious bacteria. As bacterial infection can be an underlying factor in CFS, this finding has obvious implications for CFS treatment. However, the application of Tahitian noni to CFS is more wide-reaching. According to a testimonial published in the *Health News*, Colleen Abbott, 55, had suffered with chronic fatigue syndrome for 20 years. A variety of nutritional supplements had improved her symptoms but not eliminated them. A recent accident injured her back, leaving her in pain, almost immobile, and on painkillers. Colleen reports that after taking noni for three days, she was able to "get up, walk, and climb stairs without crawling." Her sleep improved, her pain and most of her CFS symptoms went away, and instead of needing chiropractic adjustments twice daily, she had them only once a month.

"The mechanism by which noni juice accomplishes these dramatic results may be that it acts "indirectly by enhancing the immune system involving macrophages and/or lymphocytes [key cancer-fighting immune cells]," according to researcher A. Hirazumi, Ph.D.[48] Studies by R. M. Heinicke, Ph.D., at the University of Hawaii, suggest that the active ingredient in noni is xeronine, a digestive enzyme similar to bromelain in pineapple.

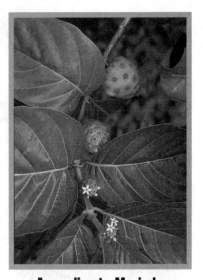

Dr. Heinicke emphasizes that noni must be consumed on an empty stomach, preferably upon rising in the morning, for the enzyme to become activated by the intestines. Dr. Heinicke believes that, once activated, xeronine helps to repair damaged cells by regulating the rigidity and shape of particular proteins comprising those cells. "Since these proteins have different functions within the cells, this explains how the administration of noni juice causes a wide range of physiological responses," states Dr. Heinicke.

According to Morinda, the product's manufacturer, about 25% of the users of noni experience a noticeable difference after using the drink for three weeks, while 50% notice benefits after three to eight weeks of daily use.

According to Morinda, the product's manufacturer, about 25% of the users of noni experience a noticeable difference after using the drink for three weeks, while 50% notice benefits after three to eight weeks of daily use. Mitchell Tate suggests a daily dosage of two tablespoons for general health maintenance, but three to four tablespoons daily for an existing health condition.

For more information about **Tahitian noni**, contact: Pascal Sureau, 5020 Lee Street, Torrance, CA 90503; tel/fax: 310-792-7275; email: pascal1@earthlink.net.

Oatstraw, Oats *(Avena sativa)*

Traditionally, oatstraw has been used to help patients recover from exhaustion and depression and it has been widely recognized as an excellent nerve tonic. Oatstraw (which is

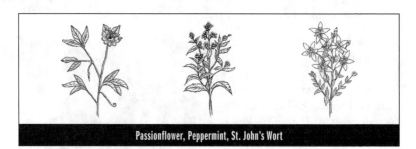

the whole oat plant including the ripe grain) contains saponins and alkaloids that stimulate and restore the nervous system. Oatstraw is also capable of providing key nutrients, including calcium, that feed a compromised nervous system. Oatstraw is sold dried and as capsules, concentrated drops, tinctures, and extracts.[49]

Passionflower *(Passiflora incarnata)*

Passionflower has enjoyed a tradition of use for its mildly sedative properties. In Germany, passionflower is approved as an over-the-counter drug for states of "nervous unrest."[50] It is often added to other calming herbs, usually valerian and hawthorn. Passionflower and hawthorn are often used together as antispasmodics for digestive spasms in cases of gastritis and colitis. It also increases circulation to the peripheries,[51] and can therefore be helpful with the CFS symptom of cold hands and feet. Pharmacological studies indicate antispasmodic, sedative, anxiety-allaying, and hypotensive (blood pressure-lowering) activity of passionflower extracts.[52] For the anxiety and digestive problems associated with CFS, this can be an effective herb.

Peppermint *(Mentha piperita)*

Peppermint has been a popular folk remedy for digestive disorders for over 200 years and is currently one of the most economically significant aromatic food/medicine crops produced in the United States.[53] Its benefits to digestive problems come from peppermint oil's relaxing effect on the smooth muscles of the bowel. It can aid in conditions from gastrointestinal cramps to irritable bowel syndrome. Peppermint oil and menthol are common ingredients in over-the-counter external pain-relieving balms and liniments. In Germany, this combination is approved for external use for muscle and nerve pain.[54]

St. John's Wort *(Hypericum perforatum)*

A remedy long used as an anti-inflammatory, wound-healer, mild sedative, and pain-reliever, St. John's Wort has recently attracted medical attention. Traditionally used to treat neuralgia, anxiety, tension, and similar problems, it is now being increasingly recommended in the treatment of depression.[55] Recent research has also suggested an antimicrobial role for this herb in viral infections from influenza to HIV.[56]

In Germany, St. John's Wort is widely prescribed for depression (66 million doses in 1994 alone). Research supports this application: in 23 separate clinical trials involving 1,757 patients who reported mild to moderately severe depression, taking between 500 and 900 mg daily of St. John's Wort extract (containing 0.75% to 2.7% hypericin, the active component of the herb) was three times more effective than a placebo and as effective as standard antidepressants such as Prozac and Zoloft.

In addition, St. John's Wort produced mild side effects in only 19% of users compared to 52.8% of those taking the conventional medications who experienced mild to severe side effects. The herb produced no toxic reactions or unfavorable interactions

> **In 23 separate clinical trials involving 1,757 patients with depression, taking 500-900 mg daily of St. John's Wort extract was three times more effective than a placebo and as effective as standard antidepressants.**

with other drugs. The researchers noted that it generally takes two to four weeks of steady use before the mood-elevating benefits of St. John's Wort take effect.[57]

Christopher Hobbs, L.Ac., founder of the American School of Herbalism, has found St. John's Wort useful in sleep disorders as well. He credits this to the same action behind the herb's antidepressant properties; that is, it maintains serotonin levels in the brain. Serotonin is a neurotransmitter (essential brain chemical) that influences mood and helps produce sleep. Dr. Hobbs also suggests adrenal-supporting herbs because compromised adrenal glands result in hormonal imbalances which can disturb sleep.[58] (See ginseng and licorice.)

Valerian (Valeriana officinalis)

The odorous root of valerian has been used in European traditional medicine as a natural tranquillizer for centuries. In Germany, valerian root and its teas and extracts are approved as over-the-counter medicines for "states of excitation" and "difficul-

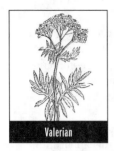

Valerian

ty in falling asleep owing to nervousness."[59]

A scientific team representing the European community has reviewed the scientific research on valerian and concluded that it is a safe nighttime sleep aid. These scientists also found that there are no major adverse reactions associated with the use of valerian and, unlike barbiturates and other conventional drugs for insomnia, valerian does not have a synergy with alcohol, meaning it is not dangerous to mix the two as is the case with the conventional medications.[60] Possessing warming qualities, valerian is also effective in easing muscle pain when applied topically.[61] Dr. Hobbs recommends a valerian-hops preparation as a daytime sedative because it will not interfere with or slow reflexive responses[62]—again, unlike conventional pharmaceuticals.

Herbs Can Be Used in Many Forms

As a result of an herbal medicine renaissance, herbs and herbal products are now available not only in natural foods stores, but also in grocery stores, drug stores, and gourmet food stores. Herbs come in many forms, including:

Whole Herbs—Whole herbs are plants or plant parts that are dried and then either cut or powdered. They can be used as teas or other products.

Teas—Teas come in either loose or teabag form. When steeped in boiled water for a few minutes, the fragrant, aromatic flavor and the herbs' medicinal properties are released.

Capsules and Tablets—One of the fastest growing markets in herbal medicine in the past 15 to 20 years has been capsules and tablets. These offer consumers convenience and, in some cases, the bonus of not having to taste the herbs, many of which have undesirable flavor profiles, from intensely bitter (e.g., goldenseal root), due to the presence of certain alkaloids, to highly astringent (e.g., oak bark), due to the presence of tannins.

Extracts and Tinctures—These offer the advantage of a high concentration in low weight and volume. They are also quickly assimilated by the body in comparison to tablets. Extracts and tinctures almost

How To Use Herbs
to Help Reverse Chronic Fatigue

For the acute infectious stage of CFS, Michael T. Murray, N.D., typically recommends:

■ echinacea, goldenseal, and licorice; three times a day of each in the following dosages:

 –as dried root (or tea), 1-2 g

 –as freeze-dried root, 500-1,000 mg

 –as tincture (1:5), 4-6 ml or 1½ teaspoons

 –as fluid extract (1:10), 0.5-2.0 ml or ¼ -½ teaspoon

 –as powdered solid extract (4:1), 250-500 mg

Note: Dr. Murray warns that if licorice is to be used for a long time, it is necessary to increase the intake of potassium-rich foods.

■ pokeweed (*Phytolacca decandra/Phytolacca americana*), dried root, 100-400 mg three times daily

■ wild indigo (*Baptisia tinctoria*), dried root, 0.5-1.0 g three times daily.

For the chronic phase of CFS, Joseph Pizzorno, N.D., president of Bastyr College in Bothell, Washington, typically recommends:

■ goldenseal and licorice, three times a day in the same dosages as used by Dr. Murray above

■ astragalus, dried root, 5-15 g three times daily

■ Siberian ginseng, three times daily in the following dosages:

 –as dried root (or tea), 2-4 g

 –as fluid extract (1:1), 2-4 ml or ½-1 teaspoon

 –as solid extract (20:1), 100-200 mg

For the recovery phase of CFS, Dr. Pizzorno typically recommends:

■ *Panax ginseng* in the following dosages:

 –as dried root, 1.5-2.0 g three times daily

 –as fluid extract, equivalent to 25-50 mg daily of ginsenosides (the biologically active ingredient)

■ Siberian ginseng, three times daily in dosages as above

always contain alcohol. The alcohol is used for two reasons: as a solvent to extract the non-water-soluble compounds from an herb and as a preservative to maintain shelf life. Properly made extracts and tinctures have virtually an indefinite shelf life. Tinctures usually contain more alcohol than extracts (sometimes 70% to 80% alcohol) depending on the particular herb and manufacturer.

Essential Oils—Essential oils are usually distilled from various parts of medicinal and aromatic plants. Some oils, however, like those from lemon, orange, and other citrus fruits, are expressed directly from fruit peels. Essential oils are highly concentrated, with one or two drops often constituting adequate dosage. Thus, they are to be used

Herbal Remedies for Fibromyalgia

According to Chanchal Cabrera, M.N.I.M.H., a clinical herbalist practicing in Vancouver, British Columbia, the following formula treats the symptoms of inflammation and helps ease the pain associated with fibromyalgia, while boosting the immune system. The blend (equal parts of each herb) should be taken three times a day, 1 tsp each time. However, before beginning any herbal protocol, Cabrera urges you to consult a qualified herbalist, as no single standard formula works for everyone.

To contact **Chanchal Cabrera, M.N.I.M.H.**: Gaia Garden Herbal Dispensary, 2672 West Broadway, Vancouver, BC, Canada V6K 2G3; tel: 604-734-4372; fax: 604-734-4376. The initials M.N.I.M.H. stand for Member of the National Institute of Medical Herbalists, a British designation indicating professional status as an herbalist. For an herbal practitioner in your area, contact: American Herbalists Guild, P.O. Box 746555, Arvada, CO 80006; tel: 303-423-8800; fax: 303-402-1564.

Equal parts of each:

- Echinacea—immune tonic
- *Cimicifuga racemosa* (black cohosh)—anti-inflammatory
- *Harpagophytum procumbens* (devil's claw)—anti-inflammatory
- *Glycyrrhiza glabra* (licorice)—adrenal tonic and anti-inflammatory
- *Taraxacum officinale* (dandelion)—used to treat all liver conditions; aids in toxin removal
- *Apium graveolens* (celery)—removes acid wastes

carefully and sparingly when employed internally. Some oils may irritate the skin and should be diluted in fatty oils or water before topical application. Notable exceptions are eucalyptus and tea tree oils which can be applied directly to the skin without concern of irritation.

Salves, Balms, and Ointments—For thousands of years, humans have used plants to treat skin irritations, wounds, and insect and snake bites. Today, a number of herbal salves, balms, and ointments, usually with a vegetable oil or petroleum jelly base, are sold in the United States and Europe to treat a variety of conditions. These products often contain aloe, marigold, chamomile, St. John's Wort, comfrey, or gotu kola.

How to Make an Herb Tea

Loose teas are usually steeped in hot water: three to five minutes for leaves and flowers (this method is called infusion), or 15 to 20 minutes at a rolling boil for denser materials like root and bark (called a decoction).

Infusions

Infusions are the simplest method of preparing an herb tea and both fresh or dried herbs may be used. Due to the higher water content of the fresh herb, three parts fresh herb replace one part of the dried

Get Anxiety Relief with Aromatherapy

Anxiety can contribute to many health problems, but aromatherapy has a quick and simple method for reducing it, according to aromatherapist Valerie Ann Worwood in her guide *The Fragrant Mind*. Aromatherapy works with the essential oils of plants, prepared in any of the following ways, says Worwood: blended with one ounce of base oil to make a massage oil; added to bath water; gently heated in a room diffuser; or inhaled from a tissue.

■ Tense Anxiety—Symptoms include bodily tension, muscle pains, aches, and a generalized soreness. Mix clary sage (10 drops), lavender (15 drops), and Roman chamomile (5 drops).

For a source of **aromatherapy blends** based on Ayurvedic medical principles and suitable for stress reduction (including Even Temper™, Worry Free™, Blissful Joy™, and Emotional Strength™), contact: Maharishi Ayur-Veda Products International, Inc., 1115 Elkton Drive, Suite 401, Colorado Springs, CO 80907; tel: 719-260-5500; fax: 719-260-7400.

■ Restless Anxiety—Here one feels dizzy, sweaty, overactive, with palpitations, the sense of a lump in the throat, frequent urination, diarrhea, or upset stomach. Worwood recommends vetiver (5 drops), juniper (10 drops), and cedarwood (15 drops).

■ Apprehensive Anxiety—Symptoms generally include worrying, brooding, unease, a sense of foreboding, even paranoia. For relief of this emotional state, try mixing bergamot (15 drops), lavender (5 drops), and geranium (10 drops).

■ Repressed Anxiety—This variant of anxiety involves feeling on edge, concentration difficulties, irritability, insomnia, or a sense of chronic exhaustion. Worwood advises a blend of neroli (10 drops), rose otto (10 drops), and bergamot (10 drops).[63]

herb. To make an infusion:

■ Put about one teaspoonful of the dried herb or herb mixture for each cup into a teapot.

■ Add boiling water and cover. Let steep for five to ten minutes. Infusions may be taken hot, cold, or iced. They may also be sweetened.

Infusions are most appropriate for plant parts such as leaves, flowers, or green stems where the medicinal properties are easily accessible. To infuse bark, root, seeds, or resin, it is best to powder them first to break down some of their cell walls before adding them to the water. Seeds like fennel and aniseed should be slightly bruised to release the volatile oils from the cells. Any aromatic herb should be infused in a pot that has a well-fitting lid, to reduce loss of the volatile oil through evaporation.

Decoctions

For hard and woody herbs (e.g., ginger root and cinnamon bark), it is best to make a decoction rather than an infusion, to ensure that the soluble contents of the herb actually reach the water. Roots, wood, bark, nuts, and certain seeds are hard and their cell walls are strong, requiring more heat to release them. These herbs need to be boiled in the water. To make a decoction:

■ Put one teaspoonful of dried herb or three teaspoonfuls of fresh material for each cup of water into a pot or saucepan. Dried herbs should be powdered or broken into small pieces, while fresh material should be cut into small pieces.

■ Add the appropriate amount of water to the herbs.

■ Bring to a boil and simmer for ten to 15 minutes.

When using a woody herb that contains a lot of volatile oil, it is best to make sure that it is powdered as finely as possible and then used in an infusion to ensure that the oils do not boil away. Decoctions can be used in the same way as an infusion.

Herbs are a practical and desirable therapy because they provide their benefits without the side effects so frequently experienced with conventional drugs. Each herb has one or more specific healing property, an advantage enabling the skilled herbalist to design a treatment program targeting specific ailments or imbalances.

Endnotes

Chapter 1

Related Epidemics: Chronic Fatigue Syndrome, Fibromyalgia, and Environmental Illness

1 U.S. Centers for Disease Control. "The Facts About Chronic Fatigue Syndrome." (August 1994). Internet: http://www.cdc.gov/ncidod. diseases/cfs/facts.htm.

2 Stoff, Jesse A., M.D., and Charles R. Pellegrino, Ph.D. *Chronic Fatigue Syndome: The Hidden Epidemic* (New York: HarperCollins, 1992).

3 U.S. Centers for Disease Control. "The Facts About Chronic Fatigue Syndrome." (August 1994). Internet: http://www.cdc.gov/ncidod. diseases/cfs/facts.htm.

4 Ibid.

5 Krieger, Lisa M. "Alarming S.F. Study of Chronic Fatigue." *San Francisco Examiner* (October 14, 1996).

6 Fukuda, Keiji, et al. "The Chronic Fatigue Syndrome: A Comprehensive Approach to its Definition and Study." *Annals of Internal Medicine* 121 (December 15, 1994), 953-959.

7 Teitelbaum, Jacob, M.D. *From Fatigued to Fantastic!* (Garden City Park, NY: Avery Publishing Group, 1996).

8 Goldenberg, Don, M.D. American College of Rheumatology meeting (1994). Dr. Goldenberg is chief of rheumatology at Newton-Wellesley Hospital in Newton, MA, and professor of medicine at Tufts University School of Medicine in Medford, MA.

9 van Why, Richard P. *Fibromyalgia Syndrome and Massage Therapy: Issues and Opportunities* (Self-published, 1994). Available from: Richard P. van Why, 123 East 8th Street, Frederick, MD 21701. Starlanyl, Devin, M.D., and Mary Ellen Copeland, M.S., M.A. *Fibromyalgia and Chronic Myofascial Pain Syndrome: A Survival Manual* (Oakland, CA: New Harbinger Publications, 1996), 8.

10 Dunstan, R.H., et al. "A Preliminary Investigation of Chlorinated Hydrocarbons and Chronic Fatigue Syndrome." *Medical Journal of Australia* 163:6 (September 18, 1995), 294-297.

11 National Institutes of Health. Internet: http://www.niaid.nih.gov/factsheets/cfs.htm

12 Stoff, Jesse A., M.D., and Charles R. Pellegrino, Ph.D. *Chronic Fatigue Syndome: The Hidden Epidemic* (New York: HarperCollins, 1992).

13 Straus, S., M.D. *Chronic Fatigue Syndrome* NIH Publication 90-3059 (Washington: U.S. Department of Health and Human Services, Public Health Service,1990), 5. Johnson, Hillary. *Osler's Web: Inside the Labyrinth of the Chronic Fatigue Syndome Epidemic* (New York: Penguin Books, 1996). *Southern Medical Journal* 88:10 (October 1995), 994-995. Cowley, Geoffrey, et al. "Chronic Fatigue Syndrome: A Modern Medical Mystery." *Newsweek* (November 12, 1990). National Institutes of Health Website: http://www.niaid.nih.gov/factsheets/cfs.htm

Chapter 2

Testing: The Key to Understanding the Causes of Your Chronic Fatigue

1 U.S. Department of Health and Human Services. *CFS: A Pamphlet for Physicians* NIH Publication 90-484 (Washington: U.S. Department of Health and Human Services,1990).

2 Rosenbaum, M., M.D., and M. Susser, M.D. *Solving the Puzzle of Chronic Fatigue Syndrome* (Tacoma, WA: Life Sciences Press, 1992), 44

3 Chaitow, L. *Post Viral Fatigue Syndrome* (London: Dents, 1989).

4 Gittleman, Ann Louise. *Guess What Came to Dinner: Parasites and Your Health* (Garden City, NY: Avery Publishing Group, 1993).

5 Galland, L., M.D. *Super-Immunity For Kids* (New York: Dell Publishing, 1989).

6 Casemore, D., M.D. "Foodborne Protozoal Infection." *The Lancet* 336 (December 1990), 1427-1432.

7 Bendig, D. W., M.D. "Diagnosis of Giardiasis in Infants and Children by Endoscopic Brush Cytology." *Journal of Pediatric Gastroenterology and Nutrition* 8:2 (1989), 204-206.

8 Straus, S., M.D. *Chronic Fatigue Syndrome* NIH Publication 90-3059 (Washington: U.S. Department of Health and Human Services, Public Health Service,1990), 5.

9 Lapp, Charles W., M.D. "Chronic Fatigue Is a Real Disease." *North Carolina Family Physician* 43:1 (Winter 1992). Dr. Lapp collaborates with Paul Cheney, M.D., the physician who treated the first cases of CFS in Incline Village, Nevada, and has since become an international author-

ity on the disorder.

10 "Diagnostic Blood Test for CFIDS?" *CFIDS Treatment News* 2:1 (Spring 1991), 3. Landay, Alan L., Carol Jessop, Evelyne Lennette, and Jay Levy. "Chronic Fatigue Syndrome: Clinical Condition Associated with Immune Activation." *The Lancet* 338:8769 (September 21, 1991), 707-712. Levy, Jay, M.D. Personal correspondence. Division of Hematology and Oncology, Department of Medicine, University of California at San Francisco (October 1997).

11 Landay, Alan L., Carol Jessop, Evelyne T. Lennette, and Jay A. Levy, "Chronic Fatigue Syndrome: Clinical Condition Associated With Immune Activation." *The Lancet* 338:8769 (September 21, 1991), 707-712.

Chapter 3
Eliminating Viruses, Infections, Candidiasis, and Parasites

1 Rosenbaum, M., M.D., and M. Susser, M.D. *Solving the Puzzle of Chronic Fatigue Syndrome* (Tacoma, WA: Life Sciences Press, 1992).

2 Ibid.

3 Editorial. "Depression, Stress and Immunity." *The Lancet* 1:8548 (June 1987), 1467-1488.

4 Galland, L., M.D., et al. *Journal of Nutritional Medicine* 1 (1990), 27-31.

5 Ostrum, Neenyah. "LEM: Exciting News for Good Health." *The New York Native* (July 31, 1989).

6 *HealthWatch* 4:3 (Summer/Fall 1994), 6. *HealthWatch* is available from: CFIDS Buyers Club, 1187 Coast Village Road, #1-280, Santa Barbara, CA 93108; tel: 800-366-6056.

7 Tyler, Allen N., M.D., N.D., D.C. "Influenza A Virus: A Possible Precipitating Factor in Fibromyalgia?" *Alternative Medicine Review* 2:2 (1997).

8 Harthoorn, A.M., and Lynda M. Martin. "The Homeopathic Treatment of Myalgic Encephalomyelitis (ME) Based on 219 Case Histories." *Biomedical Therapy* 15:2 (1997), 60-63.

9 Juven, B., et al. "Studies on the Mechanism of the Antimicrobial Action of Oleuropein." *Journal of Applied Bacteriology* 35 (1972), 559-567.

10 Walker, Morton, D.P.M. "Antimicrobial Attributes of Olive Leaf Extract." *Townsend Letter for Doctors & Patients* (July 1996), 80-85.

11 Rosenbaum, M., M.D., and M. Susser, M.D. *Solving the Puzzle of Chronic Fatigue Syndrome* (Tacoma, WA: Life Sciences Press, 1992), 131.

12 Trowbridge, J., and M. Walker. *The Yeast Syndrome* (New York: Bantam Books, 1986).

13 Pizzorno, J. E., and M.T. Murray, eds. *A Textbook of Natural Medicine* (Seattle, WA: John Bastyr College Publications, 1988-1989).

14 Chaitow, L. *Post Viral Fatigue Syndrome* (London: Dents, 1989).

15 Crinnion, W.J. *Clinical Trial Results on Neesby's Capricin* (Unpublished manuscript, September 10, 1985). Available from: Probiologic, Inc., 1803 132nd Avenue NE, Bellevue, WA 98005.

16 Pizzorno, J. E., and M.T. Murray, eds. *A Textbook of Natural Medicine* (Seattle, WA: John Bastyr College Publications, 1988-1989).

Chapter 4
Restoring Immune Vitality

1 Carrow, Donald J., M.D. "Beta-1,3-Glucan as a Primary Immune Activator." *Townsend Letter for Doctors & Patients* (June 1996), 86-91.

2 Meira, D.A., et al. "The Use of Glucan as Immunostimulant in the Treatment of Paracoccidioidomycosis." *American Journal of Tropical Medicine and Hygiene* 55:5 (November 1996), 496-503.

3 Browder, W., et al. "Synergistic Effect of Nonspecific Immunostimulation and Antibiotics in Experimental Peritonitis." *Surgery* 102:2 (August 1987), 206-214.

4 Whitaker, Julian, M.D. "Give Your Immune Cells a Natural 'Shot in the Arm'." *Health & Healing* 7:3 (March 1997), 1-3. Beardsley, Terry R., et al. "Induction of T-cell Maturation by a Cloned Line of Thymic Epithelium (TEPI)." *Proceedings of the National Academy of Sciences* 80 (1983), 6005-6009. Hays, Esther F., and Terry R. Beardsley. "Immunologic Effects of Human Thymic Stromal Grafts and Cell Lines." *Clinical Immunology and Immunopathology* 33 (1984), 381-390. Hale, Peter. "The FIV Connection." *Searchlight* (Summer 1996), 21-23. O'Brien, C.J. "In Vitro Effect of TP-1 (a Calf Thymic Extract) on Suppressor T-cell Function of Patients with Autoimmune Chronic Active Hepatitis." *International Journal of Immunopharmacology* 10:6 (1988), 651-666. Podwysocka, M., et al., "Correction of the Abnormal Ratio of OKT4+ to OKT8+ Peripheral Blood Lymphocytes in Patients Suffering Arthritis (JCA) by the Extract from Calf Thymuses." *Archivum Immunolgiae et Therapiae Experimentalis* 37:1-2 (1989), 127-132. Pontiggia, P., et al. "Effect of Treatment with Thymustimulin (TP-1) on T and B Cells in Lymphoproliferative Disorders." *Blut* 47:3 (1983), 153-156.

5 Papenburg, R., et al. "Dietary Milk Proteins Inhibit the Development of Dimethylhydrazine-induced

Malignancy." *Tumour Biology* 11:3 (1990), 129-
136. Bounous, Gustavo, M.D., et al. "Whey Proteins
as a Food Supplement in HIV-seropositive
Individuals." *Clinical and Investigative Medicine*
16:3 (1993), 204-209. Lang, C.A., et al. "Low
Blood Glutathione Levels in Healthy Aging Adults."
Journal of Laboratory and Clinical Medicine 120:5
(1992), 720-725. Julius, M., et al. "Glutathione
and Morbidity in a Community-based Sample of
Elderly." *Journal of Clinical Epidemiology* 47:9
(1994), 1021-1026.

Chapter 5
Detoxifying the Body

1 Burton Goldberg Group. *Alternative Medicine: The
Definitive Guide* (Tiburon, CA: Future Medicine
Publishing, 1995), 3.
2 Ibid., 4.
3 Elmer, Gary W., Ph.D., et al. "Biotherapeutic Agents: A
Neglected Modality for the Treatment and
Prevention of Selected Intestinal and Vaginal
Infections." *Journal of the American Medical
Association* 275:11 (March 20, 1996), 870-876.
4 Crayhon, Robert. *Health Benefits of FOS* (New
Canaan, CT: Keats Publishing, 1995).

Chapter 6
Reversing Hidden Thyroid Problems

1 McTaggart, Lynne, and Harald Gaier. "Thyroid Disease:
Overactive Medicine." *What Your Doctors Don't Tell
You* 7:7 (October 1996), 2-5. Available from: WYD-
DTY, 4 Wallace Road, London N1 2PG; tel: 0171-
354-4592.
2 *Natural Medicine Newsletter* 1:2 (March 1997).
3 Ibid.

Chapter 7
Eliminating Heavy Metal Toxicity:
Your Mercury Fillings May Be Fatiguing You

1 "Dental Mercury Hygiene: Summary of
Recommendations in 1990." *Journal of the
American Dental Association* 122 (August 1991),
112.
2 Patient records of David J. Nickel, O.M.D., L.Ac.
3 van Benschoten, M.M. "Acupoint Energetics of
Mercury Toxicity and Amalgam Removal with Case
Studies." *American Journal of Acupuncture* 22:3
(1994), 251-262.
4 "Dental Amalgam: A Scientific Review and
Recommended Public Health Service Strategy for
Research, Education and Regulation." Final Report
of the Subcommittee on Risk Management of the
Committee to Coordinate Environmental Health
and Related Programs. (Washington: U.S. Public
Health Service, 1993).
5 Lichtenberg, H. "Mercury Vapor in the Oral Cavity in
Relation to the Number of Amalgam Surfaces and
the Classic Symptoms of Chronic Mercury
Poisoning." *Journal of Orthomolecular Medicine*
11:2 (Second Quarter 1996), 87-94.
6 Ziff, S. "Consolidated Symptom Analysis of 1,569
Patients." *Bio-Probe Newsletter* 9:2 (March 1993),
7-8.
7 Melillo, W. "How Safe is Mercury in Dentistry?" *The
Washington Post Weekly Journal of Medicine,
Science and Society* (September 1991), 4.
8 Hahn, L.J., et al. "Dental 'Silver' Tooth Fillings: A Source
of Mercury Exposure Revealed by Whole-Body
Image Scan and Tissue Analysis." *FASEB Journal* 3
(1989), 2641-2646. Hahn, L.J., et al. "Whole-
Body Imaging of the Distribution of Mercury
Released from Dental Fillings into Monkey Tissues."
FASEB Journal 4 (1990), 3256-3260.
9 Vimy, M.J., Y. Takahashi, and F.L. Lorscheider.
"Maternal-Fetal Distribution of Mercury Released
from Dental Amalgam Fillings." *American
Physiological Society* 258 (1990), R939-R945.
10 For an excellent article on the subject of mercury
fillings, see: Lorscheider, Fritz, et al. "Mercury
Exposure from 'Silver' Tooth Fillings: Emerging
Evidence Questions a Traditional Dental Paradigm."
FASEB Journal 9 (1995), 504-508.

Chapter 8
Replenishing Enzyme Deficiencies

1 Howell, E., M.D. *Food Enzymes for Health and
Longevity* (Woodstock Valley, CT: Omangod Press,
1980).
2 Ibid.
3 Morley, J. E., M.B. Sterman, and J.H. Walsh, eds.
Nutritional Modulation of Neural Function. UCLA
Forum in Medical Sciences 28 (San Diego, CA:
Academica Press, 1988).
4 Jaeger, C.B., et al. "Polymer Encapsulated
Dopaminergic Cell Lines as 'Alternative Neural
Grafts'." *Progress in Brain Research* 82 (1990),
41-46.

Chapter 9
Addressing the Allergy Connection

1 Prince, T., et al. "Chronic Fatigue in a 43-year-old
Woman." *Annals of Allergy* 74 (June 1995), 474-
478.
2 Patient records of Helen Thomas, D.C., of Santa Rosa,
California.

3 "Quercetin: The Anti-Allergy Bioflavonoid." *Let's Live* (September 1992).

4 Anderson, Rosalind C., Ph.D. "Toxic Emissions from Carpets." *Journal of Nutritional & Environmental Medicine* 5:4 (1995), 375-386.

5 Hodgson, Michael, M.D., M.P.H. "The Medical Evaluation" and "The Sick Building Syndrome" in Effects of the Indoor Environment on Health. Cited in: *Occupational Medicine: State of the Art Reviews* 10:1 (January-March 1995), 167-194.

Chapter 10

Ending Nutritional Deficiencies With Supplements

1 Patient records of Guillermo Asis, M.D., of the Marino Center for Progressive Health, Cambridge, MA.

2 Kidd, Parris M., Ph.D. *Phosphatidylserine (PS): A Remarkable Brain Cell Nutrient* (Decatur, IL: Lucas Meyer, 1995). This booklet is available from: Lucas Meyer, Inc., P.O. Box 3218, Decatur, IL 62524; tel: 217-875-3660.

3 *Natural Medicine Newsletter* 1 (September 1996).

4 Murray, Michael, N.D. *Encyclopedia of Nutritional Supplements* (Rocklin, CA: Prima Publishing, 1996).

5 Murray, Michael, N.D. *Chronic Fatigue Syndrome* (Rocklin, CA: Prima Publishing, 1994), 55.

6 Ibid., 56.

7 Pao, E. M., and S. Mickle. "Problem Nutrients in the United States." *Food Technology* (September 1981), 58-79.

8 U.S. Department of Health and Human Services. *Dietary Intake Source Data: U.S. 1976-1980* DHHS Publication (PHS) 8361. (Washington: U.S. Department of Health and Human Services, 1983). Data from the National Health Survey 11:231.

9 Machlin, L. J., and M. Brin. "Vitamin E." In: *Human Nutrition— A Comprehensive Treatise*, Vol. 3, edited by R. Alfin-Slater and D. Kritchevsky (New York: Plenum Press, 1980).

10 Werbach, M.R., M.D. *Nutritional Influences on Illness* (Tarzana, CA: Third Line Press, 1993).

11 The CFIDS Information Line of the CFIDS Association of America, Inc. (P.O. Box 220398, Charlotte, NC 28222-0398; tel: 800-442-3437; fax: 704-365-9755).

12 U.S.Department of Agriculture. *Nutritive Value of American Foods in Common Units* Agriculture Handbook No. 456 (Washington: U.S. Department of Agriculture).

13 Lark, Susan M., M.D. *Chronic Fatigue Self Help Book* (Berkeley, CA: Celestial Arts, 1995).

14 Machlin, L.J., and A. Bendich. "Free Radical Tissue Damage: Protective Role of Antioxidant Nutrient." *FASEB Journal* 1:6 (1987), 441-445.

15 Cunha, Burke A., M.D. "Beta Carotene Stimulation of Natural Killer Cell Activity in Adult Patients with Chronic Fatigue Syndrome." *The CFIDS Chronicle* (Winter 1993).

16 Murray, Michael, N.D. *Encyclopedia of Nutritional Supplements* (Rocklin, CA: Prima Publishing, 1996), 36.

17 Cameron, E.T., et al. "Ascorbic Acid and Cancer: A Review." *Cancer Research* 39 (1979), 663-681.

18 Yonemoto, R.H. "Vitamin C and Immunological Response in Normal Controls and Cancer Patients." *Medico Dialogo* 5 (1979), 23-30.

19 Lombard, Jay, M.D., and Carl Germano. *The Brain Wellness Plan: Breakthrough Medical, Nutritional, and Immune-Boosting Therapies* (New York: Kensington Books, 1997), 184.

20 Werbach, M.R., M.D. *Nutritional Influences on Illness* (Tarzana, CA: Third Line Press, 1993).

21 Cheraskin, E., et al. "Daily Vitamin C Consumption and Fatigability." *Journal of the American Geriatric Society* 24:3 (1976), 136-137.

22 Cathcart, Robert, M.D. Internet: http://www.mall-net.com/cathcart/cfids.html.

23 Murray, Michael, N.D. *Encyclopedia of Nutritional Supplements* (Rocklin, CA: Prima Publishing, 1996), 438.

24 U.S.Department of Agriculture. *Nutritive Value of American Foods in Common Units* Agriculture Handbook No. 456 (Washington: U.S. Department of Agriculture).

25 Murray, Frank. "Advanced New Form of Vitamin C: Ester C." *Better Nutrition for Today's Living* (January 1993).

26 Lark, Susan M., M.D. *Chronic Fatigue Self Help Book* (Berkeley, CA: Celestial Arts, 1995).

27 Murray, Michael, N.D. *Encyclopedia of Nutritional Supplements* (Rocklin, CA: Prima Publishing, 1996), 438.

28 Werbach, M.R., M.D. *Nutritional Influences on Illness* (Tarzana, CA: Third Line Press, 1993).

29 Gridley, D.S., et al. "In Vivo and In Vitro Stimulation of Cell-mediated Immunity by Vitamin B6." *Nutrition Research* 8:2 (1988), 201-207.

30 Lark, Susan M., M.D. *Chronic Fatigue Self Help Book* (Berkeley, CA: Celestial Arts, 1995).

31 Simpson, L. "M. E. and B12." *JRS Medicine* (October 1991), 633.

32 Lapp, C.W. "Chronic Fatigue Syndrome Is a Real Disease." *North Carolina Family Physician* 443:1 (1992), 6-11.

33 Ellis, F.R., and S. Nasser. "A Pilot Study of Vitamin B12 in the Treatment of Tiredness." *British Journal*

of Nutrition 30:2 (1973), 277-283.

34 Lindenbaum, J., et al. "Neuropsychiatric Disorders Caused by Cobalamin Deficiency in the Absence of Anemia or Macrocytoses." New England Journal of Medicine 318 (1988), 1720-1728.

35 Lindenbaum, J., et al. "Prevalence of Cobalamin Deficiency in the Framingham Elderly Population." American Journal of Clinical Nutrition 60 (1994), 2-11.

36 Teitelbaum, Jacob, M.D. From Fatigued to Fantastic! (Garden City Park, NY: Avery Publishing Group, 1996), 20-21.

37 Werbach, M.R., M.D. Nutritional Influences on Illness (Tarzana, CA: Third Line Press, 1993).

38 Botez, M.I., et al. "Neuropsychological Correlates of Folic Acid Deficiency: Facts and Hypotheses." In: Folic Acid in Neurology, Psychiatry, and Internal Medicine, edited by M.I. Botez and E.H. Reynolds (New York: Raven Press, 1979).

39 Schroeder, H. The Poisons Around Us (Bloomington, IN: Indiana University Press, 1974), 126.

40 Underwood, E. Trace Elements in Human and Animal Nutrition 4th ed. (New York: Academic Press, 1977), 267.

41 Faloona, G.R., and S.A. Levine. "The Use of Organic Germanium in Chronic Epstein-Barr Virus Syndrome (CEBVS): An Example of Interferon Modulation of Herpes Reactivation." Orthomolecular Medicine 3:1 (1988), 29-31.

42 Kidd, P.M. "Germanium-132 (Ge-132): Homeostatic Normalizer and Immunostimulant. A Review of its Preventive and Therapeutic Efficacy." International Clinical Nutrition Review 7:1 (1987), 11-20.

43 Werbach, M.R., M.D. Nutritional Influences on Illness (Tarzana, CA: Third Line Press, 1993).

44 Buetler, E., et al. "Iron Therapy in Chronically Fatigued Non-Anemic Women: A Double Blind Study." Annals of Internal Medicine 52:378 (1960).

45 Cox, I.M., et al. "Red Blood Cell Magnesium and Chronic Fatigue Syndrome." The Lancet 337 (March 30, 1991), 757-760.

46 "Top CFIDS Researchers and Physicians Find Nutritional Supplement to Reduce Muscle Pain and Fatigue in Some Cases." Health Watch 4:3 (Summer/Fall 1994), 3.

47 Ibid.

48 "Management of Fibromyalgia: Rationale for the Use of Magnesium and Malic Acid." Journal of Nutritional Medicine 3 (1992), 49-59. "Alternatives: Fibromyalgia." What Doctors Don't Tell You 6:6 (September 1995), 9.

49 Keen, C.L., and S. Zidenberg-Cherr. Present Knowledge in Nutrition, 6th ed. (Washington: International Life Sciences Institute, 1990).

50 Gershwin, M.E., et al. "The Potential Impact of Nutrititional Factors on Immunological Responsiveness." In: Nutrition and Immunity (Orlando, FL: Academic Press, 1985), 201-204.

51 Werbach, M.R., M.D. Nutritional Influences on Illness (Tarzana, CA: Third Line Press, 1993).

52 Snively, W.D., and R.L. Westerman. "The Clinician Views Potassium Deficit." Minnesota Medicine (June 1965), 713-719.

53 Gaby, A.R. "Aspartic Acid Salts and Fatigue." Currents in Nutritional Therapeutics (November 1982).

54 Murray, Michael, N.D. Encyclopedia of Nutritional Supplements (Rocklin, CA: Prima Publishing, 1996), 176.

55 Fan, A.M., and K.W. Kizer. "Selenium: Nutritional, Toxicological, and Clinical Aspects." Western Journal of Medicine 153 (1990), 160-167. Burk, R.F. "Recent Developments in Trace Element Metabolism and Function: Newer Roles of Selenium in Nutrition." Journal of Nutrition 119 (1989), 1051-1054.

56 Kiremidjian-Schumacher, L., et al. "Supplementation with Selenium and Human Immune Cell Functions; II, Effect on Cytotoxic Lymphocytes and Natural Killer Cells." Biological Trace Element Research 41 (1994), 115-127.

57 Boik, John. Cancer and Natural Medicine (Princeton, MN: Oregon Medical Press, 1995), 147.

58 Werbach, M.R., M.D. Nutritional Influences on Illness (Tarzana, CA: Third Line Press, 1993).

59 Krotkiewski, M., et al. "Zinc and Muscle Strength and Endurance." Acta Physiologica Scandinavica 116:3 (1982), 309-311.

60 Kuratsune, H., et al. "Acylcarnitine Deficiency in Chronic Fatigue Syndrome." Clinical Infectious Diseases 18:Suppl. 1 (January 1994), S62-S67.

61 Eaton, K.K., and A. Hunnisett. "Abnormalities in Essential Amino Acids in Patients with Chronic Fatigue Syndrome." Journal of Nutritional Medicine 2 (1991), 369-375.

62 Kuratsune, H, et al. "Acylcarnitine Deficiency in Chronic Fatigue Syndrome." Clinical Infectious Diseases 18:Suppl. 1 (January 1994), S62-S67.

63 Plioplys, S., and A.V. Plioplys. "Serum Levels of Carnitine in Chronic Fatigue Syndrome: Clinical Correlates." Proceedings of the American Association of Chronic Fatigue Syndrome 1 (1994), 19.

64 Kuratsune, H, et al. "Acylcarnitine Deficiency in Chronic Fatigue Syndrome." Clinical Infectious Diseases 18:Suppl. 1 (January 1994), S62-S67.

65 Lombard, Jay, M.D., and Carl Germano. The Brain Wellness Plan: Breakthrough Medical, Nutritional, and Immune-Boosting Therapies (New York: Kensington Books, 1997), 188.

66 Murray, Michael, N.D. *Encyclopedia of Nutritional Supplements* (Rocklin, CA: Prima Publishing, 1996), 296.

67 Lapp, C.W. "Chronic Fatigue Syndrome Is a Real Disease." *North Carolina Family Physician* 443:1 (1992), 6-11.

68 Teitelbaum, Jacob, M.D. *From Fatigued to Fantastic!* (Garden City Park, NY: Avery Publishing Group, 1996), 57, 71.

69 Horrobin, D.F. "Post-viral Fatigue Syndrome, Viral Infections in Atopic Eczema, and Essential Fatty Acids." *Medical Hypotheses* 32:3 (1990), 211-217.

70 Behan, P.O., et al. "Effect of High Doses of Essential Fatty Acids on the Post-viral Fatigue Syndrome." *Acta Neurologica Scandinavica* 82:3 (1990), 209-216. Behan, P.O., and W. Behan. "Essential Fatty Acids in the Treatment of Post-viral Fatigue Syndrome." In: *Omega-6 Essential Fatty Acids: Pathophysiology and Roles in Clinical Medicine*, edited by D.F. Horrobin (New York: Alan R. Liss, 1990), 275-282.

71 Murray, Michael, N.D. *Encyclopedia of Nutritional Supplements* (Rocklin, CA: Prima Publishing, 1996), 438.

Chapter 11
Healing Psychological and Emotional Factors

1 Teitelbaum, Jacob, M.D. *From Fatigued to Fantastic!* (Garden City Park, NY: Avery Publishing Group, 1996), 73.

2 Stoff, Jesse A., M.D., and Charles R. Pellegrino, Ph.D. *Chronic Fatigue Syndome: The Hidden Epidemic* (New York: HarperCollins, 1992), 89.

3 Ibid., 327.

4 Teitelbaum, Jacob, M.D. *From Fatigued to Fantastic!* (Garden City Park, NY: Avery Publishing Group, 1996), 73.

5 Schellhardt, Timothy D. "Company Memo to Stressed-Out Employees: 'Deal With It'." *The Wall Street Journal* (October 2, 1996).

6 Marx, J.L. "The Immune System 'Belongs to the Body'." *Science* 277 (1985), 1190-1192.

7 White, Peter D., et al. "Randomized Controlled Trial of Graded Exercise in Patients With Chronic Fatigue Syndrome." *British Medical Journal* 314 (June 7, 1997), 1647-1652.

8 *Scandinavian Journal of Rheumatology* 15:2 (1986), 174-178.

9 Northrup, Christiane, M.D. *Health Wisdom for Women* 2:5 (1995), 3-5.

10 Cass, Hyla, M.D. "Alternative Medical Treatments for Depression." In: *Sacred Sorrows: Embracing and Transforming Depression*, edited by John E. Nelson, M.D., and Andrea Nelson, Ph.D. (New York: Jeremy P. Tarcher/Putnam, 1996), 92-101.

11 Hodgkinson, N. "'Yuppie Flu'— It is All in the Mind Say Doctors." *The Sunday Times London* (July 17, 1988).

12 Murray, Michael T., N.D. *Natural Alternatives to Prozac* (New York: William Morrow, 1996).

13 *British Homeopathic Journal* 75:3 (1986), 142-147.

14 *British Medical Journal* 299 (1989), 365-366.

Chapter 12
Correcting Chronic Fatigue With Herbs

1 Lark, Susan M., M.D. *The Chronic Fatigue Self Help Book* (Berkeley, CA: Celestial Arts, 1995).

2 McCarty, Daniel J., et al. "Treatment of Pain Due to Fibromyalgia With Topical Capsaicin: A Pilot." *Seminars in Arthritis and Rheumatism* 23:6 Suppl 3, 41-47.

3 Patient records of Dennis Zinner, D.C., of San Francisco, California.

4 Berne, Katrina, Ph.D. *Running on Empty: The Complete Guide to Chronic Fatigue Syndrome (CFIDS)* (Alameda, CA: Hunter House, 1995), 190.

5 Henry, C. J., and B. Emery. "Effect of Spiced Food on Metabolic Rate." *Human Nutrition Clinical Nutrition* 40:2 (March 1986), 165-168.

6 Glatzel, H. "Blood Circulation Effectiveness of Natural Spices." *Medizinische Klinik* 62:51 (December 1967), 1987-1989.

7 Buzzanca, G., and S. Laterza. "Clinical Trial with an Antirheumatic Ointment." *Clinica Terapeutica* 83:1 (October 1977), 71-83.

8 Mills, Simon Y., M.A. *The Dictionary of Modern Herbalism* (Rochester, VT: Healing Arts Press, 1988), 58-59.

9 ESCOP, European Scientific Cooperative for Phytotherapy. *Valerian Root* (Meppel, The Netherlands: ESCOP, European Scientific Cooperative for Phytotherapy, 1990). Foster, S. *Chamomile. Botanical Series 307* (Austin, TX: American Botanical Council, 1991).

10 Mills, Simon Y., M.A. *The Dictionary of Modern Herbalism* (Rochester, VT: Healing Arts Press, 1988), 75.

11 Puotinen, C.J. *Herbs for Detoxification* (New Canaan, CT: Keats, 1997), 67.

12 Foster, S. *Echinacea: The Purple Coneflowers. Botanical Series 301* (Austin, TX: American Botanical Council, 1991).

13 German Ministry of Health. *Echinacea purpurea Leaf. Commission E Monographs for*

Phytomedicines (Bonn, Germany: German Ministry of Health, 1989).

14 Foster, S. *Garlic. Botanical Series 311* (Austin, TX: American Botanical Council, 1991).

15 Ibid.

16 Foster, S. *Garlic. Botanical Series 311* (Austin, TX: American Botanical Council, 1991). Kleijnen, J., P. Knipschild, and G. Terriet. "Garlic, Onions and Cardiovascular Risk Factors. A Review of the Evidence from Human Experiments with Emphasis on Commercially Available Preparations." *British Journal of Clinical Pharmacology* 28:5 (November 1989), 535-544.

17 Berne, Katrina, Ph.D. *Running on Empty: The Complete Guide to Chronic Fatigue Syndrome (CFIDS)* (Alameda, CA: Hunter House, 1995), 191.

18 Braquet, P., ed. *Ginkgolides: Chemistry, Biology, Pharmacology and Clinical Perspectives, Vol. 1* (Barcelona, Spain: J. Prous Science Publishers, 1988). Braquet, P., ed. *Ginkgolides: Chemistry, Biology, Pharmacology and Clinical Perspectives, Vol. 2* (Barcelona, Spain: J. Prous Science Publishers, 1989). Fungfeld, E.W., ed. *Rokan: Ginkgo biloba* (New York: Springer Verlag, 1988).

19 Root, Jolie Martin. "16 Ways to Boost Your Brain Power." *Alternative Medicine Digest* 20 (November 1997), 17.

20 Shibata, S., et al. "Chemistry and Pharmacology of Panax." *Economic and Medicinal Plant Research* 1 (1985), 217-284.

21 Werbach, Melvyn R., M.D., and Michael T. Murray, N.D. *Botanical Influences on Illness: A Sourcebook of Clinical Research* (Tarzana, CA: Third Line Press, 1994).

22 Brekhman, I. I., and I.V. Dardymov. "Pharmacological Investigation of Glycosides From Ginseng and Eleutherococcus." *Lloydia* 32 (1969), 46-51.

23 Bombardelli, E., A. Cirstoni, and A. Lietti. "The Effect of Acute and Chronic (Panax) Ginseng Saponins Treatment on Adrenal Function; Biochemical and Pharmacological." *Proceedings of the 3rd International Ginseng Symposium* 1 (1980), 9-16. Fulder, S. J. "Ginseng and the Hypothalamic-Pituitary Control of Stress." *American Journal of Chinese Medicine* 9 (1981), 112-118.

24 Feng, L.M., H.Z. Pan, and W.W. Li. "Anti-Oxidant Action of Panax Ginseng." *Chung Hsi I Chieh Ho Tsa Chih* 7:5 (May 1987), 262, 288-290.

25 Hikino, H., et al. "Antihepatotoxic Actions of Ginsenosides From Panax Ginseng Roots." *Planta Medica* 52 (1985), 62-64.

26 Ng, T. B., and H.W. Yeung. "Hypoglycemic Constituents of Panax Ginseng." *General Pharmacology* 6 (1985), 549-552.

27 Huo, Y. S. "Anti-Senility Action of Saponin in Panax Ginseng Fruit in 327 Cases." *Chung Hsi I Chieh Ho Tsa Chih* 4:10 (October 1984), 578, 593-596.

28 Joo, C. N. "The Preventative Effect of Korean (P. Ginseng) Saponins on Aortic Atheroma Formation in Prolonged Cholesterol-Fed Rabbits." *Proceedings of the 3rd International Ginseng Symposium* (1980), 27-36.

29 Scaglione, F., et al. "Immunomodulatory Effects of Two Extracts of Panax Ginseng C.A. Meyer." *Drugs Under Experimental and Clinical Research* 16:10 (1990), 537-542.

30 Yamamoto, M., and T. Uemura. "Endocrinological and Metabolic Actions of P. Ginseng Principles." *Proceeding of the 3rd International Ginseng Symposium* (1980), 115-119.

31 Berdyshev, V. V. "Effect of the Long-Term Intake of Eleutherococcus on the Adaptation of Sailors in the Tropics." *Voenno-Meditsinskii Zhurnal* 5 (May 1981), 57-58.

32 Hoffmann, D. *The New Holistic Herbal* (Rockport, MA: Element, 1991), 204.

33 Hahn, F.E., and J. Ciak. "Berberine." *Antibiotics and Chemotherapy* 3 (1976), 577-588.

34 Choudhry, V. P., M. Sabir, and V.N. Bhide. "Berberine in Giardiasis." *Indian Pediatrics* 9:3 (March 1972), 143-146

35 Kumazawa, Y., et al. "Activation of Peritoneal Macrophages by Berberine-Alkaloids in Terms of Induction of Cytostatic Activity." *International Journal of Immunopharmacology* 6 (1984), 587-592.

36 German Ministry of Health. *Hops. Commission E Monographs for Phytomedicines* (Bonn, Germany: German Ministry of Health, 1989).

37 Lehmann, E., et al. "Efficacy of a Special Kava Extract (*Piper methysticum*) in Patients with Anxiety, Tension, and Excitedness of Non-Mental Origin." *Phytomedicine* 3 (1996), 113-119.

38 Volz, H.P., and M. Kieser. "Kava-kava Extract WS 14490 Versus Placebo in Anxiety Disorders: A Randomized Placebo-Controlled 25-Week Outpatient Trial." *Pharmacopsychiatria* 30 (1997), 1-5.

39 Mills, Simon Y., M.A. *The Dictionary of Modern Herbalism* (Rochester, VT: Healing Arts Press, 1988), 138.

40 Armanini, D., et al. "Affinity of Liquorice Derivatives for Mineralocorticoid and Glucocorticoid Receptors." *Clinical Endocrinology* 19 (November 1983), 609-612. Berne, Katrina, Ph.D. *Running on Empty: The Complete Guide to Chronic Fatigue Syndrome (CFIDS)* (Alameda, CA: Hunter House, 1995), 191.

41 Hikino, H., and Y. Kiso. "Natural Products for Liver Diseases." In: Wagner, H., H. Hikino, and N. R. Farnsworth. *Economic and Medicinal Plant Research* 2nd ed. (London: Academic Press,

1988).

42 Pompei, R., et al. "Antiviral Activity of Glycrrhizic Acid." *Experientia* 36 (March 1980), 304-305.

43 Baschetti, Riccardo. "Chronic Fatigue Syndrome and Liquorice (Letter)." *New Zealand Medical Journal* 108 (April 26, 1995), 156-157.

44 Vogel, G. "Natural Substances with Effects on the Liver." In: Wagner, H., and P. Wolff, eds. *New Natural Products and Plant Drugs with Pharmacological, Biological or Therapeutic Activity* (Heidelberg, Germany: Springer-Verlag, 1977).

45 Wagner, H., F. Willer, and B. Kreher. "Biologically Active Compounds From the Aqueous Extract of *Urtica dioica*." *Planta Medica* 55:5 (October 1989), 452-454.

46 Mittman, P. "Randomized, Double-Blind Study of Freeze-Dried *Urtica dioica* in the Treatment of Allergic Rhinitis." *Planta Medica* 56:1 (February 1990), 44-47.

47 Hoffmann, D. *The New Holistic Herbal* (Rockport, MA: Element, 1991), 218.

48 Hirazumi, A., E. Furusawa, S. C. Chou, and Y. Hokama. *Proceedings of the Western Pharmacology Society* 37 (1994), 145-146.

49 Mayell, Mark. "Increase Your Energy." *Off-the-Shelf Natural Health* (New York: Bantam Books, 1995), 123-124.

50 German Ministry of Health. *Passion Flower Leaves. Commission E Monographs for Phytomedicines* (Bonn, Germany: German Ministry of Health, 1985).

51 Mills, Simon Y., M.A. *The Dictionary of Modern Herbalism* (Rochester, VT: Healing Arts Press, 1988), 164.

52 Foster, S. *Passion Flower. Botanical Series 314* (Austin, TX: American Botanical Council, 1993).

53 Foster, S. *Peppermint. Botanical Series 306* (Austin, TX: American Botanical Council, 1991).

54 German Ministry of Health. *Peppermint Oil. Commission E Monographs for Phytomedicines* (Bonn, Germany: German Ministry of Health, 1989).

55 Suzuki, O., et al. "Inhibition of Monoamine Oxidase by Hypericin." *Planta Medica* 50 (1984), 272-274. Muldner, H., and M. Zoller. "Antidepressive Effect of a Hypericum Extract Standardized to an Active Hypericine Complex. Biochemical and Clinical Studies." *Arzneimittelforschung* 34:8 (1984), 918-920.

56 Meruelo, D., et al. "Therapeutic Agents with Dramatic Antiviral Activity and Little Toxicity at Effective Doses: Aromatic Polycyclicdiones Hypericin and Pseudohypericin." *Proceedings of the National Academy of Sciences* 85 (1988), 5230-5234.

57 De Smet, Peter, et al. "St. John's Wort as an Antidepressant." *British Medical Journal* 7052:313 (August 3, 1996), 241-242. Linde, Klaus, et al. "St. John's Wort for Depression—An Overview and Meta-Analysis of Randomized Clinical Trials." *British Medical Journal* 7052:313 (August 3, 1996), 253-258.

58 Hobbs, Christopher, L.Ac. *Stress and Natural Healing* (Loveland, CO: Interweave Press, 1997), 158-159.

59 German Ministry of Health. *Valerian. Commission E Monographs for Phytomedicines* (Bonn, Germany: German Ministry of Health, 1985).

60 ESCOP, European Scientific Cooperative for Phytotherapy. *Valerian Root* (Meppel, The Netherlands: European Scientific Cooperative for Phytotherapy, 1990).

61 Mills, Simon Y., M.A. *The Dictionary of Modern Herbalism* (Rochester, VT: Healing Arts Press, 1988), 211.

62 Hobbs, Christopher, L.Ac. "Valerian: A Literature Review." *HerbalGram* 21 (1989), 19-34.

63 Worwood, Valerie Ann. *The Fragrant Mind. Aromatherapy for Personality, Mind, Mood, and Emotions* (Novato, CA: New World Library, 1996). Available from: New World Library, 14 Pamaron Way, Novato, CA 94949; tel: 800-227-3900 or 415-884-2100; fax: 415-884-2199.

Index

BOOKS *your health* depends on

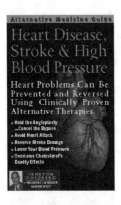
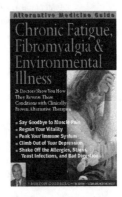
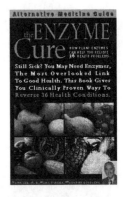
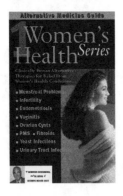
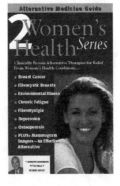
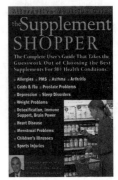